2015

The Year Book of OPHTHALMOLOGY®

Editor-in-Chief

Christopher J. Rapuano, MD

Professor of Ophthalmology, Sidney Kimmel Medical College at Thomas Jefferson University; Director, Cornea Service; Co-Director, Refractive Surgery Department, Attending Surgeon, Wills Eye Hospital, Philadelphia, Pennsylvania

Wills Eye®

ELSEVIER
MOSBY

ELSEVIER
MOSBY

Vice President, Global Medical Reference: Mary E. Gatsch
Acquisitions Editor: Jennifer Flynn-Briggs
Developmental Editor: Colleen Viola
Production Supervisor, Electronic Year Books: Donna M. Skelton
Electronic Article Manager: Mike Sheets
Illustrations and Permissions Coordinator: Dawn Vohsen

2015 EDITION

Printed in the United States of America
Composition by TNQ Books and Journals Pvt Ltd, India
Printing/binding by Sheridan Books, Inc.

Editorial Office:
Elsevier
1600 John F. Kennedy Blvd.
Suite 1800
Philadelphia, PA 19103-2899

International Standard Serial Number: 0084-392X
International Standard Book Number: 978-0-323-35548-3

Editorial Board

Carol L. Shields, MD
Professor, Sidney Kimmel Medical College at Thomas Jefferson University; Co-Director, Oncology Service; Attending Surgeon, Oncology Service, Wills Eye Hospital, Philadelphia, Pennsylvania

Kiran Talekar, MD
Assistant Professor of Radiology, Sidney Kimmel Medical College at Thomas Jefferson University, Thomas Jefferson University Hospital, Philadelphia, Pennsylvania

Contributors

Anjali Badami, BS
Medical Student, Sidney Kimmel Medical College at Thomas Jefferson University, Philadelphia, Pennsylvania

Zachary E. Daitch, BA
Medical Student, Sidney Kimmel Medical College at Thomas Jefferson University, Philadelphia, Pennsylvania

Elizabeth Blessing Elimimian, MPH
Medical Student, Sidney Kimmel Medical College at Thomas Jefferson University, Philadelphia, Pennsylvania

Robert House, BA
Medical Student, Sidney Kimmel Medical College at Thomas Jefferson University, Philadelphia, Pennsylvania

Prashanth G. Iyer, MPH
Medical Student, Sidney Kimmel Medical College at Thomas Jefferson University, Philadelphia, Pennsylvania

Benjamin J. Kim, MD
Scheie Eye Institute, University of Pennsylvania, Philadelphia, Pennsylvania

Jeffrey E. Landy, BA
Medical Student, Sidney Kimmel Medical College at Thomas Jefferson University, Philadelphia, Pennsylvania

Brendan M. Lawson, BS
Medical Student, Sidney Kimmel Medical College at Thomas Jefferson University, Philadelphia, Pennsylvania

Phoebe Mellen, BS
Medical Student, Sidney Kimmel Medical College at Thomas Jefferson University, Philadelphia, Pennsylvania

Meera Sivalingam, BA
Medical Student, Sidney Kimmel Medical College at Thomas Jefferson University, Philadelphia, Pennsylvania

Brian L. VanderBeek, MD, MPH
Scheie Eye Institute, University of Pennsylvania, Philadelphia, Pennsylvania

Yonah C. Ziemba, BTL
Medical Student, Sidney Kimmel Medical College at Thomas Jefferson University, Philadelphia, Pennsylvania

Table of Contents

Journals Represented

Journals represented in this YEAR BOOK are listed below.

AJNR American Journal of Neuroradiology
American Journal of Ophthalmology
Annals of Neurology
British Journal of Ophthalmology
Canadian Journal of Ophthalmology
Clinical Endocrinology
Cornea
Current Opinion in Ophthalmology
Current Protocols in Cytometry
Eye
Genes Chromosomes & Cancer
Indian Journal of Ophthalmology
International Journal of Dermatology
Investigative Ophthalmology & Visual Science
Journal of Cataract & Refractive Surgery
Journal of Oral and Maxillofacial Surgery
Journal of Pediatric Ophthalmology and Strabismus
Journal of Refractive Surgery
Journal of the American Association for Pediatric Ophthalmology and Strabismus
Journal of the American Medical Association
Journal of the American Medical Association Neurology
Journal of the American Medical Association Ophthalmology
Lancet Oncology
Neurology
Ocular Immunology and Inflammation
Ophthalmic Plastic and Reconstructive Surgery
Ophthalmic Surgery, Lasers & Imaging Retina
Ophthalmology
Plastic and Reconstructive Surgery
Public Library of Science One
Radiology
Retina
Thyroid

STANDARD ABBREVIATIONS

The following terms are abbreviated in this edition: acquired immunodeficiency syndrome (AIDS), cardiopulmonary resuscitation (CPR), central nervous system (CNS), cerebrospinal fluid (CSF), computed tomography (CT), deoxyribonucleic acid (DNA), diopter (D), electrocardiography (ECG), health maintenance organization (HMO), human immunodeficiency virus (HIV), intensive care unit (ICU), intramuscular (IM), intravenous (IV), magnetic resonance (MR) imaging (MRI), ribonucleic acid (RNA), ultrasound (US), and ultraviolet (UV).

NOTE

The YEAR BOOK OF OPHTHALMOLOGY® is a literature survey service providing abstracts of articles published in the professional literature. Every effort is made to assure the accuracy of the information presented in these pages. Neither the editors nor the publisher of the YEAR BOOK OF OPHTHALMOLOGY® can be responsible for errors in the original materials. The editors' comments are their own opinions. Mention of specific products within this publication does not constitute endorsement.

To facilitate the use of the YEAR BOOK OF OPHTHALMOLOGY® as a reference tool, all illustrations and tables included in this publication are now identified as they appear in the original article. This change is meant to help the reader recognize that any illustration or table appearing in the YEAR BOOK OF OPHTHALMOLOGY® may be only one of many in the original article. For this reason, figure and table numbers will often appear to be out of sequence within the YEAR BOOK OF OPHTHALMOLOGY®.

1 Cataract Surgery

A Prospective Randomized Clinical Evaluation of 3 Presbyopia-Correcting Intraocular Lenses After Cataract Extraction

Pepose JS, Qazi MA, Chu R, et al (Washington Univ School of Medicine, St Louis, MO; Chu Eye Associates, Fort Worth, TX; et al)

Am J Ophthalmol 158:436-446.e1, 2014

Purpose.—To compare contrast sensitivity, visual acuity (VA), and halos in subjects bilaterally implanted with 1 of 3 FDA-approved presbyopia-correcting intraocular lenses.

Design.—Prospective, randomized, partially masked, multicenter clinical trial.

Methods.—Seventy-eight subjects were randomized sequentially for bilateral implantation with the Crystalens AO (Bausch & Lomb Surgical), AcrySof IQ ReSTOR +3.0 (Alcon Laboratories), or Tecnis Multifocal (Abbott Medical Optics) lenses. Subjects were evaluated through visit 4 (4 to 6 months after surgery) with the following monocular and binocular assessments: high- and low-contrast VA, contrast sensitivity without glare, halos or starbursts, defocus curves, optical scatter, retinal point spread function, and safety.

Results.—The Crystalens AO and ReSTOR +3.0 demonstrated better monocular and binocular contrast sensitivity without glare at low to mid spatial frequencies compared with the Tecnis Multifocal lens. Binocular uncorrected distance VA was not significantly different between the 3 lenses. The Crystalens AO had significantly better binocular low-contrast distance-corrected VA than the ReSTOR +3.0 and better mean monocular low-contrast DCVA than the Tecnis Multifocal lens. The Crystalens AO demonstrated significantly better monocular and binocular uncorrected and distance-corrected intermediate VA than the ReSTOR +3.0 or Tecnis Multifocal lenses. The ReSTOR +3.0 lens had significantly better monocular and binocular uncorrected and distance-corrected near VA tested at 40 cm compared with the Crystalens AO and Tecnis Multifocal lens. The Crystalens AO elicited significantly less halos than the Tecnis Multifocal lens and less optical scatter than the ReSTOR +3.0 or Tecnis Multifocal lens.

Conclusions.—The Crystalens AO had statistically better uncorrected intermediate VA and distance-corrected intermediate VA than the ReSTOR +3.0 or Tecnis Multifocal lenses and fewer photic phenomenon than the Tecnis Multifocal lens. Both multifocals had better distance-corrected near VA and uncorrected near VA than the Crystalens AO.

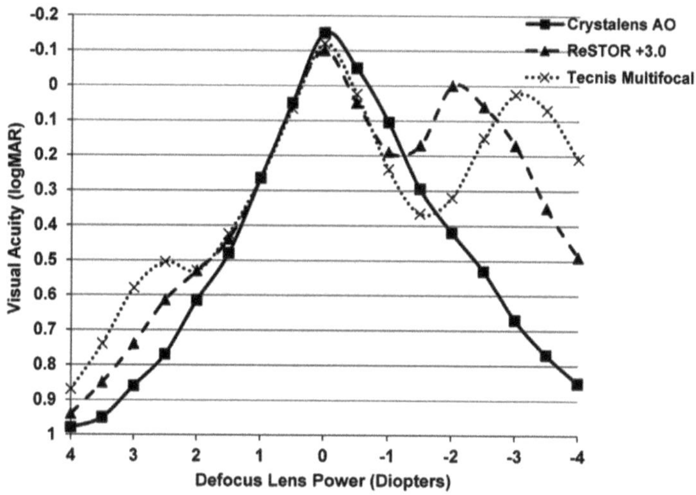

FIGURE 7.—Overlay of monocular defocus curves showing the mean logarithm of the minimal angle of resolution (logMAR) visual acuity versus defocus lens power (in diopters) by lens type at visit 4 for 3 presbyopia-correcting intraocular lenses. (Reprinted from American Journal of Ophthalmology. Pepose JS, Qazi MA, Chu R, et al. A prospective randomized clinical evaluation of 3 presbyopia-correcting intraocular lenses after cataract extraction. *Am J Ophthalmol.* 2014;158:436-446.e1, Copyright 2014, with permission from Elsevier.)

These findings may guide intraocular lens selection for individual patients seeking to optimize vision at specific vergences or lighting conditions (Fig 7).

▶ This randomized study comparing the most updated versions of the 3 presbyopia-correcting intraocular lenses (IOLs) available in the United States today provides useful information for surgeons who are selecting these lenses for their patients. As could be expected, all 3 lenses performed well as per their labeled indications when implanted in ideal candidates, with highly accurate biometry and tightly controlled refractive error. In general, the Crystalens AO had fewer photic phenomena and better intermediate vision than the 2 multifocal IOLs. Both multifocal IOLs had better near vision compared with Crystalens AO. The Restor +3 had a slight advantage over the Tecnis multifocal for near and intermediate visual acuity at the distances tested (Fig 7) and for subjective perception of halos.

One limitation of this study is lack of long-term follow-up, as refractive stability may be lower in Crystalens longer term. Also, subjective patient ratings regarding quality of uncorrected vision at all distances and the need for spectacle use, which could be important for patient satisfaction, were not collected.

M. F. Pyfer, MD

Comparison of near vision, intraocular lens movement, and depth of focus with accommodating and monofocal intraocular lenses

Dhital A, Spalton DJ, Gala KB (St. Thomas' Hosp, London, UK)

J Cataract Refract Surg 39:1872-1878, 2013

Purpose.—To compare visual acuity, intraocular lens (IOL) movement, and depth of focus with the Crystalens HD single-optic accommodating IOL and the Tecnis ZCB00 aspheric monofocal IOL.

Setting.—St. Thomas' Hospital, London, United Kingdom.

Design.—Prospective randomized controlled trial.

Methods.—Patients with bilateral symptomatic cataract had bilateral sequential cataract surgery within 6 weeks with randomized implantation of the accommodating or monofocal IOL in both eyes. Exclusion criteria included other ocular conditions and corneal astigmatism greater than 2.00 diopters. The primary outcome was uniocular distance-corrected near visual acuity (DCNVA). Secondary measures were IOL movement, depth of focus, intermediate and distance vision, objective refraction, and pupil size at distance and near fixation. Results from 3 months postoperatively are presented.

Results.—Three months postoperatively, 64 patients (32 in each group) were available for study. The distance vision was not statistically significantly different between the accommodating IOL and monofocal IOL (mean 0.05 logMAR versus 0.06 logMAR). The mean DCNVA (0.48

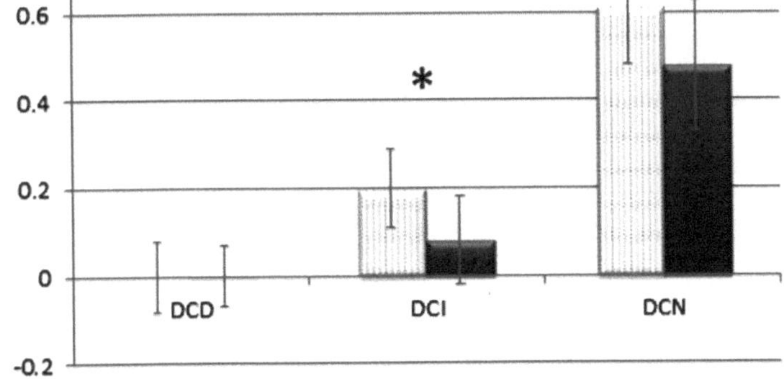

FIGURE 1.—Comparison of uniocular distance-corrected near, intermediate, and distance logMAR acuities between the accommodating IOL and monofocal IOL. *Asterisk* indicates $P < .001$. Error bars indicate standard deviation (DCD = distance-corrected distance acuity, DCI = distance corrected intermediate acuity, DCN = distance-corrected near visual acuity). (Reprinted from Journal of Cataract & Refractive Surgery. Dhital A, Spalton DJ, Gala KB. Comparison of near vision, intraocular lens movement, and depth of focus with accommodating and monofocal intraocular lenses. *J Cataract Refract Surg* 2013;39:1872-1878, Copyright 2013, with permission from ASCRS and ESCRS.)

logMAR ± 0.15 [SD] versus 0.61 ± 0.13 logMAR) and intermediate visual acuity (0.08 ± 0.1 logMAR versus 0.20 ± 0.09 logMAR) were significantly better with the accommodating IOL ($P < .001$). Neither IOL had clinically significant movement, and near vision did not directly correlate with movement of the accommodating IOL. The accommodating IOL provided greater depth of focus.

Conclusions.—Near and intermediate acuities were better with the accommodating IOL. This effect was not directly linked to IOL movement but was at least partly due to depth of focus (Fig 1).

▶ This is a well-controlled randomized study comparing bilateral implantation of the Crystalens HD accommodating intraocular lens (IOL) versus the AMO Tecnis one-piece monofocal IOL. Best-corrected monocular distance vision measured was similar in both groups. However, distance-corrected near and intermediate visual acuities were better in patients with the accommodating lens (Fig 1). This is the expected result, as the accommodating lens is designed for improved depth of focus, although the mechanism for this is uncertain. This study also measured movement of both IOLs under accommodative effort and in response to pharmacologic pupil dilatation and constriction. There was minimal movement in both groups, indicating that accommodation or pseudoaccomodation is not achieved by axial lens position changes.

Most patients who opt for an accommodating IOL and corneal relaxing incisions for correction of astigmatism are interested in optimal uncorrected visual acuity for both distance and near. The authors state that about 0.5 diopters of mini-monovision was targeted in both groups. However, the uncorrected binocular visual results are not provided, which is a limitation of the study. In my experience, one potential shortcoming of the accommodating IOL is greater variation in final refractive error, which may also drift over time. This could not be assessed in this study, as the achieved postoperative refractive error in each group was not published.

M. F. Pyfer, MD

Impact of Personality Characteristics on Patient Satisfaction After Multifocal Intraocular Lens Implantation: Results From the "Happy Patient Study"

Mester U, Vaterrodt T, Goes F, et al (Augenzentrum im Medizeum, Saarbrücken, Germany; SHG Klinik, Saarbrücken, Germany; Goes Eye Ctr, Antwerp, Belgium; et al)

J Refract Surg 30:674-678, 2014

Purpose.—This prospective multicenter study assessed personality characteristics that may influence patient satisfaction after implantation of multifocal intraocular lenses (MIOLs).

Methods.—One hundred eighty-three patients who underwent bilateral implantation of different MIOLs were enrolled. Uncorrected and corrected distance visual acuity for distance and near (ie, UDVA, UNVA, CDVA, and CNVA) were assessed preoperatively and 3 and 6 months after implantation. Before surgery, personality characteristics were evaluated using a questionnaire based on the NEO Personality Inventory Test and the Compulsiveness Inventory Test. At the 3- and 6-month postoperative visits, patients answered a questionnaire concerning overall satisfaction, need for spectacles at different distances, visual function at different distances and lighting conditions, photic phenomena, and ease of performing daily activities.

Results.—Three months after surgery (n = 163), mean CDVA was 0.03 ± 0.09 logMAR, UDVA was 0.05 ± 0.09 logMAR, and UNVA was 0.04 ± 0.11 logMAR. At the 6-month visit (n = 131), mean CDVA was 0.02 ± 0.07 logMAR, UDVA was 0.06 ± 0.09 logMAR, and UNVA was 0.05 ± 0.01 logMAR. Most patients (82.2%) would opt for an MIOL again, 3.7% would not, and 14.1% were uncertain. Overall satisfaction with the procedure was correlated to low astigmatism, good visual function, low spectacle dependence, and less halos or glare. The personality characteristics of compulsive checking, orderliness, competence, and dutifulness were statistically significantly correlated to subjective disturbance by glare and halos.

Conclusions.—Postoperative patient satisfaction after MIOL implantation is correlated to visual performance, spectacle independence, and less photic phenomena. Personality characteristics have an impact on subjective disturbance by photic phenomena and thus are important for patient satisfaction.

▶ This study examines patient satisfaction with bilateral multifocal intraocular lens (MFIOL) implantation in more than 150 subjects. The results confirm some common conceptions and refute others. Here, as expected, better uncorrected distance visual acuity and lower postoperative refractive cylinder were correlated with higher satisfaction. Interestingly, type of MFIOL, preoperative expectations, and patient sex were not correlated to satisfaction. Subjective perception of glare and halos was related to dissatisfaction, and the personality traits of compulsive checking and orderliness were highly correlated to perception of glare and halos.

Surgeons who use the Dell Index or some variation to prescreen patients for MFIOL are already asking patients about perfectionist tendencies. Patients who score high in compulsive checking and orderliness are likely to rate themselves as more "perfectionistic," so this study in a sense supports use of the Dell Index questionnaire.

Future modifications of MFIOL prescreening tools should include a question regarding compulsive checking. In fact, some have suggested asking, "How many times a day do you clean your spectacles?" as a measure of compulsive or perfectionistic behavior.

M. F. Pyfer, MD

Multifocal Intraocular Lens Explantation: A Case Series of 50 Eyes

Kamiya K, on Behalf of the Survey Working Group of the Japanese Society of Cataract and Refractive Surgery (Univ of Kitasato School of Medicine, Kanagawa, Japan; et al)

Am J Ophthalmol 158:215-220.e1, 2014

Objective.—To assess the visual complaints, reasons, and patient satisfaction for multifocal intraocular lens (IOL) explantation.

Design.—Retrospective observational case series.

Methods.—This study evaluated 50 eyes of 37 patients who underwent multifocal IOL explantation followed by IOL implantation. Before and 3 months after IOL exchange surgery, we investigated the symptoms, reasons, patient demographics, clinical results, and patient satisfaction in eyes undergoing multifocal IOL explantation. Data collected included preoperative subjective and objective findings, reasons, IOL type, postoperative course, and patient satisfaction.

Results.—The most common complaints for IOL explantation were waxy vision, followed by glare and halos, blurred vision at far, dysphotopsia, blurred vision at near, and blurred vision at intermediate. The most common reasons for IOL explantation were decreased contrast sensitivity, followed by photic phenomenon, unknown origin including neuroadaptation failure, incorrect IOL power, preoperative excessive expectation, IOL dislocation/decentration, and anisometropia. The axial length was 25.13 ± 1.83 mm. Of the explanted multifocal IOLs, 84% were diffractive and 16% were refractive. Monofocal IOLs accounted for 90% of the exchanged IOLs. Patient satisfaction was significantly improved from 1.22 ± 0.55 preoperatively to 3.78 ± 0.97 postoperatively, which was graded on a scale of 1 (very dissatisfied) to 5 (very satisfied) (Wilcoxon signed-rank test, $P < .001$).

Conclusions.—Multifocal IOL explantation was required in some patients undergoing multifocal IOL implantation. IOL exchange surgery appears to be a feasible surgical option for dissatisfied patients with persistent visual symptoms after multifocal IOL implantation (Table 2).

▶ This study retrospectively examined reasons for and outcomes of intraocular lens (IOL) exchange performed after implantation of a multifocal IOL. Fifty patients were included, and during the same period, about 4200 multifocal IOLs were implanted at the centers involved in the study. This finding indicates an approximate risk for IOL exchange of 1.2% for this population, although this was not controlled in the study, and some patients may have gone elsewhere for exchange. Reasons for dissatisfaction with multifocal IOLs were primarily waxy vision and photic phenomena such as glare and halos (Table 2). The explanted IOLs were primarily diffractive, although the exact models were not reported, and the replacement IOL was primarily monofocal. After exchange, patient satisfaction on a 5-point scale increased to essentially the same as that of primary monofocal IOL patients.

TABLE 2.—Visual Complaints Before and After Multifocal Intraocular Lens (N = 50 Eyes)

Visual Complaints Before Multifocal IOL Explantation	
Blurred vision	
At far	12 eyes (24%)
At intermediate	3 eyes (6%)
At near	9 eyes (18%)
Waxy vision	29 eyes (58%)
Photic phenomena	
Glare/halos	15 eyes (30%)
Dysphotopsia	10 eyes (20%)
Visual Complaints of Dissatisfied Patients After Multifocal IOL Explantation	
Blurred vision	
At far	1 eye (2%)
Waxy vision	2 eyes (4%)

IOL = intraocular lens.

Reprinted from American Journal of Ophthalmology. Kamiya K. Multifocal Intraocular Lens Explantation: A Case Series of 50 Eyes. *Am J Ophthalmol.* 2014;158:215–220.e1, Copyright 2014, with permission from Elsevier.

This study indicates that, despite good refractive outcome in uncomplicated surgery, surgeons can expect about 1% to 2% of multifocal IOL patients to be dissatisfied with vision enough to require surgical replacement with a monofocal lens. This is consistent with my experience. Patients implanted with presbyopia-correcting lenses should be advised of possible need for IOL exchange, and surgeons should be prepared to handle this eventuality.

M. F. Pyfer, MD

Cortex Removal After Laser Cataract Surgery and Standard Phacoemulsification: A Critical Analysis of 800 Consecutive Cases

Conrad-Hengerer I, Schultz T, Jones JJ, et al (Ruhr Univ Eye Clinic, Bochum, Germany)

J Refract Surg 30:516-520, 2014

Purpose.—To evaluate the ease of anterior cortex removal and hydrodissection of the lens in femtosecond laser-assisted cataract surgery compared with standard phacoemulsification.

Methods.—In the femtosecond laser-assisted cataract surgery group (400 eyes), a femtosecond laser was used for capsulotomy and followed by lens fragmentation. In the standard group, the capsulorhexis was performed manually. In both groups, a normal hydrodissection was set, the nucleus was aspirated with or without ultrasound phacoemulsification energy, and residual cortex removal and posterior capsule polishing were performed using bimanual irrigation/aspiration. The primary end point was the time (in seconds) required for the removal of the cortex from instrument insertion in the eye until aspiration tip removal. Secondary end points were the effective phacoemulsification time, quality of the anterior capsule, and anterior or posterior capsule ruptures.

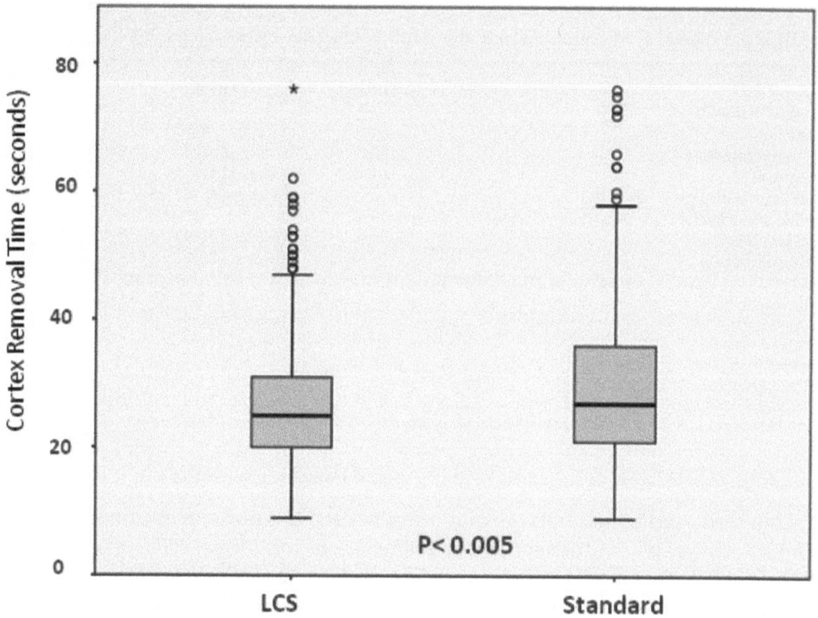

FIGURE 1.—Boxplot of cortex removal time. The bottom and top of the box are the 25th and 75th percentiles, respectively; the band near the center is the 50th percentile (median). The bars outside the box indicate the maximum and minimum of all data. A minor outlier (denoted by a small circle) is an observation 1.5× interquartile range outside the central box. A major outlier (denoted by *) is an observation 3.0× interquartile range outside the central box. The difference between the femtosecond laser-assisted cataract surgery (LCS) and standard groups is statistically significant ($P < .005$), but clinically irrelevant. (Reprinted with permission from SLACK Incorporated: Conrad-Hengerer I, Schultz T, Jones JJ, et al. Cortex removal after laser cataract surgery and standard phacoemulsification: a critical analysis of 800 consecutive cases. *J Refract Surg*. 2014;30:516-520, with permission from SLACK Incorporated.)

Results.—Cortex removal time measured 30 ± 13 seconds (range: 10 to 76 seconds) for the standard group and 27 ± 10 seconds (range: 9 to 72 seconds) for the femtosecond laser-assisted cataract surgery group ($P < .005$). After laser-assisted capsulotomy, one capsule was still adherent following removal by forceps. No anterior or posterior capsular tears were observed in either group.

Conclusions.—In femtosecond laser-assisted cataract surgery, the biaxial cortex removal time was comparable with the time in standard phacoemulsification (Fig 1).

▶ As femtosecond laser-assisted cataract surgery (FLACS) becomes more widely used, surgeons, as expected, have adjusted their techniques to obtain the best results from this tool compared with completely manual phacoemulsification cataract surgery (MCS). One portion of cataract surgery that has been reported to require a change in technique in FLACS is lens cortex aspiration. The cortex has been reported to be more adherent to the capsule, or "stickier" and, therefore, more difficult to remove with FLACS.

This study, by a single very experienced FLACS surgeon over a large number of cases, found that when using bimanual cortex aspiration, there was no difference in time required for this surgical step between FLACS and MCS (Fig 1). This finding seems to refute the notion that cortical removal in FLACS is more difficult.

Certainly, and I can verify this through personal experience, there is a learning curve for an experienced surgeon when adopting FLACS. My opinion is that 50 to 100 FLACS cases are required before one is truly comfortable and facile with the technique. I suggest withholding any opinion about the advantages or disadvantages of FLACS until you have performed at least 50 cases. Lens cortical removal in FLACS may initially be more challenging for several reasons: progressive intraoperative mitosis, lack of cortical tags extending beyond the anterior capsule edge, and some compression of cortex by gas bubble formation that makes cortical cleaving hydrodissection more difficult. This is somewhat counterbalanced by the "pneumo-dissection" effect of the gas bubbles in FLACS that helps achieve nuclear mobility with little or no hydrodissection. I use intracameral epinephrine or phenylephrine on every FLACS case to maintain pupil dilation and have switched to a curved soft-tipped coaxial irrigation-aspiration instrument. These adjustments have made cortical cleanup with FLACS as efficient as that in MCS in my hands. My personal experience is, therefore, consistent with the results of this study.

M. F. Pyfer, MD

Higher-Order Aberrations Associated With Better Near Visual Acuity in Eyes With Aspheric Monofocal IOLs

Song IS, Kim MJ, Yoon SY, et al (Hanyang Univ Med Ctr, Seoul, Korea; Univ of Ulsan College of Medicine, Seoul, Korea; et al)

J Refract Surg 30:442-446, 2014

Purpose.—To investigate higher-order aberrations (HOAs) related to increased uncorrected near visual acuity in eyes with aspheric monofocal intraocular lenses.

Methods.—All patients underwent phacoemulsification followed by implantation of aspheric monofocal intraocular lenses with a negative spherical aberration (Tecnis one-piece, ZCB00; Abbott Medical Optics, Inc., Milpitas, CA). The distance-corrected near visual acuity (DCNVA), corrected near visual acuity, uncorrected near visual acuity, corrected distance visual acuity, uncorrected distance visual acuity, defocus curve, and ocular and corneal HOAs were examined 1 month after surgery. All near visual acuity measurements were taken with a 4-mm external aperture after pharmacologic dilation. Eyes were divided into two groups according to the DCNVA: eyes with DCNVA of 0.4 logMAR (20/50 Snellen) or better (0.4 logMAR or better group) and eyes with DCNVA worse than 0.4 logMAR (0.4 logMAR or worse group). The HOAs for a 4-mm pupil between the two groups were compared.

TABLE 2.—Ocular Higher-Order Aberrations Over a 4-mm Pupil in Both Groups

Aberrometric Data	0.4 logMAR or Better Group (μm)	0.4 logMAR or Worse Group (μm)	P[a]
Z_3^{-3}	-0.056 ± 0.187	-0.061 ± 0.170	.86
Z_3^{-1}	-0.038 ± 0.043	0.015 ± 0.061	.01
Z_3^{+1}	-0.014 ± 0.068	-0.003 ± 0.037	.38
Z_3^{+3}	0.040 ± 0.128	-0.025 ± 0.116	.17
Z_4^{-4}	0.011 ± 0.024	-0.001 ± 0.036	.31
Z_4^{-2}	-0.003 ± 0.024	-0.009 ± 0.018	.53
Z_4^{0}	-0.010 ± 0.033	-0.012 ± 0.023	.28
Z_4^{+2}	0.004 ± 0.026	0.004 ± 0.290	.89
Z_4^{+4}	-0.036 ± 0.032	-0.028 ± 0.037	.51
Coma-like RMS	0.215 ± 0.119	0.198 ± 0.107	.71
Spherical-like RMS	0.064 ± 0.035	0.068 ± 0.024	.51
Higher-order RMS	0.232 ± 0.119	0.219 ± 0.101	.84

RMS = root mean square
[a]*Mann–Whitney U test.*
Reprinted with permission from SLACK Incorporated: Song IS, Kim MJ, Yoon SY, et al. Higher-Order Aberrations Associated With Better Near Visual Acuity in Eyes With Aspheric Monofocal IOLs. *J Refract Surg.* 2014;30:442-446.

Results.—A total of 37 eyes of 36 patients were included. The mean ocular spherical aberration was -0.010 ± 0.033 μm in the 0.4 logMAR or better group and -0.012 ± 0.023 μm in the 0.4 logMAR or worse group ($P = .28$). Among ocular HOAs, only vertical coma Z_3^{-1} showed a significant difference between the groups, with a mean ocular vertical coma of -0.038 ± 0.043 μm in the 0.4 logMAR or better group and 0.015 ± 0.061 μm in the 0.4 logMAR or worse group ($P = .01$). In corneal HOAs, no components showed a significant difference between the groups.

Conclusions.—In cases of aspheric intraocular lens implantation, ocular vertical coma may be a major HOA associated with better near visual acuity. Although corneal aberrations are major determinants of ocular aberrations after cataract surgery, aberrations from internal optics may still play an important role in visual performance (Table 2).

► This study found that negative vertical coma in patients with 1 type of aspheric intraocular lens (IOL) helps increase pseudo-accommodation, resulting in better near acuity with distance correction in place or without correction in most emmetropic eyes. No other higher-order aberration was correlated with better near vision in these eyes (Table 2). Significantly, increased negative coma in the better near-vision group was not detected on the anterior corneal surface but was noted only when whole eye aberrations were measured. This indicates that the coma likely comes from either the posterior cornea or the IOL itself. Tilt and decentration of IOLs has been shown to influence vertical coma, but that was not measured in this study. Also, there was no attempt to measure movement of the IOL during near vision testing; however, all measurements were done after pharmacologic pupil dilation and cycloplegia, so the effect of ciliary muscle contraction should be minimal.

This result agrees with the anecdotal experience of many surgeons including myself, who have found that a significant percentage of patients implanted with monofocal aspheric IOLs achieve better uncorrected near vision than would be expected based on their refraction alone. As has been discussed before in relation to astigmatism correction, there is a significant need for reliable posterior corneal measurements during preoperative evaluation for cataract surgery. No instrument in common use today fulfills this need, but high-resolution anterior segment ocular coherence tomography appears promising. An instrument with this capability will be an important part of a cataract surgeon's armamentarium in the near future.

M. F. Pyfer, MD

The Impact on Vision of Aspheric to Spherical Monofocal Intraocular Lenses in Cataract Surgery: A Systematic Review with Meta-Analysis

Schuster AK, Tesarz J, Vossmerbaeumer U (Univ of Heidelberg, Germany; et al)

Ophthalmology 120:2166-2175, 2013

Purpose.—To provide a summary of the impact on vision of an aspheric intraocular lens (IOL) compared with a spherical IOL in cataract surgery.

Design.—Systematic review with meta-analysis.

Participants.—Patients from published randomized controlled trials (RCTs) of cataract surgery with aspheric compared with spherical monofocal IOL implantation.

Methods.—We systematically searched the peer-reviewed literature in MEDLINE, EMBASE, Web of Science, BIOSIS, and the Cochrane Library according to the Cochrane Collaboration method to identify relevant RCTs. The inclusion criteria were RCTs on cataract surgery comparing the use of aspheric versus spherical IOL implantation that assessed visual acuity, contrast sensitivity, or quality of vision. The effects were calculated as mean differences or standardized mean differences (Hedges' g) and pooled using random-effect models.

Main Outcome Measures.—Best-corrected visual acuity (BCVA), contrast sensitivity, and subjective perception of the quality of vision.

Results.—Forty-three studies provided data and were included, comprising 2076 eyes implanted with aspheric IOLs and 2034 eyes implanted with spherical IOLs. The BCVA showed a significant difference for aspheric IOLs (−0.01 logarithm of the minimum angle of resolution; 95% confidence interval [CI], −0.02 to −0.00). For contrast sensitivity, a significant advantage for aspheric IOLs was found under photopic and mesopic light conditions (photopic: Hedges' g 0.42, 95% CI 0.24−0.61 (3 cycles per degree [cpd]) to 0.53, 95% CI 0.33−0.73 (12 cpd); mesopic: Hedges' g 0.49, 95% CI 0.23−0.75 (1.5 cpd) to 0.76, 95% CI 0.52−1.00 (18 cpd)). Questionnaires targeting the subjective perception of quality of vision yielded less conclusive results.

Conclusions.—Overall, a patient may achieve better contrast sensitivity with an aspheric IOL than with a spherical IOL, especially under dim light. There was no clinically relevant difference in BCVA between aspheric and spherical IOL implantation. The findings on the subjective perception of visual quality were heterogeneous with no clear result favoring either option.

▶ This is an extensive meta-analysis of the existing literature comparing visual outcomes of aspheric intraocular lenses (IOLs) with those of spherical IOLs. The analysis included 43 studies and more than 4000 eyes in good quality randomized trials. Even though most of the individual studies concluded an advantage for aspheric IOLs, this analysis combining data from all the studies found an advantage only in mesopic contrast sensitivity. Best-corrected visual acuity and subjective quality of vision were essentially equivalent between aspheric and spherical IOLs.

Because asphericity is almost universally accepted now as a desirable quality for an IOL, this finding may be a moot point. Almost all foldable IOLs in common use now have an aspheric modified optic designed to minimize total eye spherical aberration. Current aspheric IOLs either attempt to balance the estimated positive spherical aberration of the cornea by adding negative spherical aberration or are designed with zero spherical aberration. The theoretical benefit of an aspheric IOL is greater through a larger pupil aperture but requires excellent centration of the IOL. In fact, a negative aspheric IOL may even degrade vision compared with an old standard spherical IOL if decentered more than 0.4 mm.[1] This analysis did not address these principles, and it may not have been addressed by the prior studies included in the meta-analysis here.

M. F. Pyfer, MD

Reference

1. Roshdy MM, Riad RF, Morkos FF, Hassouna AK, Wahba SS. Effect of a single-piece aspheric hydrophobic acrylic intraocular lens design on centration and rotation. *J Cataract Refract Surg*. 2013;39:408-413.

Using continuous intraoperative optical coherence tomography measurements of the aphakic eye for intraocular lens power calculation

Hirnschall N, Norrby S, Weber M, et al (Hanusch Hosp, Vienna, Austria; Leek, The Netherlands)

Br J Ophthalmol 99:7-10, 2015

Background/Aims.—To include intraoperative measurements of the anterior lens capsule of the aphakic eye into the intraocular lens power calculation (IPC) process and to compare the refractive outcome with conventional IPC formulae.

Methods.—In this prospective study, a prototype operating microscope with an integrated continuous optical coherence tomography (OCT) device (Visante attached to OPMI VISU 200, Carl Zeiss Meditec AG, Germany) was used to measure the anterior lens capsule position after implanting a capsular tension ring (CTR). Optical biometry (intraocular lens (IOL) Master 500) and ACMaster measurements (Carl Zeiss Meditec AG, Germany) were performed before surgery. Autorefraction and subjective refraction were performed 3 months after surgery. Conventional IPC formulae were compared with a new intraoperatively measured anterior chamber depth (ACD) ($ACD_{IntraOP}$) partial least squares regression (PLSR) model for prediction of the postoperative refractive outcome.

Results.—In total, 70 eyes of 70 patients were included. Mean axial eye length (AL) was 23.3 mm (range: 20.6– 29.5 mm). Predictive power of the intraoperative measurements was found to be slightly better compared to conventional IOL power calculations. Refractive error dependency on AL for Holladay I, HofferQ, SRK/T, Haigis and $ACD_{intraOP}$ PLSR was $r^2 = -0.42$ ($p < 0.0001$), $r^2 = -0.5$ ($p < 0.0001$), $r^2 = -0.34$ ($p = 0.010$), $r^2 = -0.28$ ($p = 0.049$) and $r^2 < 0.001$ ($p = 0.866$), respectively.

Conclusions.—$ACD_{IntraOP}$ measurements help to better predict the refractive outcome and could be useful, if implemented in fourth-generation IPC formulae.

▶ This report describes a novel technique to enhance the accuracy of intraocular lens (IOL) power calculation by using intraoperative biometry. Specifically, the final IOL position is estimated by measuring the exact axial location of the anterior lens capsule using intraoperative ocular coherence tomography (OCT). The only other intraoperative IOL power calculation system in use today involves wavefront aberrometry through the aphakic eye during surgery. This system still requires estimation of the IOL position to predict the overall refractive error.

Here the authors measured the exact anterior chamber depth after placement of a capsular tension ring but prior to IOL insertion. They used a commercial OCT system integrated with the operating microscope. This information was then used to create a regression formula including axial length and IOL power to estimate the final spherical equivalent refraction. The authors state that keratometry did not affect the estimation, so it was not included. The method showed a slight improvement compared with the standard third- and fourth-generation IOL power calculation formulas.

This is the first attempt published to measure true IOL position during surgery to improve power calculation accuracy. The main significance of this work in my opinion is that it could be combined with intraoperative wavefront aberrometry to enhance the accuracy of that technique. Estimation of final IOL position remains the greatest source of error in IOL power calculation today, and performing intraoperative measurement as described here has the potential to reduce that error.

M. F. Pyfer, MD

Achieving Target Refraction after Cataract Surgery

Simon SS, Chee YE, Haddadin RI, et al (Massachusetts Eye and Ear Infirmary, Boston)

Ophthalmology 121:440-444, 2014

Purpose.—To evaluate the difference between target and actual refraction after phacoemulsification and intraocular lens implantation at an academic teaching institution's Comprehensive Ophthalmology Service.

Design.—Retrospective study.

Participants.—We examined 1275 eye surgeries for this study.

Methods.—All consecutive cataract surgeries were included if they were performed by an attending or resident surgeon from January through December 2010. Postoperative refractions were compared with preoperative target refractions. Patients were excluded if they did not have a preoperative target refraction documented or if they did not have a recorded postoperative manifest refraction within 90 days.

Main Outcome Measures.—The main outcome measure was percentage of cases achieving a postoperative spherical equivalent ± 1.0 diopter (D) of target spherical equivalent.

Results.—We performed 1368 cataract surgeries from January through December of 2010. Of these, 1275 (93%) had sufficient information for analysis. Of the included cases, 94% (1196 of 1275) achieved ±1.0 D of target refraction by 90 days after cataract surgery.

Conclusions.—This paper establishes a new benchmark for a teaching hospital, where 94% of patients achieved within 1.0 D of target refraction after cataract surgery. The refractive outcomes after cataract surgery at this academic teaching institution were higher than average international benchmarks.

▶ This retrospective review of refractive outcome from cataract surgery over a 1-year period at a large teaching hospital proposes a new benchmark for this metric. The authors are to be commended for achieving 94% within 1 diopter (D) and 67% within 0.5 D of the target refraction. It is a testament to an organized preoperative evaluation and measurement process, careful lens calculation and selection, and meticulous surgery and is higher than previously reported benchmarks for refractive outcome.[1]

However, I do not agree that refractive outcome is a better measure of the outcome of cataract surgery than final visual acuity. Accuracy in achieving target refraction is only one aspect of quality in cataract surgery and should be evaluated along with other metrics. Complications that may be more common for surgeons in training, such as prolonged corneal edema, retained lens fragments, vitreous loss, and postoperative cystoid macular edema, are more likely to affect visual acuity than refractive outcome. These were not reported, and neither was final visual acuity. Also, since refraction is a manual process that is somewhat subjective, a standardized impartial and preferably masked observer should perform it. Because this study was retrospective in nature, perhaps auto refraction without subjective refinement or wavefront aberrometry could be added as an objective measure. Other outcome measures, such as time to achieve refractive stability at final visual acuity, and intraoperative parameters, such as operating time and total ultrasound power used, are also critical in any proposed quality metric for cataract surgical outcomes.

M. F. Pyfer, MD

Reference

1. Gale RP, Saldana M, Johnston RL, Zuberbuhler B, McKibbin M. Benchmark standards for refractive outcomes after NHS cataract surgery. *Eye (Lond)*. 2009; 23:149-152.

Three-Year Incidence and Factors Associated With Posterior Capsule Opacification After Cataract Surgery: The Australian Prospective Cataract Surgery and Age-related Macular Degeneration Study

Fong CS-U, Mitchell P, Rochtchina E, et al (Univ of Sydney, Australia; et al)
Am J Ophthalmol 157:171-179.e1, 2014

Purpose.—To assess 3-year incidence and associated factors of posterior capsule opacification (PCO) after phacoemulsification surgery.

Design.—Cohort study.

Methods.—A total of 1934 consecutive patients aged ≥64 years undergoing phacoemulsification surgery at Westmead Hospital were recruited, of whom 1495 (77.3%) had retroillumination anterior segment images taken of the surgical eyes after 1 month and at a further postoperative visit within 3 years. Severe PCO was defined if the view of the optic disc was obscured, or neodymium-yttrium-aluminum-garnet capsulotomy was performed. Cumulative incidence of PCO was estimated using Kaplan-Meier methods. Associations of PCO with surgeon groups and different types of implanted intraocular lenses (IOLs) were assessed, adjusting for age, sex, diabetes, and ethnicity.

Results.—Three-year cumulative incidence of PCO was 38.5% (95% confidence interval [CI] 36.1%-40.9%) among the 1495 patients, including 4.7% (95% CI 3.5%-5.8%) with severe PCO. PCO incidence was higher in: (1) eyes operated on by junior trainees (49%) compared to those by senior ophthalmologist surgeons (36%) (adjusted odds ratio [OR] 1.6, 95% CI 1.2-2.0); and (2) eyes with hydrophobic, 3-piece (either square-edged [51%, OR 2.3, 95% CI 1.4-3.6] or partial-round-edged [39%, OR 1.5, 95% CI 1.1-2.1]), or hydrophilic IOLs (64%, OR 2.9, 95% CI 1.9-4.4) compared to those with single-piece, square-edged, hydrophobic IOLs (34%), after additional adjustment for surgeon group.

Conclusions.—Predominantly mild PCO occurred in one-third of eyes after phacoemulsification surgery. Possible predisposing factors associated with PCO development include surgery performed by ophthalmologic

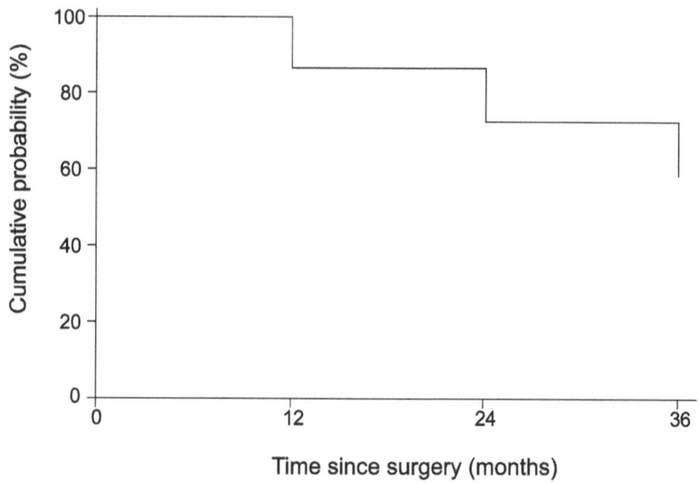

FIGURE 5.—Kaplan-Meier survival plot of patients not having any (both mild and severe) posterior capsule opacification 1-3 years after cataract surgery in the Australian Prospective Cataract Surgery and Age-related Macular Degeneration study. (Reprinted from American Journal of Ophthalmology. Fong CS-U, Mitchell P, Rochtchina E, et al. Three-year incidence and factors associated with posterior capsule opacification after cataract surgery: the Australian prospective cataract surgery and age-related macular degeneration study. *Am J Ophthalmol.* 2014;157:171-179.e1, Copyright 2014, with permission from Elsevier.)

trainees and the use of hydrophilic or other hydrophobic IOLs apart from the single-piece, square-edged one (Fig 5).

▶ This large prospective study across multiple surgeons including residents in training that shows posterior capsule opacification (PCO) after cataract surgery is quite common. The overall incidence of PCO is approximately 35% within 3 years after surgery. It is much more common with hydrophilic intraocular lenses (IOLs) (64%) and for junior trainees (49%), presumably because of incomplete cortical cleanup and lens epithelial cell removal. Although only 5% to 10% of the IOLs used in this study were lenses other than single-piece square-edged hydrophobic acrylic, the large cohort makes comparisons between groups statistically valid. The reported higher biocompatibility of hydrophilic acrylic lenses may predispose this type to greater incidence of PCO, but the cause was not examined in this study.

This publication confirms prior reports that PCO is lower for single-piece square-edged hydrophobic acrylic lenses. It is the first large study to compare rates of PCO between experienced surgeons and those in the first 2 years of training.

In reference to this article, experienced surgeons using the most popular lens implants may inform their cataract surgery patients that about one-third will have some PCO within 3 years after surgery. The timing of YAG laser capsulotomy of course is quite variable, based on patient symptoms and surgical judgment, but from this study would not be expected to be more than 35% over the first 3 postoperative years.

M. F. Pyfer, MD

Effect of total lens epithelial cell destruction on intraocular lens fixation in the human capsular bag

Spalton DJ, Russell SL, Evans-Gowing R, et al (King Edward VII Hosp, London, UK; Univ of East Anglia, Norwich, UK)

J Cataract Refract Surg 40:306-312, 2014

Purpose.—To evaluate the effect of complete destruction of lens epithelial cells (LECs) in the capsular bag on intraocular lens (IOL) stability.

Setting.—School of Biological Sciences, University of East Anglia, Norwich, United Kingdom.

Design.—Comparative evaluation.

Methods.—An in vitro organ culture model using the bag-zonule-ciliary body complex isolated from fellow human donor eyes was prepared. A capsulorhexis and fiber extraction were performed, and an Acrysof IOL was implanted. Preparations were secured by pinning the ciliary body to a silicone ring and maintaining it in 6 mL Eagle minimum essential medium supplemented with 5% v/v fetal calf serum and 10 ng/mL transforming growth factor-β2 for 3 weeks or more. One bag of each pair was treated with 1 μM thapsigargin to destroy all LECs. Observations of LEC growth were captured by phase-contrast microscopy, IOL stability by video microscopy, and endpoint analysis through scanning electron microscopy and immunocytochemistry.

Results.—The LECs in control capsular bags migrated centrally, closing the bag and fixating the IOL between the anterior and posterior capsules, as seen clinically. These events were not observed in the thapsigargin-treated group. After a period of controlled orbital movement, the IOL in the control group stabilized quicker than in the treated bags. There was no IOL rotation in the bag; however, the IOLs in the treated group rocked with axial movement.

Conclusions.—The LECs appeared to aid stabilization of current IOL designs in the capsular bag. The results have clinical implications for IOL design and for strategies to prevent posterior capsule opacification (Fig 2).

▶ Prevention of posterior capsule opacification (PCO) is likely critical for successful function of advanced intraocular lens (IOL) designs such as accommodating lenses. This study shows that complete chemical elimination of lens epithelial cells (LECs) not only prevents PCO formation but also allows standard single-piece IOLs to remain somewhat mobile within the capsular bag owing to lack of adhesive "shrink wrap" effect of the capsule around the implant (Fig 2). Thus, it may be more desirable to prevent LEC proliferation and migration rather than to completely eliminate them during cataract surgery. New IOL designs have been tested that keep the capsular bag open after surgery, and it has been found that contact with aqueous fluid seems to inhibit LEC proliferation.[1] This report supports the notion that this is a better technique to prevent capsular fibrosis and PCO formation than complete elimination of LECs.

M. F. Pyfer, MD

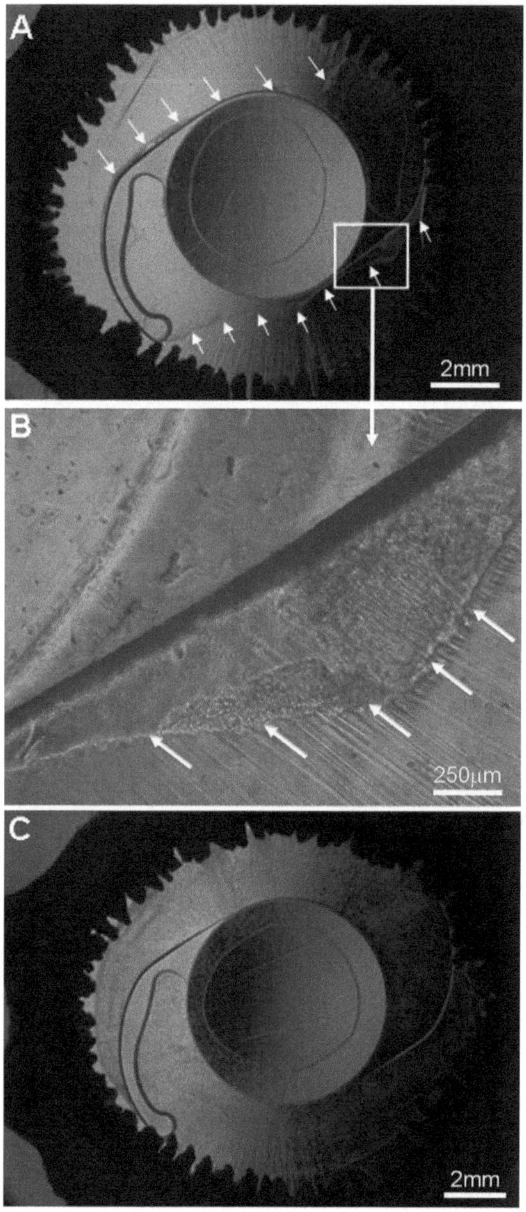

FIGURE 2.—Low-power modified dark-field images showing gross changes in control and thapsigargin-treated capsular bags. *A* and *B*: Distinct regions of adhesion (*arrows*) between the anterior capsule and posterior capsule can be observed in control preparations. *C*: No adhesion between opposing capsule surfaces can be seen in thapsigargin-treated capsular bags. (Reprinted from Journal of Cataract & Refractive Surgery. Spalton DJ, Russell SL, Evans-Gowing R, et al. Effect of total lens epithelial cell destruction on intraocular lens fixation in the human capsular bag. *J Cataract Refract Surg.* 2014;40:306-312, Copyright 2014, with permission from ASCRS and ESCRS.)

Reference

1. Floyd AM, Werner L, Liu E, et al. Capsular bag opacification with a new accommodating intraocular lens. *J Cataract Refract Surg.* 2013;39:1415-1420.

Light transmittance of 1-piece hydrophobic acrylic intraocular lenses with surface light scattering removed from cadaver eyes

Werner L, Morris C, Liu E, et al (Univ of Utah, Salt Lake City)

J Cataract Refract Surg 40:114-120, 2014

Purpose.—To assess the potential effect of surface light scattering on light transmittance of 1-piece hydrophobic acrylic intraocular lenses (IOLs) with or without a blue-light filter.

Setting.—John A. Moran Eye Center, University of Utah, Salt Lake City, Utah, USA.

Design.—Experimental study.

Methods.—Intraocular lenses were obtained from human cadavers (49 IOLs total; 36 with blue-light filter) and from finished-goods inventory (controls). The IOLs were removed from cadaver eyes and the power and model matched to unused controls. After surface proteins were removed, the IOLs were hydrated for 24 hours at room temperature. Surface light scattering was measured with a Scheimpflug camera (EAS-1000 Anterior Segment Analysis System). Light transmittance was measured with a Lambda 35 UV/V is spectrophotometer (single-beam configuration; RSA-PE-20 integrating sphere).

Results.—Hydrated scatter values ranged from 4.8 to 202.5 computer-compatible tape (CCT) units for explanted IOLs with blue-light filter and 1.5 to 11.8 CCT units for controls; values ranged from 6.0 to 137.5 CCT units for explanted IOLs without a blue-light filter and 3.5 to 9.6 CCT units for controls. In both groups, there was a tendency toward increasing scatter values with increasing postoperative time. No differences in light transmittance were observed between explanted IOLs and controls in both groups (IOLs with blue-light filter: $P = .407$; IOL with no blue-light filter: $P = .487$; both paired t test).

Conclusions.—Although surface light scattering of explanted IOLs was significantly higher than that of controls and appeared to increase with time, no effect was observed on light transmittance of 1-piece hydrophobic acrylic IOLs with or without a blue-light filter. (Figs 1 and 2).

▶ Subsurface nanoglistenings in hydrophobic acrylic intraocular lenses (IOLs) that develop months to years after implantation have been described and extensively studied. This phenomenon is particularly evident in the Acrysof line of IOLs and is commonly visible on slit lamp examination. What is not known, but has been debated, is the visual significance of IOL glistenings. Case reports of IOL explantation owing to decreased visual acuity attributed to glistenings

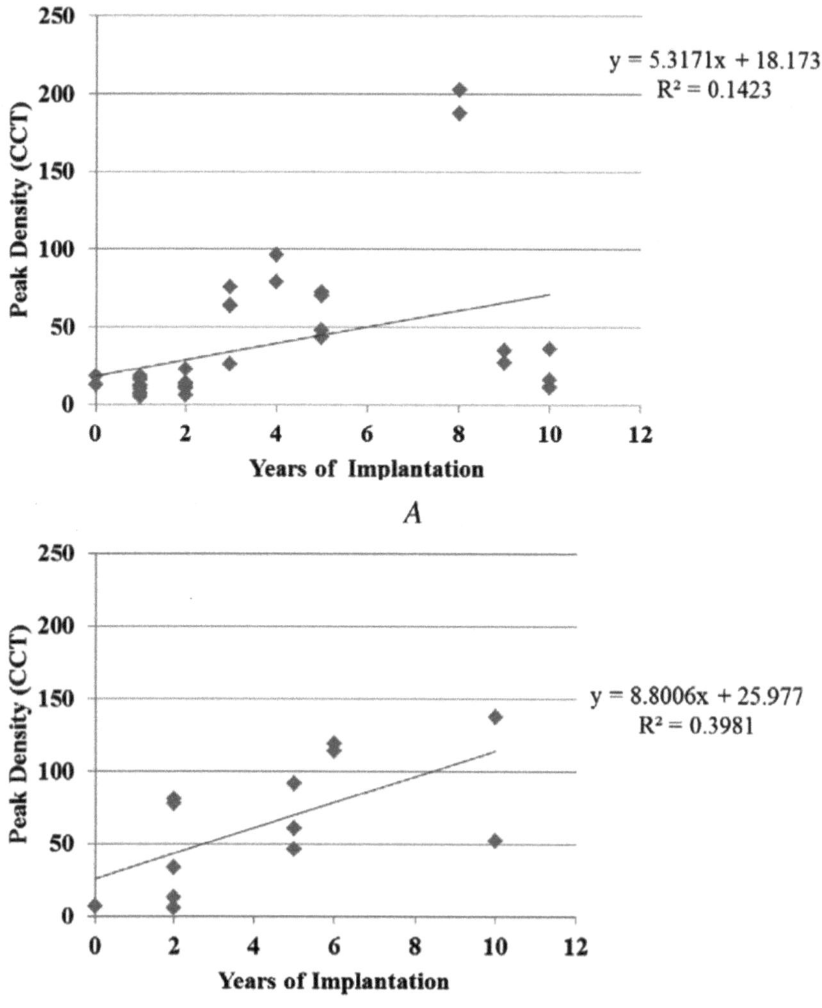

FIGURE 1.—Surface light scattering as a function of postoperative time. *A*: Group of IOLs with a blue-light filter (n = 36) (correlation coefficient [R^1] = 0.377; P = .023). *B*: Non-blue-light filtering IOL group (n = 13) (R^2 = 0.631; P = .019). Correlation coefficient comparison (R^1 versus R^2) P = .338; slope comparison P = .432 using analysis of covariance (CCT = computer-compatible tape). (Reprinted from Journal of Cataract & Refractive Surgery. Werner L, Morris C, Liu E, et al. Light transmittance of 1-piece hydrophobic acrylic intraocular lenses with surface light scattering removed from cadaver eyes. *J Cataract Refract Surg*. 2014;40:114-120, Copyright 2014, with permission from ASCRS and ESCRS.)

have been published, but larger studies have not found a measurable effect on visual acuity or contrast sensitivity to date.

This well-controlled postmortem IOL analysis shows that single-piece Acrysof acrylic IOLs, with a blue-light filter or without, have no significant loss of light transmittance or change in spectral transmission up to 10 years

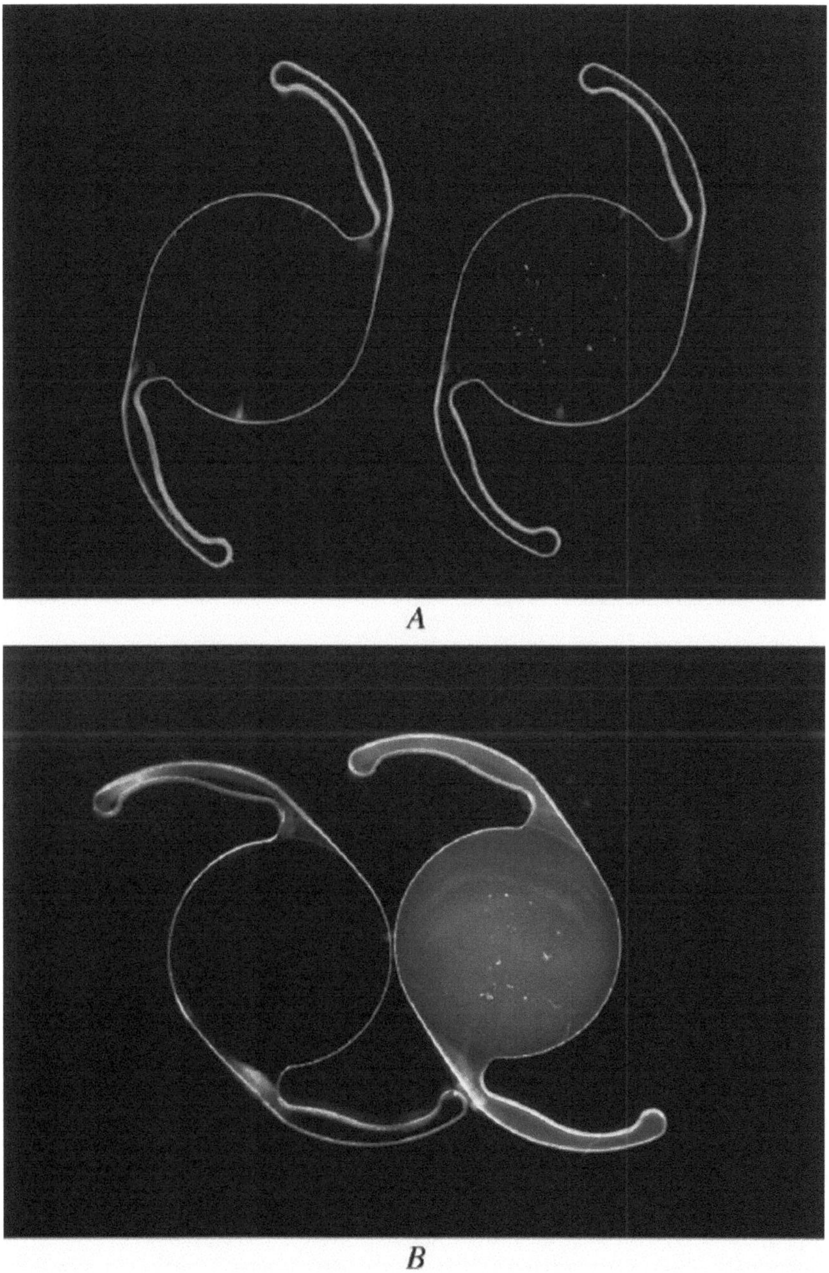

FIGURE 2.—Gross photographs (dark-field images with a 90-degree off-axis illumination) of a cadaver-eye-removed blue light–filtering IOL (*right*) with corresponding control IOL (*left*). *A*: In the dry state, no optic haziness is observed. *B*: In the hydrated state, the IOLs are immersed in a balanced salt solution. The explanted IOL shows overall haziness compared with the control IOL. Optic pits, probably caused by neodymium:YAG laser application, can also be observed on the explant. (Reprinted from Journal of Cataract & Refractive Surgery. Werner L, Morris C, Liu E, et al. Light transmittance of 1-piece hydrophobic acrylic intraocular lenses with surface light scattering removed from cadaver eyes. *J Cataract Refract Surg*. 2014;40:114-120, Copyright 2014, with permission from ASCRS and ESCRS.)

after implantation. However, there is a significant increase in surface light scattering that trends higher with implantation time (Figs 1 and 2). The visual significance of light scattering at lower levels is not well known. Higher levels of scattering (greater than 50 on a 0–255 scale) were found to be visually significant in another report.[1] This study also showed no difference in transmittance or scattering after implantation between blue-blocking and non blue-blocking Acrysof IOLs.

Millions of these IOLs have been implanted worldwide over the last 20 years, and this study supports the expectation of continued good visual performance for patients with them in place, based on light transmission stability over time. What remains to be shown is whether light scattering continues to increase beyond 10 years, and is this visually significant and measurable in vivo. Other hydrophobic acrylic lenses should be examined similarly.

M. F. Pyfer, MD

Reference

1. Miyata K, Honbo M, Otani S, Nejima R, Minami K. Effect on visual acuity of increased surface light scattering in intraocular lenses. *J Cataract Refract Surg.* 2012;38:221-226.

Influence of Ocular Features and Incision Width on Surgically Induced Astigmatism After Cataract Surgery

Chang S-W, Su T-Y, Chen Y-L (Far Eastern Memorial Hosp, New Taipei City, Taiwan; Natl Yang-Ming Univ, Taipei, Taiwan; Natl Taiwan Univ, Taipei; et al)
J Refrac Surg 31:82-88, 2015

Purpose.—To identify factors associated with surgically induced astigmatism (SIA) following phacoemulsification.

Methods.—Six hundred five eyes underwent phaco-emulsification with a 2.2-mm (the 2.2-mm group, n = 248) or 2.75-mm (the 2.75-mm group, n = 357) superior limbal incision. Preoperative axial length, anterior chamber depth, corneal curvature, and intraocular pressure were measured. Corneal curvature and intraocular pressure were measured at 1 day, 1 week, and 1, 2, and 3 months postoperatively. SIA, corneal flattening, and torque were calculated using the Alpins method. The effect of preoperative corneal astigmatism meridian on SIA was also examined. Differences in SIA between the 2.2- and 2.75-mm groups were explored, and correlations between SIA and preoperative corneal astigmatism, anterior chamber depth, axial length, age, and intraocular pressure were analyzed.

Results.—SIA, corneal flattening, and torque were smaller in the 2.2-mm group than in the 2.75-mm group at 1 week (P = .003, .006, and .014, respectively), but not statistically different thereafter. Higher preoperative corneal astigmatism, older age, and shallower anterior chamber depth were associated with greater SIA in both groups. The effect of astigmatism meridian on SIA was more noticeable in the 2.75-mm group.

TABLE 2.—Summary of Significant Correlations Between SIA and Other Dactors

	Incision Size			
	2.75 mm		2.2 mm	
Time Postoperatively	*r*	*P*	*r*	*P*
1 day				
Preoperative corneal astigmatism	0.244	.004	0.311	< .001
Age	0.348	< .001	0.255	< .001
ACD	−0.234	.028	−0.222	.003
Preoperative axial length	−0.215	.003	–	–
Preoperative IOP	−0.340	.006	–	–
1 week				
Preoperative corneal astigmatism	0.315	.001	0.188	.006
Age	0.243	< .001	0.267	< .001
ACD	−0.220	.002	−0.194	.014
Preoperative axial length	−0.184	.006	–	–
Preoperative IOP	−0.355	.02	–	–
1 month				
Preoperative corneal astigmatism	0.205	.021	0.236	.001
Age	0.344	< .001	0.22	.002
ACD	−0.220	.029	−0.192	.024
Preoperative axial length	0.184	.040	–	–
Preoperative IOP	−0.278	.005	–	–
IOP 3 months postoperatively	−0.271	.033	–	–
2 months				
Preoperative corneal astigmatism	0.205	.001	0.251	.005
Age	0.293	< .001	–	–
ACD	0.273	.001	–	–
Preoperative axial length	−0.146	.016	–	–
Preoperative IOP	−0.223	.030	–	–
IOP 3 months postoperatively	−0.317	.012	–	–
3 months				
Preoperative corneal astigmatism	0.185	.006	–	–
Age	0.297	< .001	–	–
ACD	−0.214	.006	–	–
Preoperative axial length	0.203	.003	–	–
Preoperative	−0.233	.046	–	–
IOP 3 months postoperatively	−0.256	.044	–	–

SIA = surgically induced astigmatism; ACD = anterior chamber depth; IOP = intraocular pressure.
Reprinted with permission from SLACK Incorporated: Chang S-W, Su T-Y, Chen Y-L. Influence of Ocular Features and Incision Width on Surgically Induced Astigmatism After Cataract Surgery. *J Refrac Surg*. 2015;31:82–88.

Shorter axial length and lower intraocular pressures were associated with greater SIA in the 2.75-mm group but not in the 2.2-mm group.

Conclusions.—Reducing limbal incision width and considering patient age, the meridian and magnitude of corneal astigmatism, anterior chamber depth, axial length, and intraocular pressure, and adjusting the flattening component of SIA input for toric intraocular lens power calculation could potentially improve the astigmatism control in refractive lens surgery (Table 2).

▶ This study evaluated surgically induced astigmatism (SIA) in several hundred patients for a single surgeon. The use of a superior limbal incision is a drawback, as most surgeons operate temporally or on the axis of the steep corneal meridian. However, the most significant result here is that after

1 week, there is no significant difference in SIA between a 2.2-mm incision and a 2.75-mm incision. Many surgeons have converted to 2.2-mm temporal corneal incisions to reduce SIA, and this study indicates that it may not be necessary. I recommend that if a surgeon is more comfortable or efficient using a 2.75-mm incision, then there is no compelling reason to reduce this to 2.2 mm.

In a further subgroup analysis, it was found that in the 2.75-mm incision group, certain factors had more effect on SIA than in the 2.2-mm group. These factors included patient age, preoperative intraocular pressure, preexisting corneal astigmatism, and anterior chamber depth (Table 2). For surgeons interested in fine tuning their SIA adjustment for toric intraocular lens calculations, it may be useful to adjust for these preoperative measurements in your personal nomogram.

M. F. Pyfer, MD

Post-cataract Prevention of Inflammation and Macular Edema by Steroid and Nonsteroidal Anti-inflammatory Eye Drops: A Systematic Review

Kessel L, Tendal B, Jørgensen KJ, et al (Copenhagen Univ Hosp Glostrup, Denmark; Danish Health and Medicines Authority, Copenhagen, Denmark; et al)

Ophthalmology 121:1915-1924, 2014

Purpose.—Favorable outcome after cataract surgery depends on proper control of the inflammatory response induced by cataract surgery. Pseudophakic cystoid macular edema is an important cause of visual decline after uncomplicated cataract surgery.

Design.—We compared the efficacy of topical steroids with topical nonsteroidal anti-inflammatory drugs (NSAIDs) in controlling inflammation and preventing pseudophakic cystoid macular edema (PCME) after uncomplicated cataract surgery.

Participants.—Patients undergoing uncomplicated surgery for age-related cataract.

Methods.—We performed a systematic literature search in Medline, CINAHL, Cochrane, and EMBASE databases to identify randomized trials published from 1996 onward comparing topical steroids with topical NSAIDs in controlling inflammation and preventing PCME in patients undergoing phacoemulsification with posterior chamber intraocular lens implantation for age-related cataract.

Main Outcome Measures.—Postoperative inflammation and pseudophakic cystoid macular edema.

Results.—Fifteen randomized trials were identified. Postoperative inflammation was less in patients randomized to NSAIDs. The prevalence of PCME was significantly higher in the steroid group than in the NSAID group: 3.8% versus 25.3% of patients, risk ratio 5.35 (95% confidence interval, 2.94–9.76). There was no statistically significant difference in the number of adverse events in the 2 treatment groups.

Conclusions.—We found low to moderate quality of evidence that topical NSAIDs are more effective in controlling postoperative inflammation after cataract surgery. We found high-quality evidence that topical NSAIDs are more effective than topical steroids in preventing PCME. The use of topical NSAIDs was not associated with an increased events. We recommend using topical NSAIDs to prevent inflammation and PCME after routine cataract surgery.

▶ This meta-analysis of 15 randomized, controlled trials comparing topical steroid with nonsteroidal anti-inflammatory drug (NSAID) use after routine cataract surgery concludes that there is strong evidence to recommend the use of NSAIDs to prevent postoperative cystoid macular edema (CME). The definition of CME in these studies is by ocular coherence tomography or intravenous fluorescein angiography at 4 to 5 weeks after surgery. Only low-risk eyes were included in the underlying studies, and 7 studies with 521 eyes were suitable for inclusion in the CME endpoint. Four of those used fluorometholone as the steroid, and none used prednisolone or difluprednate, which are more potent steroids in common use in the United States. This finding may explain the higher than expected incidence of CME in the steroid-only arm (25%).

Prior published studies comparing steroid alone with steroid plus NSAID were equivocal, some showing reduced CME[1] and others showing no difference.[2] Incidence of CME with prednisolone alone in prior studies was about 3% to 12%, much lower than in this report.[3]

The question of whether NSAIDs provide an added benefit after cataract surgery has been one of the most studied and controversial issues in ophthalmology in recent years. This topic takes on added impact as the cost of medications increases, even alternative generic formulations. Most cataract surgeons prescribe at least a topical steroid for patients after cataract surgery, typically prednisolone in the United States. If used, NSAIDs are usually added during the perioperative period, started up to 3 days before surgery to help prevent intraoperative miosis and to reduce postoperative discomfort. If continued more than 1 to 2 weeks after surgery, NSAIDs are used off label for control of inflammation and prevention of CME.

This study adds evidence that topical NSAIDs are more effective than a low potency steroid for prevention of CME. Because CME frequently results in decreased visual acuity and contrast sensitivity that may be difficult to eradicate and is sometimes permanent, it makes sense on a case-by-case basis to use NSAIDs plus a potent steroid after cataract surgery. This is especially true in patients at higher risk for CME (epiretinal membrane, diabetic, previous CME in fellow eye, chronic uveitis). This is my practice, until a definitive, large, well-controlled, randomized trial is published that shows otherwise.

M. F. Pyfer, MD

References

1. Wittpenn JR, Silverstein S, Heier J, Kenyon KR, Hunkeler JD, Earl M, Acular LS for Cystoid Macular Edema (ACME) Study Group. A randomized, masked comparison of topical ketorolac 0.4% plus steroid vs steroid alone in low-risk cataract surgery patients. *Am J Ophthalmol.* 2008;146:554-560.

2. Almeida DR, Khan Z, Xing L, et al. Prophylactic nepafenac and ketorolac versus placebo in preventing postoperative macular edema after uneventful phacoemulsification. *J Cataract Refract Surg*. 2012;38:1537-1543.
3. Yilmaz T, Cordero-Coma M, Gallagher MJ. Ketorolac therapy for the prevention of acute pseudophakic cystoid macular edema: a systematic review. *Eye (Lond)*. 2012;26:252-258.

Incidence of postoperative endophthalmitis from 1990 to 2009 using povidone–iodine but no intracameral antibiotics at a single academic institution

Nentwich MM, Ta CN, Kreutzer TC, et al (Ludwig-Maximilians-Univ, Munich, Germany; Stanford Univ, CA)
J Cataract Refract Surg 41:58-66, 2015

Purpose.—To correlate the incidence of postoperative endophthalmitis with changes in the preoperative prophylaxis over a 20-year period.

Setting.—Department of Ophthalmology, Ludwig-Maximilians-University, Munich, Germany.

Design.—Retrospective chart review.

Methods.—Patients diagnosed with postoperative endophthalmitis from 1990 to 2009 after intraocular surgery performed at the same institution were included. Because of changes in the preoperative prophylaxis during the study period, 3 groups were formed for data analysis: Period 1 (1990 to 1992), no standardized prophylaxis regimen; period 2 (1993 to 1998), preoperative topical medication, povidone–iodine 10.0% periorbitally, and 1 drop of povidone–iodine 1.0% in the conjunctiva sac; and period 3 (1999 to 2009), similar to period 2 except with irrigation of the conjunctival sac with 10 mL of povidone–iodine 1.0%.

Results.—The overall rate of postoperative endophthalmitis was 0.113% (77/68 323) for all intraocular surgeries. It decreased significantly from 0.291% (16/5505) in period 1 to 0.170% (33/19 413) in period 2 to 0.065% (28/43 405) in period 3 ($P < .001$). In cataract surgery, the overall rate of postoperative endophthalmitis was 0.125% (30/24 034). It decreased in each subsequent period, from 0.338% (9/2662) in period 1 to 0.224% (15/6696) in period 2 to 0.041% (6/14 676) in period 3 ($P < .001$). Coagulase-negative *Staphylococcus* was the most commonly isolated organism (47.4%).

Conclusions.—The rate of postoperative endophthalmitis decreased over a 20-year period at a single academic institution. Although multiple factors might have contributed to this decline, implementation of a preoperative prophylaxis protocol using copious povidone–iodine might have been the most important contributor (Fig 1).

▶ This study demonstrates a significant reduction in postoperative endophthalmitis at a single institution over a 20-year period. Standardized perioperative preparation was introduced in year 3, then changed in year 9 to combine

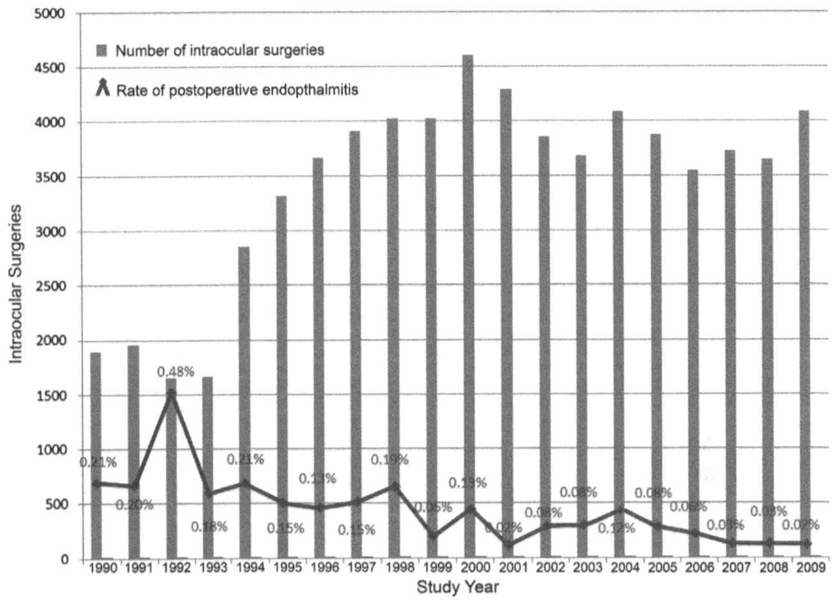

FIGURE 1.—Number of intraocular surgeries and rate of postoperative endophthalmitis. (Reprinted from Journal of Cataract & Refractive Surgery. Nentwich MM, Ta CN, Kreutzer TC, et al. Incidence of postoperative endophthalmitis from 1990 to 2009 using povidone–iodine but no intracameral antibiotics at a single academic institution. *J Cataract Refract Surg*. 2015;41:58-66, Copyright 2015, with permission from ASCRS and ESCRS.)

irrigation of the conjunctival fornices with 1% povidone–iodine solution plus the usual topical and eyelid povidone–iodine prep. A corresponding 2.5-fold drop in endophthalmitis rate coincided with this change (Fig 1). No intracameral antibiotic was used, and the authors state that the pre- and postoperative topical antibiotic regimen remained constant. One limitation of this study is that evolution in surgical technique undoubtedly occurred during this time, including a trend toward smaller incision sizes, but this was not analyzed or controlled.

The main conclusion of this observational study with historical control is that with preoperative povidone–iodine irrigation in addition to the usual prophylactic measures for cataract surgery, the rate of endophthalmitis (0.049%) was as low as those reported in other large studies using intracameral cefuroxime (0.062%).[1]

This evidence is strong enough to recommend that all eye surgeons begin preoperative flushing of the fornices with dilute povidone–iodine in addition to their standard surgical prep, especially if not using intracameral antibiotics. Most centers dispense dilute povidone–iodine drops topically from a syringe or prepackaged vial and then waste the excess. This excess could be used for fornix irrigation, so there should be no added cost to this measure.

M. F. Pyfer, MD

Reference

1. Endophthalmitis Study Group, European Society of Cataract & Refractive Surgeons. Prophylaxis of postoperative endophthalmitis following cataract surgery: results of the ESCRS multicenter study and identification of risk factors. *J Cataract Refract Surg*. 2007;33:978-988.

Intraocular Pressure and Wound Status in Eyes Immediately After Scleral Tunnel Incision and Clear Corneal Incision Cataract Surgery

Hayashi K, Tsuru T, Yoshida M, et al (Hayashi Eye Hosp, Fukuoka, Japan)
Am J Ophthalmol 158:232-241, 2014

Purpose.—To compare intraocular pressure (IOP) and wound architecture immediately after cataract surgery using a scleral tunnel incision or clear corneal incision.

Design.—Prospective randomized clinical trial.

Methods.—Bilateral eyes of 64 patients undergoing phacoemulsification were randomized to 2 groups: 2.4 mm scleral tunnel incision or 2.4 mm clear corneal incision. IOP was adjusted upon completion of surgery to between 15 and 30 mm Hg. The wound was hydrated in 87.5% of eyes in the clear corneal incision group. IOP was measured using a rebound tonometer preoperatively; at the conclusion of surgery; and at 5, 10, 15, 30, and 60 minutes postoperatively. The Seidel test and anterior segment optical coherence tomography (AS OCT) were performed at 30 minutes postoperatively.

Results.—In the scleral tunnel incision group, mean IOP decreased to the preoperative level within 15 minutes postoperatively and did not change significantly for up to 60 minutes. In the clear corneal incision group, IOP decreased to lower than the preoperative IOP at 30 minutes postoperatively. Mean IOP was significantly higher in the scleral tunnel incision group than in the clear corneal incision group throughout the postoperative period ($P \leq 0339$). Hypotony (<10 mm Hg) was observed in 7 eyes (10.9%) that underwent clear corneal incision and in no eyes that underwent scleral tunnel incision ($P = .0131$). Wound leakage and loss of wound coaptation were not observed in any eyes.

Conclusions.—IOP was significantly higher immediately after scleral tunnel incision without hydration than after clear corneal incision with hydration, and both incisions closed within 30 minutes postoperatively without leakage based on AS OCT (Fig 3).

▶ A previous study showed that transient hypotony after sutureless clear corneal incision (CCI) surgery may allow bacteria-sized particles on the surface to enter the eye.[1] Also, several studies have found a somewhat higher incidence of postoperative endophthalmitis in CCI cataract surgery compared with scleral tunnel incision.[2] It is well established that the intraocular pressure (IOP) normalizes in

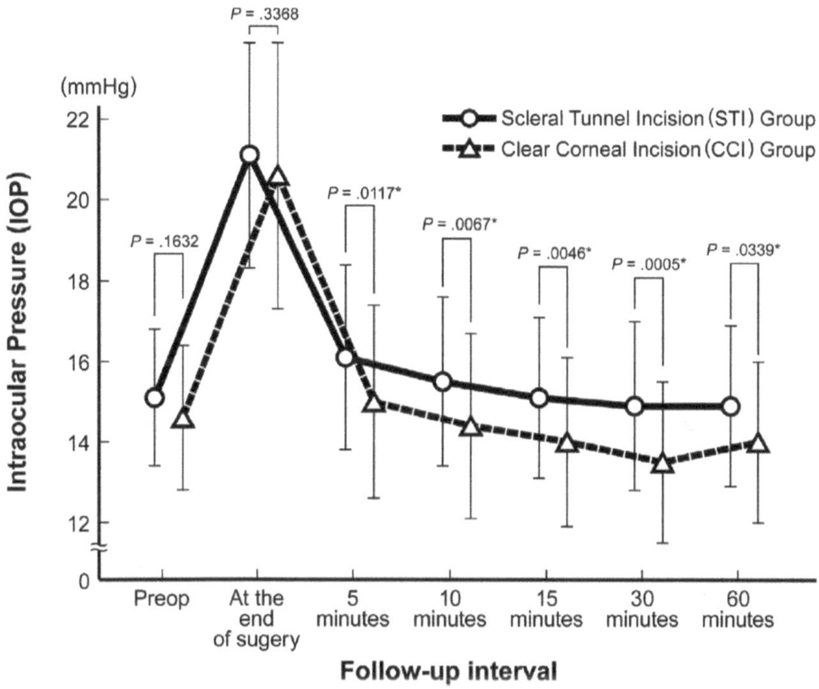

FIGURE 3.—Comparison of mean (± standard deviation) intraocular pressure (IOP) between eyes that underwent 2.4 mm scleral tunnel incision or a 2.4 mm clear corneal incision. Mean postoperative IOP was significantly higher in the scleral tunnel incision group than in the clear corneal incision group throughout the follow-up period. *Statistically significant difference between the 2 time intervals. (Reprinted from American Journal of Ophthalmology. American Journal of Ophthalmology. Hayashi K, Tsuru T, Yoshida M, et al. Intraocular pressure and wound status in eyes immediately after scleral tunnel incision and clear corneal incision cataract surgery. *Am J Ophthalmol.* 2014;158:232-241, Copyright 2014, with permission from Elsevier.)

healthy eyes 30 to 60 minutes after uncomplicated cataract surgery, even though elevated IOP may occur later owing to retained viscoelastic or inflammation.

This randomized trial found that during the first hour after surgery, eyes undergoing CCI cataract surgery frequently had an IOP lower than baseline compared with those eyes undergoing scleral tunnel incisions, which do not (Fig 3). No incision leakage or lack of apposition was found to explain this period of relative hypotony. However, at least theoretically, low IOP may allow for ingress of bacteria from the ocular surface and increase the risk of infection.

Many surgeons intentionally overpressurize the eye at the conclusion of surgery when using a sutureless CCI. The authors did not study whether this maneuver can prevent the early period of low pressure. Because most cataract surgeons currently use sutureless clear corneal incisions in most cases, it is unlikely they will revert to scleral tunnel incisions as the authors suggest for more difficult or complex cases. However, the addition of suture closure or an adhesive sealant is certainly prudent in such cases to prevent early leakage from transient low IOP.

M. F. Pyfer, MD

References

1. Chawdhary S, Anand A. Early post-phacoemulsification hypotony as a risk factor for intraocular contamination: in vivo model. *J Cataract Refract Surg*. 2006;32: 609-613.
2. Cooper BA, Holekamp NM, Bohgian G, Thompson PA. Case-control study of endophthalmitis after cataract surgery comparing scleral tunnel and clear corneal wounds. *Am J Ophthalmol*. 2003;136:300-305.

Increase in microbial contamination risk with compression of the lid margin in eyes having cataract surgery

Ye T, Chen W, Congdon N, et al (Sun Yat-sen Univ, Guangzhou, China)
J Cataract Refract Surg 40:1377-1381, 2014

Purpose.—To assess the bacterial contamination risk in cataract surgery associated with mechanical compression of the lid margin immediately after sterilization of the ocular surface.

Setting.—Department of Cataract, Zhongshan Ophthalmic Center, Sun Yat-sen University, Guangzhou, China.

Design.—Prospective randomized controlled double-masked trial.

Methods.—Patients with age-related cataract were randomly assigned to 1 of 2 groups. In Group A (153 eyes), the lid margin was compressed and scrubbed for 360 degrees 5 times with a dry sterile cotton-tipped applicator immediately after ocular sterilization and before povidone–iodine irrigation of the conjunctival sac. Group B (153 eyes) had identical sterilization but no lid scrubbing. Samples from the lid margin, liquid in the collecting bag, and aqueous humor were collected for bacterial culture. Primary outcome measures included the rate of positive bacterial culture for the above samples. The species of bacteria isolated were recorded.

Results.—Group A and Group B each comprised 153 eyes. The positive rate of lid margin cultures was 54.24%. The positive rate of cultures for liquid in the collecting bag was significantly higher in Group A (23.53%) than in Group B (9.80%) ($P = .001$).The bacterial species cultured from the collecting bag in Group B were the same as those from the lid margin in Group A. The positive culture rate of aqueous humor in both groups was 0%.

Conclusion.—Mechanical compression of the lid margin immediately before and during cataract surgery increased the risk for bacterial contamination of the surgical field, perhaps due to secretions from the lid margin glands.

▶ In this randomized trial of performing eyelid margin scrubbing as part of the standard preoperative surgical preparation before cataract surgery, the authors found that this maneuver actually increased the risk of bacterial contamination of the surgical field. The study is too small to assess endophthalmitis risk directly, but contamination of the field is a reasonable surrogate measure that likely increases the risk for infection.

Pretreatment of blepharitis and lid margin disease before surgery has been recommended, and the authors speculate that this could reduce the rate of contamination despite unavoidable mechanical eyelid compression during surgery. This was not tested but would be an excellent extension to the current study.

My current practice is to institute eyelid hygiene at least 1 month prior to surgery in all patients found to have even mild blepharitis on preoperative examination. Regardless of whether eyelid hygiene measures have been performed ahead of time, this study supports avoidance of compressing or scrubbing the lids immediately prior to surgery.

M. F. Pyfer, MD

Lens-based glaucoma surgery: Using cataract surgery to reduce intraocular pressure

Brown RH, Zhong L, Lynch MG (Atlanta Ophthalmology Associates, GA; Emory Univ Eye Ctr, Atlanta, GA; Univ of Miami Miller School of Medicine, FL)

J Cataract Refract Surg 40:1255-1262, 2014

Cataract surgery has been demonstrated to lower intraocular pressure (IOP) in eyes with glaucoma. The evidence is strong in angle-closure patients that cataract surgery improves IOP and dramatically reduces the future risk for IOP spikes and acute attacks. Randomized controlled trials (RCTs) have shown that cataract surgery may be preferable to laser iridotomy or phacotrabeculectomy. The data are so convincing that an RCT has been undertaken to assess whether clear lens extraction may be appropriate following acute attacks and in cases of uncontrolled IOP. The case favoring cataract surgery in open-angle glaucoma (OAG) is more controversial. Impressive IOP reduction has been shown in OAG patients when the patients are stratified by preoperative IOP. The patients with the highest preoperative IOPs have pressure reductions up to 8.5 mm Hg. However, these findings have been criticized for methodological weaknesses. Combining cataract surgery with microinvasive glaucoma surgery in phaco-plus procedures provides further options for lens-based glaucoma surgery (Fig 2).

▶ This concise review updates the indications for cataract surgery in patients with open-angle glaucoma (OAG) based on current surgical techniques (Fig 2). Modern small-incision phacoemulsification cataract surgery alone usually results in intraocular pressure (IOP) reduction in proportion to the preoperative IOP. New microinvasive glaucoma surgery (MIGS) procedures combined with cataract surgery allow for further IOP reduction, in what the author calls "phaco-plus" procedures.

Lens extraction is now well established as an effective treatment for primary-angle closure glaucoma. The role of early cataract surgery in the management of OAG is also expanding, as evidence mounts of its effectiveness at reducing IOP. This gradual paradigm shift is a direct result of modern, minimally invasive cataract surgical techniques using small incisions, atraumatic pupil expansion,

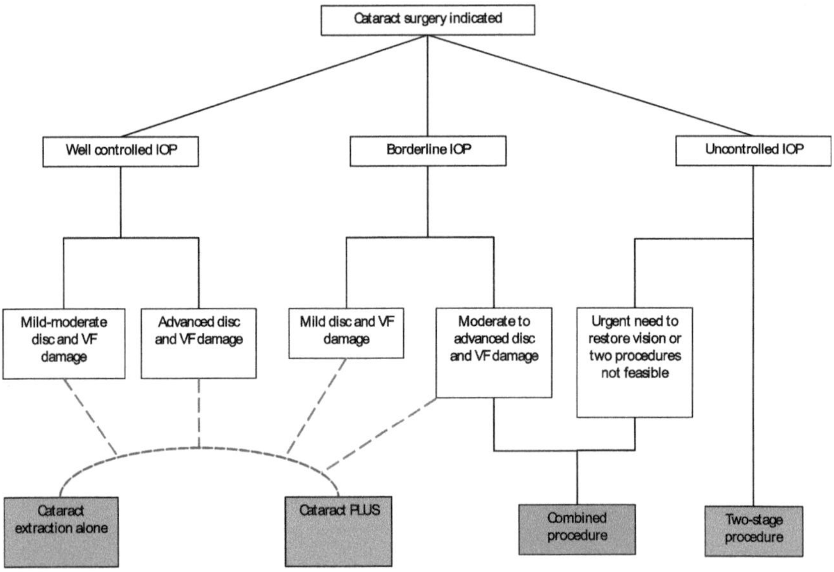

FIGURE 2.—Surgical options for a patient with cataract and glaucoma in 2013. "Uncontrolled IOP" means an IOP that is greater than either cataract surgery alone or phacoplus surgery would be expected to achieve. Dotted lines indicate options that must be weighed individually for each patient. (Reprinted from Journal of Cataract & Refractive Surgery. Brown RH, Zhong L, Lynch MG, Lens-based glaucoma surgery: using cataract surgery to reduce intraocular pressure. *J Cataract Refract Surg.* 2014;40:1255-1262, Copyright 2014, with permission from ASCRS and ESCRS.)

minimal ultrasound energy, complete cortical removal, and fully in-the-bag intraocular lens placement. Also, effective prevention of postoperative inflammation with potent topical steroid and nonsteroidal medications help maintain normal-angle anatomy and function after cataract surgery.

It is reasonable to expect that phaco-plus procedures using MIGS, along with sustained-release IOP-lowering medications, will lead to further reductions in the need for trabeculectomy and aqueous tube shunt procedures.

M. F. Pyfer, MD

Cataract Surgery in Patients with Fuchs' Endothelial Corneal Dystrophy: When to Consider a Triple Procedure

van Cleynenbreugel H, Remeijer L, Hillenaar T (The Rotterdam Eye Hosp, The Netherlands; Rotterdam Ophthalmic Inst, The Netherlands)
Ophthalmology 121:445-453, 2014

Purpose.—To ascertain preoperative and intraoperative factors that predict the need for endothelial keratoplasty (EK) in patients with Fuchs' endothelial corneal dystrophy (FECD) undergoing cataract surgery.

Design.—Prospective, observational cohort study.

Participants.—Eighty-nine patients (89 eyes) with FECD who require cataract surgery.

Methods.—One month before cataract surgery, we assessed best-corrected visual acuity, contrast sensitivity, straylight, keratometry, ultrasonic pachymetry, intraocular pressure, 7 corneal features of FECD and cataract density at slit-lamp examination, and corneal backscatter using in vivo confocal microscopy (IVCM; Confoscan 4, NIDEK Technologies, Padova, Italy). After surgery, measurements were repeated at 1, 2, and 12 months. We used stepwise binary logistic regression analysis to evaluate 30 preoperative and 5 intraoperative parameters for their ability to predict the postoperative need for EK. Receiver operating characteristic (ROC) curves of the predictive factors were used to identify their optimal cutoff points.

Main Outcome Measures.—Central corneal thickness (CCT) and backscatter at the basal epithelial cell layer (EV).

Results.—After cataract surgery, 35 (39%) of 89 eyes underwent EK to restore vision. Of all preoperative and intraoperative parameters, only CCT and EV were identified as significant factors, predictive of the need for EK. The area under the ROC curve of EV was significantly higher than that of CCT ($P = 0.003$), whereas a combination of both factors in a linear discriminant function did not improve the predictive value ($P = 0.66$). As optimal cutoff points, we chose 1894 scatter units for EV and 630 μm for CCT. Both cutoff points correspond with a specificity of 94% and represent sensitivity of 63% for EV and 40% for CCT.

Conclusions.—Backscatter at the basal epithelial cell layer measured by IVCM predicts the need for EK after cataract surgery in patients with FECD. As an indicator for the corneal hydration state, the EV improves patient selection for combined cataract surgery and EK. In deciding whether to perform a triple procedure, CCT remains a less effective, but adequate, alternative. Regardless of the predictive factor used, a tailor-made approach is recommended accounting for individuals' expectations (Table 4).

▶ This prospective cohort study in patients with Fuchs' endothelial corneal dystrophy (FECD) undergoing phacoemulsification cataract extraction (CE), sought to determine predictive factors for requiring endothelial keratoplasty (EK) 2 months after cataract surgery. An extensive set of preoperative and intraoperative parameters were evaluated (Table 4). The authors confirmed that central corneal thickness (CCT) remains useful with high specificity at a cutoff of 630 μm. However, epithelial membrane backscatter (EV) on confocal microscopy was even better, with high specificity and sensitivity at a cutoff of 1894, which is outside the range for normal eyes. CCT has been used for this purpose for years but is limited by a wide range of normal values that overlaps the cutoff. CCT also fluctuates with time of day and corneal hydration status, but EV does not. One limitation of using confocal microscopy for preoperative evaluation of FECD patients is that the instrument is expensive and technically challenging to use compared with ultrasound pachymetry.

TABLE 4.—Preoperative and Intraoperative Characteristics of Fuchs' Endothelial Corneal Dystrophy Patients Undergoing Cataract Surgery with Corresponding Area under the Receiver Operating Characteristic Curves

	Preoperative or Intraoperative	Area under the Receiver Operating Characteristic Curve	95% Confidence Interval	*P* Value*
Patient characteristics				
Age, yrs	72±8.3	0.700	0.589–0.811	<0.001
Morning blur, n (%)	52 (58)	0.678	0.583–0.773	<0.001
Female, n (%)	54 (61)	0.576	0.471–0.681	0.16
Family history of FECD, n (%)	12 (14)	0.554	0.476–0.631	0.18
Right eye, n (%)	45 (51)	0.554	0.447–0.661	0.32
Slit-lamp examination				
Folds in posterior stroma, n (%)	37 (42)	0.746	0.652–0.840	<0.001
Subepithelial fibrosis, n (%)	15 (17)	0.644	0.558–0.729	0.001
Peripheral guttae, n (%)	65 (73)	0.628	0.544–0.712	0.003
Diffuse endothelial pigment granules, n (%)	40 (45)	0.577	0.471–0.683	0.16
Epithelial microcystic edema, n (%)	3 (3)	0.543	0.496–0.590	0.074
Epithelial bullae, n (%)	2 (2)	0.529	0.490–0.568	0.15
Endothelial pigment island, n (%)	17 (19)	0.516	0.433–0.600	0.70
LOCS III				
Cortical cataract	1.5±1.4	0.705	0.602–0.808	<0.001
Nuclear opalescence	3.2±0.8	0.634	0.517–0.751	0.025
Nuclear color	3.9±0.8	0.598	0.476–0.720	0.12
Subcapsular cataract	0.4±0.9	0.546	0.484–0.608	0.15
Additional examinations				
Central corneal thickness, μm	597±52	0.807	0.717–0.898	<0.001
Best-corrected visual acuity, logMAR	0.33±0.18	0.710	0.603–0.816	<0.001
Endothelial cell density, n (%)	25 (28)	0.637	0.553–0.722	0.002
Contrast sensitivity, logCS	1.17±0.22	0.629	0.510–0.749	0.034
Refractive astigmatism, D	1.5±1.1	0.573	0.447–0.699	0.25
Intraocular straylight, log(s)	1.51±0.26	0.567	0.439–0.694	0.31
Average keratometry, D	44.0±1.6	0.560	0.433–0.686	0.35
Applanation tonometry, mmHg	14.9±3.2	0.528	0.406–0.650	0.65
Corneal backscatter, SU				
Epithelial valley	1773±835	0.914	0.855–0.973	<0.001
Subepithelial peak	3071±1400	0.885	0.815–0.955	<0.001
Anterior stroma	1709±551	0.824	0.740–0.908	<0.001
Cornea	1526±385	0.820	0.734–0.906	<0.001
Mid stroma	1156±297	0.727	0.617–0.837	<0.001
Posterior stroma	1258±315	0.628	0.501–0.756	0.049
Intraoperative parameters				
Ultrasound time, seconds	51.1±25.0	0.692	0.574–0.811	0.002
Cumulative dissipated energy	11.5±6.9	0.665	0.549–0.780	0.005
Torsional amplitude	54.6±7.3	0.592	0.458–0.725	0.18
Balanced salt solution use, ml	67.8±18.8	0.516	0.385–0.648	0.81
Aspiration time, seconds	212±90	0.511	0.378–0.643	0.87

D = diopters; FECD = Fuchs' Endothelial Corneal Dystrophy; LOCS III = Lens Opacities Classification System, version III; logCS = logarithm of contrast sensitivity; logMAR = logarithm of the minimum angle of resolution; log(s) = logarithm of the straylight parameter; SU = scatter units.

Data are mean ± standard deviation unless otherwise stated.

*$P \leq 0.05$ indicates the area under the receiver operating characteristic curve is significantly different from chance discrimination (i.e., area under the receiver operating characteristic curve, 0.500).

This study also looked at intraoperative cataract surgical parameters and found that total ultrasound energy and time were correlated with need for EK, but aspiration time and total irrigation fluid used were not. This is useful information for cataract surgeons who operate on these high-risk patients and indicates that techniques that minimize total ultrasound use, such as pulsed modulation modes and femtosecond laser prefragmentation, may help decrease the rate of endothelial decompensation in FECD patients after cataract surgery. This should hold true even if those techniques increase aspiration time and fluid volume.

This is an excellent report to guide cataract surgeons who do not perform EK and specialist consultants who are asked to evaluate FECD patients prior to cataract surgery. For the cataract surgeon, a confocal microscope is not required, and a CCT cutoff of 630 μm can be used to trigger referral for combined EK/CE as long as the patient is willing to accept up to 60% chance of requiring EK later for full visual rehabilitation. For corneal specialists, confocal microscopy should be considered as measurement of EV can provide a more sensitive test, especially since central endothelial cell density usually cannot be determined in these patients because of confluent guttata.

M. F. Pyfer, MD

Severe Bilateral Ischemic Retinal Vasculitis Following Cataract Surgery

Nicholson LB, Kim BT, Jardón J, et al (Harvard Med School, Boston, MA; Univ of Miami Miller School of Medicine, FL; Univ of Puerto Rico School of Medicine, San Juan; et al)

Ophthalmic Surg Lasers Imaging Retina 45:338-342, 2014

This report describes two cases of severe, bilateral ischemic retinal vasculitis following cataract surgeries at different surgical centers. In both cases, the patient underwent bilateral cataract surgeries, performed 1 week apart for each eye. In the perioperative period following the second of the two surgeries, both patients developed severe, bilateral intraocular inflammation and profound vision loss. The underlying cause of this adverse response remains unknown. The authors suggest that the severe inflammatory reaction could be related to an intraoperative intracameral vancomycin injection (Fig 3).

▶ This report documents 2 cases of idiopathic profound bilateral vision loss after routine delayed sequential second eye cataract surgery. This is a devastating outcome due to severe inflammation and ischemic retinal vasculitis (Fig 3) and may be related to a delayed immune reaction to intracameral vancomycin. One patient had a previous incidence of acute renal failure after a single dose of intravenous vancomycin several years earlier, which is suggestive of a systemic immune hypersensitivity reaction to the drug.

More cases and further study are required to determine the specific cause of this fortunately rare event. This report illustrates that widespread use of intracameral antibiotic injection during cataract surgery may lead to rare but unexpected complications. This and other uncommon problems, such as toxic anterior

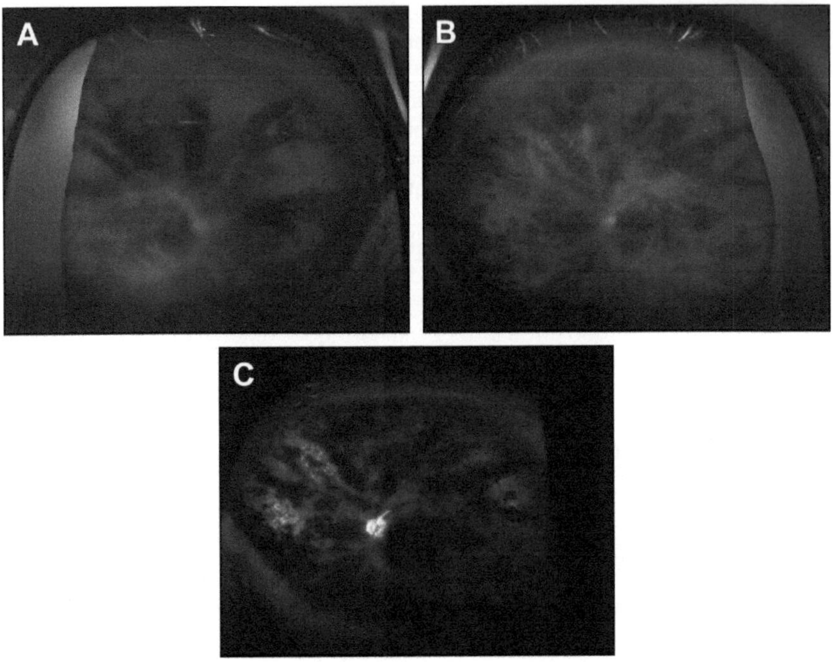

FIGURE 3.—Patient 2: Fundus photographs of right (A) and left (B) eyes illustrating bilateral diffuse perivascular exudates and hemorrhages consistent with hemorrhagic retinal vasculitis. Fluorescein angiogram of the left eye (C) illustrating severe nonperfusion of retinal vessels and vascular leakage. (Reprinted with permission from SLACK Incorporated: Nicholson LB, Kim BT, Jardón J, et al, Severe bilateral ischemic retinal vasculitis following cataract surgery. *Ophthalmic Surg Lasers Imaging Retina.* 2014;45:338-342.)

segment syndrome, need to be included in any economic cost—benefit analysis of intracameral antibiotic use for prevention of endophthalmitis after cataract surgery.

M. F. Pyfer, MD

2 Refractive Surgery

Twenty-Year Follow-Up of a Randomized Prospective Clinical Trial of Excimer Laser Photorefractive Keratectomy

O'Brart DPS, Shalchi Z, McDonald RJ, et al (St. Thomas' Hosp, London, UK; et al)

Am J Ophthalmol 158:651-663, 2014

Purpose.—To investigate the 20-year efficacy and safety of photorefractive keratectomy (PRK).

Design.—Long-term observational case series.

Methods.—In the setting of a university hospital, a study population of 42 patients (42 eyes) who had, as part of a randomized prospective trial, undergone PRK 20 years previously were studied. All had received −3.0 or −6.0 diopter (D) corrections with either 5.0 or 6.0 mm optical zones or a multizone treatment. The mean preoperative spherical equivalent refractive error (SEQ) was −5.13 D (range, −2.75 to −8.0 D). The outcome measures included visual acuity, refractive error, corneal topography and axial length.

Results.—Between 1 and 20 years there was an increase in mean myopic SEQ of −0.54 D ($P < 0.02$). In patients younger than 40 years of age at time of correction, this increase was −0.92 D ($P < 0.002$) with an accompanying increase in variance ($P < 0.02$), whereas in those older than 40 it was −0.08 D ($P = 0.8$). In female patients the change was −0.69 D ($P < 0.01$), while in males it was −0.26 D ($P = 0.6$). The efficacy index at 20 years was 0.49, and the safety index was 0.97. Corrected distance visual acuity improved between 1 and 20 years ($P < 0.01$); 93% of corneas were clear at 20 years; 3 eyes had trace haze. There was an improvement in haze scores between 1 and 20 years ($P < 0.02$). Cornea power remained unchanged between 6 months and 20 years ($P = 0.4$). Axial length increased by a mean of 0.84 mm ($P < 0.0001$). There was no ectasia.

Conclusions.—There was a slight but significant increase in myopic SEQ after PRK between 1 and 20 years, particularly in those under 40 at the time of treatment and in female patients. Corneal power remained unchanged, but axial length increased. The procedure was safe, with no long-term sight-threatening complications and with improvements in corrected distance visual acuity and corneal transparency with time (Table 1).

▶ Although the authors included only 42 of the 100 original patients in the study, that's not bad 20 years postoperatively. It is also nice to know that the demographics of the 58 patients they did not include were similar to the

TABLE 1.—Refractive Outcomes in Diopters ± 1 Standard Deviation Preoperatively and at 1 and 20 Years After Photorefractive Keratectomy for the Whole Cohort and for Subgroups, Including Patients Younger Than and Older Than 40 Years of Age at Time of Surgery*

	Pre-Op	1 Year	20 Years	*P* Value Change in SEQ†	*P* Value Change in Variance†
Whole cohort n = 42	−5.13 ± 1.86	−1.18 ± 1.35	−1.72 ± 1.69	*P* < 0.02	*P* = 0.1
<40 at surgery n = 23	−5.1 ± 1.76	−1.21 ± 1.04	−2.12 ± 1.78	*P* < 0.005	*P* < 0.02
>40 at surgery n = 19	−5.17 ± 2.02	−1.14 ± 1.68	−1.23 ± 1.46	*P* = 0.8	*P* = 0.6
Female patients n = 28	−5.08 ± 1.92	−1.16 ± 1.25	−1.83 ± 1.63	*P* < 0.01	*P* = 0.2
Male patients n = 14	−5.23 ± 1.78	−1.22 ± −1.57	−1.48 ± 1.85	*P* = 0.6	*P* = 0.6
−3.0 D Corrections n = 20	−3.31 ± −0.54	−0.39 ± 0.46	−0.86 ± −1.1	*P* < 0.05	*P* < 0.0005
−6.0 D Corrections n = 22	−6.8 ± 0.62	−1.89 ± 1.5	−2.5 ± 1.78	*P* = 0.09	*P* = 0.5
5.0 mm optical zones n = 17	−4.78 ± 1.75	−1.21 ± 1.69	−1.85 ± 1.85	*P* = 0.08	*P* = 0.8
6.0 mm optical zones n = 18	−4.68 ± 1.79	−0.86 ± 1.03	−1.21 ± 1.46	*P* = 0.2	*P* = 0.2
Multizone treatment n = 7	−7.16 ± 0.71	−1.99 ± 0.89	−2.7 ± 1.59	*P* = 0.2	*P* = 0.2

SEQ = spherical equivalent refractive error.
*Female and male patients, −3.0 and −6.0 diopter corrections and 5.0 mm, 6.0 mm and multizone treatment groups.
†*P* value for changes between 1 and 20 years.
Reprinted from American Journal of Ophthalmology. O'Brart DPS, Shalchi Z, McDonald RJ, et al. Twenty-Year Follow-Up of a Randomized Prospective Clinical Trial of Excimer Laser Photorefractive Keratectomy. *Am J Ophthalmol.* 2014;158:651-663, Copyright 2014, with permission from Elsevier.

patients whom they did include. The most important findings a long-term study such as this one (which used first-generation excimer laser technology) can provide are delayed complications that might be inherent to the procedure, such as corneal scarring, edema, or ectasia. Fortunately, they did not find any such problems. In fact, corrected distance vision and corneal haze continued to improve with time.

They did find some myopic regression, greater in patients under age 40 years at the time of the surgery and more in female than male patients (Table 1). Interestingly, the corneal powers remained stable from 6 months to 20 years, while the axial lengths increased (mean increase of 0.84 mm, $P < .0001$). So in patients with apparently stable refractions for 2 years (as required to participate in the study), the eyes may not actually be perfectly stable from a refractive standpoint. This is good to keep in mind when discussing long-term expectations with patients.

C. J. Rapuano, MD

The U.S. Army Surface Ablation Study: Comparison of PRK, MMC-PRK, and LASEK in Moderate to High Myopia

Sia RK, Ryan DS, Edwards JD, et al (Warfighter Refractive Eye Surgery Program and Res Ctr at Fort Belvoir, VA; Tulane Univ, New Orleans, LA; et al)
J Refract Surg 30:256-264, 2014

Purpose.—To compare visual outcomes following photorefractive keratectomy (PRK), PRK with mitomycin C (MMC-PRK), and LASEK in moderate and high myopia in military personnel.

Methods.—This prospective, randomized contralateral eye study included 167 patients 21 years or older with manifest spherical equivalent −5.99 ± 1.40 diopters (D) (range: −3.88 to −9.38 D) randomized to either MMC-PRK or LASEK treatment in their dominant eye and conventional PRK without MMC in the fellow eye. All procedures were performed using the LADARVision 4000 Excimer Laser System (Alcon Surgical Inc., Ft. Worth, TX). High- and low-contrast visual acuities, manifest refraction, endothelial cell count, and corneal haze were evaluated up to 12 months postoperatively.

Results.—At 12 months postoperatively, visual outcomes were comparable among the treatment groups. Corneal haze of any grade was less common in MMC-PRK compared to PRK at 1 month (21.4% vs 31.0%; $P < .01$) and 3 months (12.8% vs 35.9%; $P = .03$) postoperatively; it was also less common in MMC-PRK compared to LASEK at 1 month (21.4% vs 55.9%; $P < .01$), 3 months (12.8% vs 42.4%; $P < .01$), and 6 months (12.2% vs 36.4%; $P = .03$) postoperatively. Haze rate (grade 0.5 or higher) was comparable between LASEK and PRK. Clinically significant haze (grade 2 or higher) developed after PRK (4 eyes) and LASEK (2 eyes), but not after MMC-PRK.

Conclusions.—MMC-PRK showed some benefits in minimizing corneal haze formation. One year after surgery, there was no discernible difference in the postoperative refractive outcomes among the three methods.

▶ For a variety of reasons that the authors discuss, "laser refractive surgery is the preferred method of vision correction on the modern battlefield." They note that approximately three-quarters of the refractive procedures in the U.S. Army are surface ablation procedures. The well-known disadvantages of surface ablation compared with LASIK are more pain, slower visual acuity, and more haze. Laser-assisted sub-epithelial keratectomy (LASEK), where the epithelium is loosened from the corneal surface with alcohol, moved to the side for the excimer laser ablation, and then repositioned, was thought to help with these 3 issues. Intraoperative mitomycin C (MMC) has been shown to decrease haze after surface ablation. The authors performed a nice controlled bilateral eye study comparing each of these surface ablation variants to standard photorefractive keratectomy (PRK) without MMC.

Mean spherical equivalent was −4D. Conventional excimer laser treatments with a 6.5-mm optical zone were performed in all eyes. MMC 0.02% was used for 60 seconds. Postoperative fluorometholone 0.1% drops were used in all of eyes for a 10-week taper. Interestingly, the authors had planned to enroll almost 500 patients but underwent an unanticipated change in their laser platform, so they closed the study after 167 patients. Ninety-one percent of patients were seen at 6 months, and 79% of patients were seen at 1 year.

Overall, the results were rather similar for the 3 groups, including postoperative pain, uncorrected and best corrected visual acuity, and endothelial cell counts. In the first week, the epithelial defects in the LASEK eyes did not heal as quickly as the PRK or PRK-MMC eyes. Corneal haze (0.5 or greater) was seen in statistically significantly fewer PRK-MMC eyes than PRK eyes or

LASEK eyes up to 6 months postoperatively (Fig 6 in the original article). Four PRK and 2 LASEK eyes had grade 2 haze, and no PRK-MMC eyes had grade 2 haze. A small subset of eyes treated for > 6D of myopia was looked at and the PRK-MMC eyes tended to have less haze than the PRK and LASEK eyes. Although all 3 variations of surface ablation worked well, the take-home message for me supports using what I believe is the most common surface ablation technique—namely, PRK with MMC. Given MMC's excellent safety profile and the fact that haze is much easier to prevent than to treat, this is my preferred surface ablation technique. Whether 60 seconds of MMC is the optimal duration of treatment is not addressed by this study. I personally use MMC 0.02% for 12 seconds in eyes with over ~2D of myopia and all eyes with moderate to high degrees of astigmatism.

C. J. Rapuano, MD

Outcomes of Photorefractive Keratectomy Enhancement After LASIK

Lee BS, Gupta PK, Davis EA, et al (Univ of Washington, Seattle; Minnesota Eye Consultants, Minneapolis)

J Refract Surg 30:549-556, 2014

Purpose.—To report the outcomes of photorefractive keratectomy (PRK) enhancement after LASIK for patients diagnosed as having hyperopic and myopic refractive errors.

Methods.—In this retrospective case series at a single private practice in the United States, all patients undergoing PRK enhancement after LASIK were identified. Patients with visually significant cataract, non-plano targets, and follow-up of fewer than 226 days were excluded. The primary outcome measure was uncorrected distance visual acuity (UDVA) with secondary measures of corrected distance visual acuity (CDVA) and postoperative refractive error. Linear regression analysis was performed for actual versus targeted change in spherical equivalent.

Results.—Mean UDVA improved from 20/39 to 20/24 for hyperopes ($n = 14$; $P < .002$) and from 20/45 to 20/22 for myopes ($n = 29$; $P < .0000001$) after enhancement. All patients had a UDVA of 20/40 or better at their most recent follow-up visit. Fifty percent of hyperopes and 65.5% of myopes were 20/20 or better. The mean refractive error for hyperopes changed from +1.10 ± 0.71 (range: +0.13 to +2.25 diopters [D]) to +0.38 ± 0.66 D (range: −0.75 to +1.38 D) and from −1.21 ± 0.61 (range: −3.25 to −0.38 D) to +0.34 ± 0.45 D (range: −0.25 to +1.75 D) for myopes. The manifest refraction cylinder decreased from 0.84 to 0.46 D in hyperopes ($P = .02$) and from 0.64 to 0.26 D in myopes ($P < .002$). CDVA was maintained in both groups, with only one patient in each worse than 20/20. There was a nonsignificant trend toward less haze in the patients receiving mitomycin C (5.1% vs 25%, $P = .14$). Linear regression showed a tendency toward overtreatment in the myopic group.

Conclusions.—PRK is safe and highly effective for patients who previously underwent LASIK and in whom the surgeon would prefer not to perform a flap-lift enhancement.

► This is the largest series I know of reviewing refractive results of photorefractive keratectomy (PRK) after laser in situ keratomileusis (LASIK). Given the increased difficulty of lifting LASIK flaps the longer it is after surgery, combined with the fact that femtosecond laser flaps are more difficult to lift than microkeratome flaps, as well as the greater recognition of the dangers of epithelial ingrowth after LASIK flap lift enhancements, surface ablation is being done more and more for LASIK enhancements. I personally haven't lifted a LASIK flap for an enhancement in years. I do PRK using alcohol to remove the epithelium. The authors used alcohol or performed transepithelial PRK in this series. It is important to mention that epi-LASIK should not be performed given the increased risk of damaging the LASIK flap.

The authors used a wavefront-guided treatment with the VISX laser for all of their procedures. They used an average of 0.21-diopter nomogram undercorrection for the hyperopic eyes and a 0.17-diopter nomogram undercorrection for the myopic eyes. They found an approximately 0.2-diopter undercorrection in the hyperopic eyes and thus recommended not using a nomogram adjustment for hyperopes. They also did not achieve much refractive effect in the eyes with low amounts of hyperopia and state that "enhancements for a refractive errors less than +1 diopter may not be effective." Only 7.4% of the myopic eyes were undercorrected. The authors recommend a correction factor based on linear regression from their results (Fig 6 in the original article).

Almost all of their patients had adjunctive mitomycin C (MMC) with good results (application times varied). I too use MMC on my PRK eyes after LASIK (0.02% for 30 seconds). Additionally, the authors had 4 eyes with stage 1 and 1 eye with stage 2 diffuse lamellar keratitis, but none required a flap lift. For me the short-term downsides of PRK after LASIK do not outweigh the risks of lifting a LASIK flap, especially if it has been more than a year after the LASIK.

C. J. Rapuano, MD

Patient satisfaction and clinical outcomes with laser refractive surgery performed by surgeons in training

Nehls SM, Ghoghawala SY, Hwang FS, et al (Univ of Wisconsin, Madison; Wayne State Univ, Detroit, MI)

J Cataract Refract Surg 40:1131-1138, 2014

Purpose.—To evaluate the refractive error quality of life (RQL) improvement, patient satisfaction, and clinical results of laser refractive surgery performed by residents or fellows.

Setting.—Department of Ophthalmology and Visual Sciences, University of Wisconsin, Madison, USA.

Design.—Case series.

Methods.—This study reviewed the clinical results of consecutive refractive surgery cases performed between March 2010 and February 2012 by ophthalmology residents or fellows. One-year postoperative analysis of the RQL and patient satisfaction in a subgroup of patients was completed using the National Eye Institute Refractive Error Correction Quality of Life-42 instrument (NEI RQL-42), and a comparison with NEI published normative data and post-refractive data was performed.

Results.—Data were obtained from 138 eyes that had laser in situ keratomileusis and 4 eyes that had photorefractive keratectomy. The 1-year postoperative analysis of the RQL and patient satisfaction was completed in 34 patients. After 6 months postoperatively, the mean uncorrected distance visual acuity was 0.01 logMAR (95% confidence interval [CI], −0.012 to 0.023). The mean postoperative residual refractive error spherical equivalent was −0.20 diopter (D) (95% CI, −0.26 to −0.13). No eye lost corrected distance visual acuity. Equivalent or better satisfaction in the RQL was found in all but 1 of the 13 scale scores of the NEI RQL-42 compared with previously published NEI data.

Conclusions.—Laser refractive surgery performed by residents and fellows showed high patient satisfaction and an improved RQL 1-year postoperatively. Clinical outcomes validated the safety and efficacy of refractive surgery performed by surgeons in training.

▶ As someone who routinely supervises refractive surgery procedures performed by residents and cornea fellows, I was happy to read the results of this article. The authors' findings confirm my clinical impression that residents and fellows can perform safe and effective refractive surgery under proper supervision. I have found the refractive surgery results, complication rates, and patient satisfaction are basically the same when performed by surgeons in training compared with practicing surgeons. At Wills Eye Hospital, the price for refractive surgery performed by residents and fellows is about half of the "normal" price (in addition to the refractive surgery evaluation being free). The authors of this article asked patients about their primary motivation to have their surgery performed by a physician in training and found 76.5% said it was "price." In my experience, it is closer to 90% to 100%.

This study did have a few limitations. One is that of the 71 patients who had surgery by residents and fellows during the study period, fewer than half (34) completed the 1-year questionnaire. Another is the questionnaire was not given preoperatively and could therefore not be compared with the 1-year results. The bottom line is that patients did well and were overall happy. Eighty-five percent reported it they were "very likely" to refer others for a resident or fellow to do their refractive surgery.

C. J. Rapuano, MD

Change in keratometry after myopic laser in situ keratomileusis and photorefractive keratectomy

Kim G, Christiansen SM, Moshirfar M (Univ of Utah, Salt Lake City)

J Cataract Refract Surg 40:564-574, 2014

Purpose.—To compare the change in keratometry (K), spherical equivalent (SE), and visual acuity after myopic laser in situ keratomileusis (LASIK) and photorefractive keratectomy (PRK).

Setting.—Academic tertiary care center.

Design.—Retrospective review.

Methods.—The postoperative K, SE, and uncorrected and corrected distance visual acuities were measured 6 months, 9 months, 1 year, 2 years, 3 years, 4 to 5 years, 6 to 7 years, and 8+ years postoperatively. A difference (Δ) for each variable was calculated from its 6-month postoperative baseline. The rates of change were grouped based on the magnitude of myopic correction (0.00 to 2.99 diopters [D]; 3.00 to 5.99 D; 6.00 to 8.99 D), type of surgery (LASIK versus PRK), and age (<34 years; 34 to 45 years; >45 years).

Results.—Statistically significant differences were found in the rates of change between low and moderate corrections to high corrections for ΔK_{avg} ($P = .0472$ and $P = .0091$, respectively) and ΔSE (both $P < .0001$). Statistically significant differences were found in the rate of change in ΔK_{avg} between all 3 ages groups ($P = .0330$, $P = .0051$, and $P < .0001$) and in ΔSE between ages less than 34 years and 34 to 45 years to ages over 45 years ($P = .0158$ and $P = .0015$, respectively). There was no significant difference in the rate of change in ΔK_{avg} and ΔSE between LASIK and PRK ($P = .3599$ and $P = .9403$, respectively).

Conclusion.—There was keratometric and refractive regression for myopic LASIK, with the rate of regression depending on treatment magnitude and age (Table 1).

▶ Refractive regression after hyperopic laser in situ keratomileusis (LASIK) and photorefractive keratectomy (PRK) is common and well known. Regression after myopic LASIK and PRK is much less common and less well studied. These authors used their large database of myopic LASIK and PRK patients to look at this issue. Inclusion criteria included an examination during the "baseline period," which was defined as 6 to 8 months postoperatively and a minimum of 2 years follow-up. Of the records of 7826 eyes they reviewed, 475 eyes met all of the eligibility criteria. They divided eyes by myopic spherical equivalent into 3 groups: 0 to > 3 D, 3 to < 6 D, and 6 to 9 D. They divided patients by age into < 34 years old, 34 to 45 years old, and > 45 years old.

As might be expected, the K readings, although overall fairly stable, regressed most in the high-myopia group and least in the low-myopia group. Similarly, the keratometry readings regressed most in the younger age group and least in the older age group (Table 1). The results were no different when comparing the LASIK and PRK eyes. When the authors analyzed their data, they concluded that the refractive regression in older patients was related to lenticular changes.

TABLE 1.—Outcome Variables at Each Follow-up Visit by Age Group

		ΔK (D)		ΔSE (D)		ΔUDVA (Lines)		ΔCDVA (Lines)	
Age/FU Visit	Eyes (n)	n	Mean ± SD	n	Mean ± SD	n	Mean ± SD	n	Mean ± SD
Age <35 years									
9 months	151	96	0.05 ± 0.54	146	−0.03 ± 0.37	151	−0.02 ± 0.98	145	0.01 ± 0.74
1 year	113	70	−0.05 ± 0.78	112	−0.03 ± 0.36	113	0.02 ± 0.98	106	0.05 ± 0.66
2 year	139	93	0.14 ± 0.70	138	−0.09 ± 0.39	138	−0.14 ± 1.12	136	−0.03 ± 0.83
3 years	60	35	0.23 ± 0.60	59	−0.10 ± 0.32	60	−0.09 ± 0.84	58	0.07 ± 0.77
4–5 years	46	24	0.06 ± 0.94	46	−0.23 ± 0.43	46	−0.24 ± 1.10	44	0.24 ± 1.80
6–7 years	22	9	0.14 ± 1.39	21	−0.34 ± 0.68	22	−0.64 ± 1.93	22	−0.17 ± 0.70
>8 years	9	4	0.53 ± 0.36	9	−0.15 ± 0.31	9	−0.60 ± 1.15	8	−0.78 ± 0.65
Age 35–45 years									
9 months	185	89	0.11 ± 0.59	183	−0.03 ± 0.29	185	0.01 ± 0.88	173	−0.07 ± 0.68
1 year	158	73	0.17 ± 0.67	154	−0.06 ± 0.36	158	0.00 ± 1.00	148	−0.02 ± 1.16
2 year	183	92	0.01 ± 0.66	177	−0.07 ± 0.4	183	−0.15 ± 1.07	172	−0.04 ± 0.79
3 years	81	33	0.05 ± 0.81	79	−0.10 ± 0.48	81	−0.18 ± 1.11	77	−0.13 ± 0.91
4–5 years	94	54	−0.04 ± 1.27	92	−0.13 ± 0.50	94	−0.46 ± 1.18	89	−0.09 ± 0.86
6–7 years	55	24	−0.38 ± 1.24	54	−0.25 ± 0.54	55	−0.83 ± 1.71	51	−0.10 ± 0.89
>8 years	28	10	−0.15 ± 0.34	28	−0.44 ± 0.72	28	−1.71 ± 2.85	27	0.26 ± 0.89
Age >45 years									
9 months	181	91	0.02 ± 0.75	176	−0.05 ± 0.35	181	0.08 ± 1.26	177	0.08 ± 0.97
1 year	156	67	0.24 ± 0.61	151	−0.01 ± 0.41	155	−0.18 ± 1.68	149	0.18 ± 1.00
2 year	165	77	0.00 ± 0.76	161	−0.03 ± 0.52	164	0.04 ± 1.84	160	0.05 ± 1.09
3 years	106	51	0.07 ± 0.82	104	−0.03 ± 0.45	105	−0.17 ± 1.49	105	−0.10 ± 0.99
4–5 years	115	50	−0.01 ± 0.86	112	−0.02 ± 0.56	115	−0.31 ± 2.22	111	−0.08 ± 1.03
6–7 years	66	26	0.17 ± 1.04	65	−0.05 ± 0.62	65	−0.65 ± 1.95	66	−0.34 ± 1.79
>8 years	42	16	−0.06 ± 0.79	42	−0.07 ± 0.52	42	−0.42 ± 1.59	42	−0.31 ± 0.73

Δ = change from baseline; CDVA = corrected distance visual acuity; FU = follow-up; K = keratometry; SE = spherical equivalent; UDVA = uncorrected distance visual acuity.

Reprinted from Kim G, Christiansen SM, Moshirfar M. Change in keratometry after myopic in situ keratomileusis and photorefractive keratectomy. *J Cataract Surg*. 2014;40:564-574.

They noted, "The decreasing accommodative tone among presbyopic patients slows the myopic regression rate of the spherical equivalent with increased age." The authors also pointed out that a little myopia as we get older isn't always all that bad.

C. J. Rapuano, MD

The Subject-Fixated Coaxially Sighted Corneal Light Reflex: A Clinical Marker for Centration of Refractive Treatments and Devices

Chang DH, Waring GO IV (Empire Eye and Laser Ctr, Bakersfield, CA; Med Univ of South Carolina, Charleston)
Am J Ophthalmol 158:863-874, 2014

Purpose.—To describe the inconsistencies in definition, application, and usage of the ocular reference axes (optical axis, visual axis, line of sight, pupillary axis, and topographic axis) and angles (angle kappa, lambda, and alpha) and to propose a precise, reproducible, clinically defined reference marker and axis for centration of refractive treatments and devices.

Design.—Perspective.

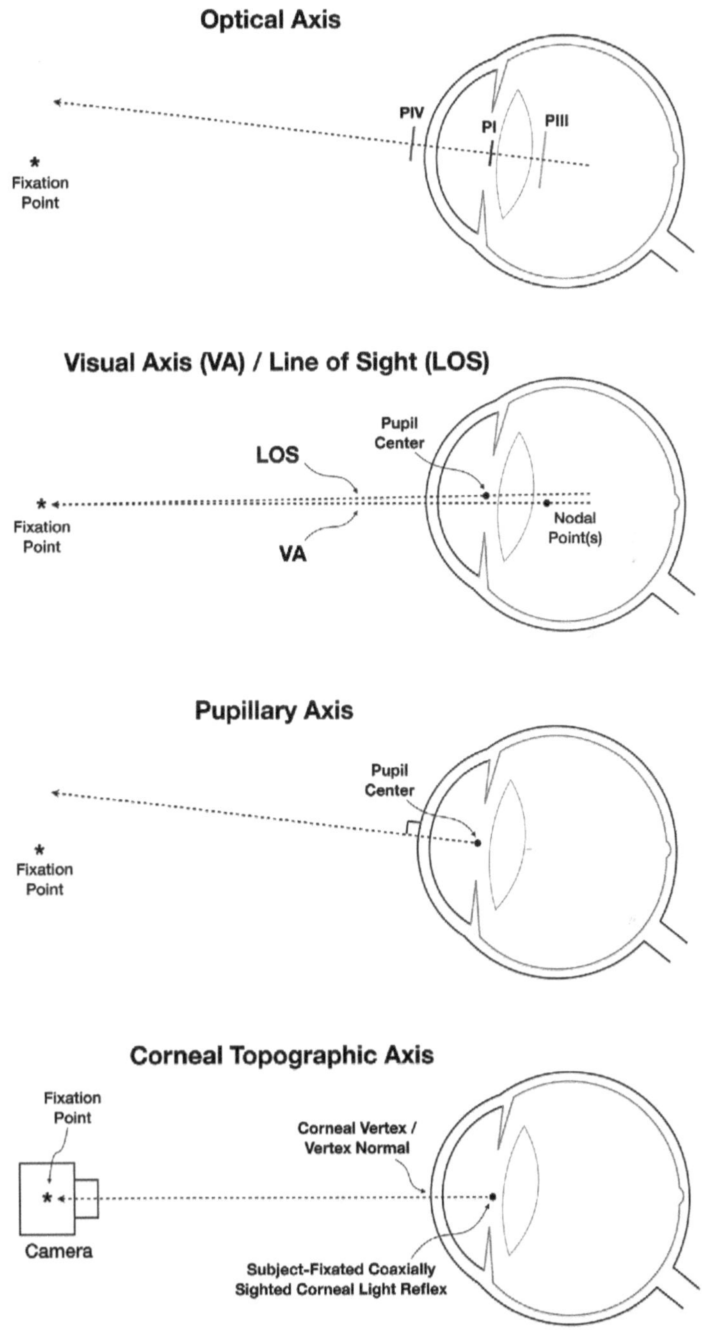

FIGURE 1.—Diagrammatic representation of different ocular reference axes. (Top) Optical axis: a line that most closely connects the three Purkinje images. (Second from top) Visual axis and line of sight: Both visual axis and line of sight originate at the fixation point and travel on different pathways (through the nodal point[s] and center of the pupil, respectively) toward the fovea. (Third from top) Pupillary axis: a line perpendicular to the cornea that passes through the center of the entrance pupil. (Bottom) Corneal topographic axis: line connecting the fixation point in the topographer to the vertex normal on the cornea. (Reprinted from American Journal of Ophthalmology. Chang DH, Waring GO IV. The subject-fixated coaxially sighted corneal light reflex: a clinical marker for centration of refractive treatments and devices. *Am J Ophthalmol.* 2014;158:863-874, Copyright 2014, with permission from Elsevier.)

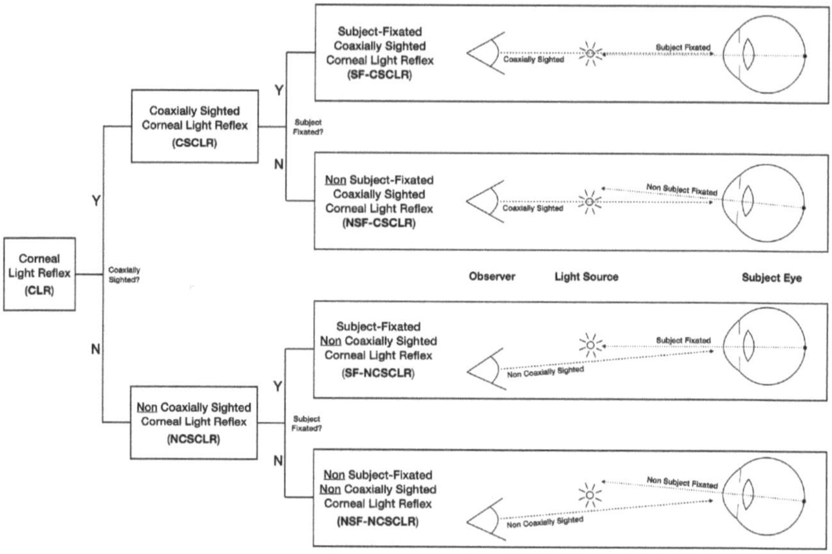

FIGURE 4.—The 4 possible relationships between the observer, the light source, and the subject eye. Using the example of an observer looking at a subject eye through a stereo coaxial light source (eg, the Zeiss Lumera microscope) with the subject fixated on the right light: subject-fixated coaxially sighted corneal light reflex (observer using right eye to view right corneal light reflex), non-subject-fixated coaxially sighted corneal light reflex (observer using left eye to view left corneal light reflex), subject-fixated non—coaxially sighted corneal light reflex (observer using left eye to view right corneal light reflex), and non-subject-fixated non—coaxially sighted corneal light reflex (observer using right eye to view left corneal light reflex). The subject-fixated non—coaxially sighted corneal light reflex is also the corneal light reflex seen when a subject fixates at the fixation light of a surgical keratoscope mounted on the microscope objective lens, at the headlight mounted in the middle of binocular loupes, or at the light source of a slit-lamp biomicroscope. The non-subject-fixated non—coaxially sighted corneal light reflex is also the corneal light reflex seen when the subject eye is fixated between the stereo coaxial lights on a Lumera or at the observer's ear at a slit-lamp biomicroscope. (Reprinted from American Journal of Ophthalmology. Chang DH, Waring GO IV. The subject-fixated coaxially sighted corneal light reflex: a clinical marker for centration of refractive treatments and devices. *Am J Ophthalmol.* 2014;158:863-874, Copyright 2014, with permission from Elsevier.)

Methods.—Literature review of papers dealing with ocular reference axes, angles, and centration.

Results.—The inconsistent definitions and usage of the current ocular axes, as derived from eye models, limit their clinical utility. With a clear understanding of Purkinje images and a defined alignment of the observer, light source/fixation target, and subject eye, the subject-fixated coaxially sighted corneal light reflex can be a clinically useful reference marker. The axis formed by connecting the subject-fixated coaxially sighted corneal light reflex and the fixation point, the subject-fixated coaxially sighted corneal light reflex axis, is independent of pupillary dilation and phakic status of the eye. The relationship of the subject-fixated coaxially sighted corneal light reflex axis to a refined definition of the visual axis without reference to nodal points, the foveal-fixation axis, is discussed. The displacement between the subject-fixated coaxially sighted corneal light reflex and pupil center is described not by an angle, but by a chord, here termed chord mu. The application of the subject-fixated coaxially sighted corneal light reflex to the surgical centration of refractive treatments and devices is discussed.

Conclusion.—As a clinically defined reference marker, the subject-fixated coaxially sighted corneal light reflex avoids the shortcomings of current ocular axes for clinical application and may contribute to better consensus in the literature and improved patient outcomes (Figs 1 and 4).

▶ Reading about the numerous ocular reference axes, such as optical axis, visual axis, line of sight, pupillary axis, has always been quite confusing to me (Fig 1). While the typically small differences in these various concepts are not hugely important when deciding where to center a corneal transplant (given the many other variables affecting vision after a graft), it did become much more important when we started doing radial keratotomy and excimer laser refractive surgery and, more recently, premium intraocular lens procedures.

The authors do an admirable job in attempting to review the pros and cons of many of the traditional ocular reference axes and make the case for a subject-fixated coaxially sighted corneal light reflex as perhaps the best landmark on which to center our refractive surgery and intraocular lens procedures (Fig 4). The debate is certainly not over, but this article is a good place for those interested in it to start.

C. J. Rapuano, MD

The Role of the Mesopic Pupil on Patient-Reported Outcomes in Young Patients With Myopia 1 Month After Wavefront-Guided LASIK

Schallhorn S, Brown M, Venter J, et al (Univ of California–San Francisco; Optical Express, San Diego, CA; Optical Express, London, UK; et al)

J Refract Surg 30:159-165, 2014

Purpose.—To determine the relationship between low-light pupil size and patient-reported outcomes 1 month after wavefront-guided LASIK in young patients with myopia.

Methods.—Retrospective case series of 10,944 eyes of 5,563 young patients with myopia who underwent wavefront-guided LASIK (6.0-mm optical zone). Preoperative pupil size was measured under low-light conditions with an infrared pupillometer. Visual and refractive outcomes were evaluated at 1 month postoperatively. A questionnaire was administered to assess patient-reported outcomes including satisfaction with the procedure, night driving, and glare and halo visual symptoms.

Results.—The average patient age was 29.8 years (range: 18 to 40 years). The mean preoperative manifest spherical equivalent of −3.49 diopters (D) (range: −0.50 to −11.75 D) was reduced to −0.04 ± 0.29 D at 1 month, with 94% of eyes achieving an uncorrected distance visual acuity of 20/20 or better. The mean low-light pupil diameter was 6.6 mm (range: 4 to 9 mm) and 1,514 patients (27.2%) had a

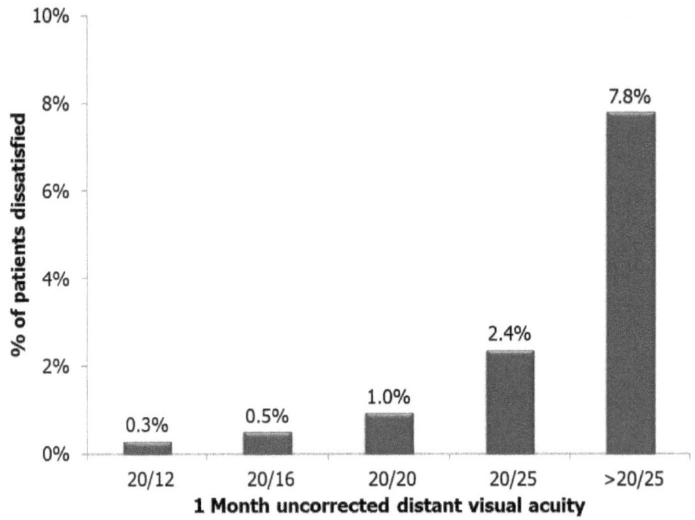

FIGURE 6.—Surgery dissatisfaction ("dissatisfied" or "very dissatisfied") stratified by postoperative uncorrected distance visual acuity. (Reprinted from Schallhorn S, Brown M, Venter J, et al. The role of the mesopic pupil on patient-reported outcomes in young patients with myopia 1 month after wavefront-guided LASIK. *J Refract Surg*. 2014;30:159-165.)

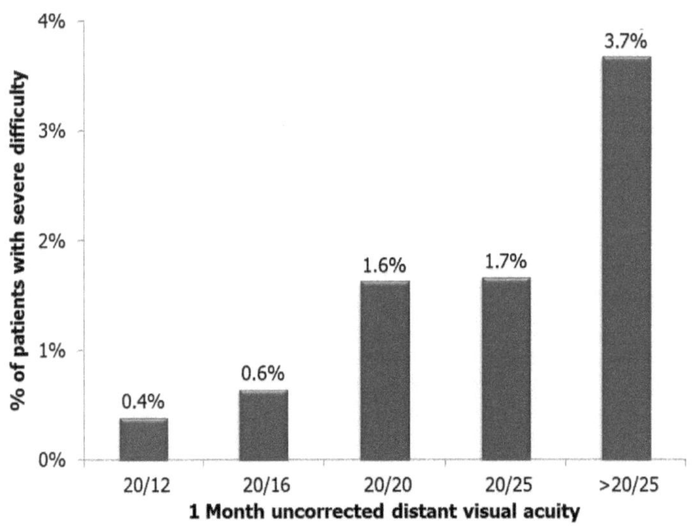

FIGURE 7.—Severe halo or starburst difficulty stratified by postoperative uncorrected distance visual acuity. (Reprinted from Schallhorn S, Brown M, Venter J, et al. The role of the mesopic pupil on patient-reported outcomes in young patients with myopia 1 month after wavefront-guided LASIK. *J Refract Surg*. 2014;30:159-165.)

TABLE 1.—Demographic Data and 1-Month Postoperative Results

Variables	Attended 1-Month Exam, Questionnaire	Consecutive Treatments	Did Not Attend 1-Month Exam	Attended 1-Month Exam, No Questionnaire
No. of patients (eyes)	5,563 (10,944)	13,481 (26,446)	2,789 (5,459)	5,129 (10,043)
% of total	41.3	100	20.7	38.0
% of attending 1 month	52.0	79.3	–	48.0
Age (y)	29.8	29.8	29.2	30.1
Gender (M/F) (%)	45.7/54.3	45.7/54.3	51.1/48.9	42.9/57.1
Mean preop MSE (D) (range)	-3.49 (-0.50 to -11.75)	-3.47 (-0.38 to -12.5)	-3.34 (-0.38 to -11.75)	-3.52 (-0.50 to -12.5)
Mean pupil diameter (mm) (range)	6.59 (4.0 to 9.0)	6.59 (4.0 to 9.0)	6.57 (4.0 to 9.0)	6.59 (4.0 to 9.0)
Mean 1-month MSE ± SD	-0.04 ± 0.29	-0.04 ± 0.30	–	-0.05 ± 0.30
% 20/20 UDVA at 1 month	94.0	93.2	–	92.4

preop = preoperative; MSE = mean spherical equivalent; D = diopters; SD = standard deviation; UDVA = uncorrected distance visual acuity.

Reprinted from Schallhorn S, Brown M, Venter J, et al. The role of the mesopic pupil on patient- reported outcomes in young patients with myopia 1 month after wavefront-guided LASIK. *J Refract Surg*. 2014;30:159-165.

diameter of 8 mm or larger. No correlation between pupil diameter and patient-reported outcomes was found (r range: −0.02 to 0.07). Logistic regression analysis identified postoperative uncorrected distance visual acuity and postoperative manifest refraction as significant predictors of night halo complaints after wavefront-guided LASIK ($P < .01$).

Conclusions.—In this large series of young patients with myopia treated with wavefront-guided LASIK, low-light pupil diameter was not predictive of surgery satisfaction, ability to perform activities, or visual symptoms at 1 month postoperatively (Figs 6 and 7, Table 1).

▶ The teaching for many years, which often continues today, is that the low-light pupil size correlates with unwanted visual symptoms, such as glare and halos and difficulty with night driving after refractive surgery. The authors report results of a retrospective review of their large database of LASIK patients. Inclusion criteria were consecutive wavefront-guided LASIK with a VISX laser and Intralase flap for myopia with or without astigmatism in patients up to age 40 years from 2008 to 2010. Patients had to be examined and complete the questionnaire 1 month postoperatively. Low-light pupil size was measured with the Colvard pupillometer. It should be noted that only 41% of patients eligible to be included in the study were actually examined and completed the questionnaire at 1 month. Although that was still a huge number of patients (> 5500), it was not everyone. The authors appropriately compared patients who completed the study and those who did not as far as age, gender, preoperative mean spherical equivalent, and mean pupil diameter (and also postoperative mean spherical equivalent and 20/20 results for those who were examined at 1 month but did not complete the questionnaire), and there were no differences between the groups (Table 1).

They found no relationship between low-light pupil size and patient satisfaction, ability to perform activities such as night driving, or visual symptoms at 1 month. Not unexpectedly, patient satisfaction and symptoms of halo correlated with worse postoperative uncorrected vision (Figs 6 and 7). Dissatisfaction was also correlated with the degree of postoperative cylinder. Halos were also correlated with the amount of preoperative sphere and preoperative cylinder. As is quite evident in Figs 6 and 7, the degree of patient dissatisfaction increases dramatically when you go from 20/25 or better to worse than 20/25 uncorrected vision. Having said that, patients were even happier with better uncorrected vision than 20/25.

C. J. Rapuano, MD

Indications for and Outcomes of Tertiary Referrals in Refractive Surgery

Patryn EK, Vrijman V, Nieuwendaal CP, et al (Academic Med Centre, Amsterdam, The Netherlands)

J Refract Surg 30:54-61, 2014

Purpose.—To review the spectrum of disease, symptomatology, and management offered to patients referred for a second opinion after refractive surgery.

Methods.—A prospective cohort study was done on all patients referred from October 1, 2006, to September 30, 2011, to a tertiary eye clinic after refractive surgery of any kind (ie, corneal laser surgery, conductive keratoplasty, radial keratotomy, phakic implants, refractive lens exchanges, or any combination thereof). Data analysis was performed on all demographic and clinical aspects of this cohort, including the initial complaint, type of referral, number of complaints, procedure previously performed, diagnosis at our center, type of advice given, and rate and type of surgical intervention.

Results.—One hundred thirty-one eyes (69 patients) were included. Corneal refractive surgery was performed in 82% (108 eyes), and 11% (14 eyes) were seen after phakic intraocular lens (PIOL) implantation and 7% (9 eyes) after refractive lens exchange. The most common diagnoses were tear film dysfunction (30 eyes, 23%), residual refractive error (25 eyes, 19%), and cataract (20 eyes, 15%). Most patients (42 patients, 61%) were treated conservatively. In 27 patients (39%), 36 eyes (28%) were managed surgically. Severe visual loss was seen in 1 eye.

Conclusions.—No major problems were found in most second opinions after refractive surgery referral. Dry eyes, small residual refractive error, or higher-order aberrations were the most common complaints. Surgical intervention was needed in 36 eyes (28%), almost half of which were cataract extractions. Severe visual loss was seen in 1 eye with a PIOL. There

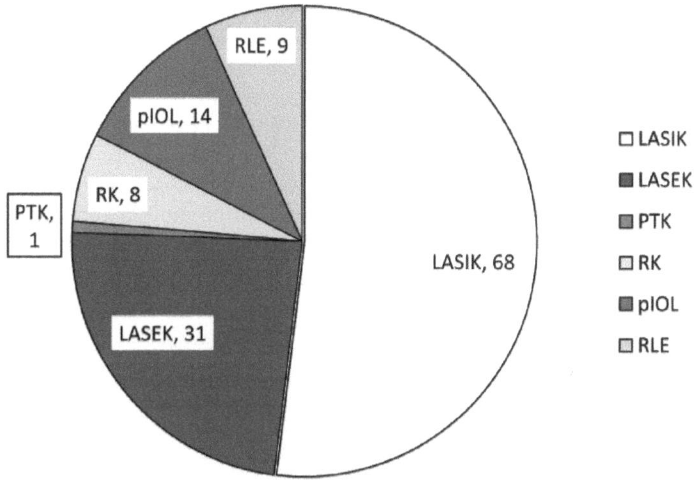

FIGURE 2.—Distribution of type of refractive surgery in this cohort. Corneal laser surgery accounted for more than 82% of referrals. Phakic intraocular lens surgery accounted for 10.6% or referrals, and 6.9% had refractive surgery. PIOL = phakic intraocular lens; RK = radial keratectomy; PTK = phototherapeutic keratectomy; RLE = refractive lens exchange. (Reprinted from Patryn EK, Vrijman V, Nieuwendaal CP, et al. Indications for and outcomes of tertiary referrals in refractive surgery. *J Refract Surg.* 2014;30:54-61, with permission from SLACK Incorporated.)

was no incidence of severe visual loss in keratorefractive and refractive lens exchange procedures (Fig 2).

▶ I selected this article for 2 reasons: (1) it looks at the interesting question of second opinions after refractive surgery in Europe and (2) to question whether it is a "prospective cohort study" as stated in the article.

The authors looked at patients, seen in their clinic in the Netherlands, complaining of problems after a variety of refractive surgery procedures including laser in situ keratomileusis (LASIK), surface ablation, conductive keratoplasty, radial keratotomy, phakic intraocular lenses (PIOL), and refractive lens exchanges. There is a fine line between refractive lens exchange and routine cataract surgery, which the authors did not define. More than half of the eyes had previously undergone LASIK, and one-quarter had previously undergone surface ablation (Fig 2). Interestingly, the results were very similar to our study out of Wills Eye Institute, published in 2008,[1] which looked at referrals for patients who were unhappy after LASIK. However, they also looked at eyes after other refractive surgical procedures. The following comment in the authors' discussion is interesting: "In our opinion, a disproportionate amount of severe complications occurred after PIOL implantations, requiring complicated solutions such as glaucoma implant surgery, lens extraction, and Descemet's membrane endothelial keratoplasty. Significantly more interventions were needed in the PIOL vs the corneal surgery and lens exchange groups." Perhaps there is a good reason for the relatively small numbers of PIOL procedures performed in the United States compared with Europe.

My second reason for selecting this study was to discuss the use of "prospective cohort study," which is what the authors called their study. To me "prospective" means the investigators had a specific question that they were trying to answer from the beginning. With this specific question in mind, a study is designed, institutional review board (IRB) approval is obtained, and patients are enrolled with their knowledge and informed consent from the beginning. From my reading, this study did not do these things. There was no mention of IRB approval or patients signing informed consent. To me that sounds like a retrospective study, which is fine, but just call it what it is.

C. J. Rapuano, MD

Reference

1. Levinson BA, Rapuano CJ, Cohen EJ, Hammersmith KM, Ayres BD, Laibson PR. Referrals to the Wills Eye Institute Cornea Service after laser in situ keratomileusis: reasons for patient dissatisfaction. *J Cataract Refract Surg*. 2008;34:32-39.

Corneal Sensation and Dry Eye Symptoms after Conventional versus Inverted Side-Cut Femtosecond LASIK: A Prospective Randomized Study

Kung JS, Sáles CS, Manche EE, et al (Stanford Univ School of Medicine, CA)

Ophthalmology 121:2311-2316, 2014

Purpose.—To compare corneal sensation and self-reported dry eye symptoms after femtosecond-assisted LASIK with conventional versus inverted side cuts.

Design.—Prospective, randomized, eye-to-eye study.

Participants.—A total of 120 eyes in 60 participants with myopia.

Methods.—Fellow eyes were randomized to receive femtosecond-assisted LASIK with a conventional 70-degree side cut made with the 60 kHz IntraLase FS (Abbott Medical Optics, Santa Ana, CA) or an inverted 130-degree side cut made with the 150 kHz IntraLase iFS (Abbott Medical Optics). Cochet–Bonnet aesthesiometry (Luneau Ophthalmologia, Chartes, France) measured corneal sensation (60 mm = normal sensation; <60 mm = depressed sensation) preoperatively and at postoperative months 1, 3, 6, and 12. Participants also completed serial dry eye surveys using the same subscales (frequency, severity, bothersome) as the validated, Rasch-tested, linear-scaled Quality of Vision questionnaire.

Main Outcome Measures.—Objective corneal sensation and self-reported light sensitivity, dryness, foreign body sensation, and pain/discomfort.

Results.—Preoperative corneal sensation as measured by mean Cochet–Bonnet aethesiometry was equal between the inverted and conventional side cut groups but was better in eyes with an inverted side cut compared with a conventional side cut at all postoperative months (inverted vs. conventional: 1 month, 14.5 vs. 13.2 mm; 3 months, 24.9 vs. 18.4 mm; 6 months, 51.2 vs. 42.6 mm; 12 months, 59.8 vs. 58.3 mm; all $P \leq 0.02$).

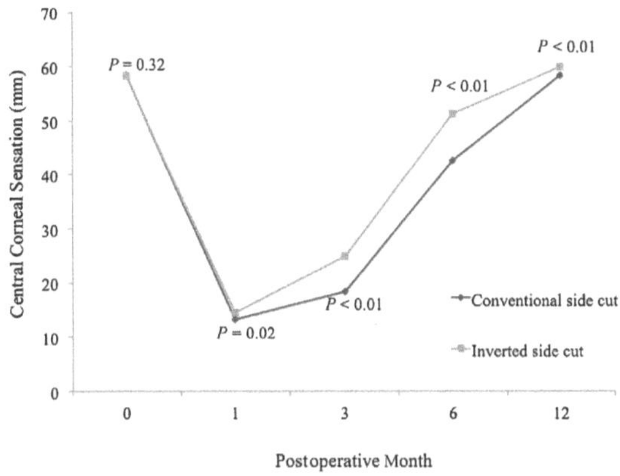

FIGURE 2.—Mean corneal sensation: Cochet–Bonnet. (Reprinted from Ophthalmology. Kung JS, Sáles CS, Manche EE, et al. Corneal sensation and dry eye symptoms after conventional versus inverted side-cut femtosecond LASIK: a prospective randomized study. *Ophthalmology.* 2014;121:2311-2316, Copyright 2014, with permission from the American Academy of Ophthalmology.)

None of the subjective dry eye parameters demonstrated statistically significant differences between the groups at any time point.

Conclusions.—The LASIK flaps with an inverted side cut are associated with superior recovery of corneal sensation compared with flaps with a conventional side cut during the first postoperative year; however, this may not translate to significant improvements in subjective dry eye symptoms (Fig 2).

▶ In theory, an inverted side-cut for laser-assisted in situ keratomileusis (LASIK) flap seems like a good idea. The flap edge should tuck into position and ideally stay in place better than with a more vertical side-cut. If the flap edge aligns well with its preoperative position, the severed peripheral corneal nerves should be more able to find their way across the "gap" to more rapidly reenervate the central cornea. That is the question evaluated by this nicely done study.

Decreased corneal sensation after LASIK is thought to be one of the main factors causing dry eye problems. Manche and colleagues performed LASIK with a conventional side-cut in 1 eye and an inverted side-cut in the fellow eye and looked at corneal sensation and dry eye symptoms. In both groups, they found a huge decrease in corneal sensation at the 1-month postoperative visit, which returned to near normal by 1 year. Although corneal sensation was "statistically significantly" worse at the 1-, 3-, 6-, and 12-month time points in the conventional side-cut group compared with the inverted side-cut group, it is unclear to me that the small differences were clinically significant. The authors state in their discussion that significantly more eyes returned to full corneal sensation in the inverted side-cut group than the conventional side-cut group at 1 year, but looking at Fig 2, this may not be clinically significant either.

Interestingly, the statistically significant superiority of the inverted side-cut did not translate into statistically significantly improved dry eye symptoms compared with the conventional side-cut at any point in the study. I am all in favor of anatomic improvements, even without definitive clinical advantages, as long as we do not oversell it to our patients, our colleagues, and ourselves.

C. J. Rapuano, MD

Combination Therapy With Diquafosol Tetrasodium and Sodium Hyaluronate in Patients With Dry Eye After Laser In Situ Keratomileusis

Toda I, Ide T, Fukumoto T, et al (Minamiaoyama Eye Clinic, Tokyo, Japan; et al)
Am J Ophthalmol 157:616-622, 2014

Purpose.—To evaluate the possible advantages of combination therapy with diquafosol tetrasodium and sodium hyaluronate for dry eye after laser in situ keratomileusis (LASIK).

Design.—Prospective randomized comparative trial.

Methods.—A total of 206 eyes of 105 patients who underwent LASIK were enrolled in this study. Patients were randomly assigned to 1 of 4 treatment groups according to the postoperative treatment: artificial tears, sodium hyaluronate, diquafosol tetrasodium, and a combination of hyaluronate and diquafosol. Questionnaire responses reflecting subjective dry eye symptoms, uncorrected and corrected visual acuity, functional visual acuity, manifest refraction, tear break-up time, fluorescein corneal staining, Schirmer test, and corneal sensitivity were examined before and 1 week and 1 month after LASIK.

Results.—Distance uncorrected visual acuity was significantly better in the combination group than in the hyaluronate group 1 week and 1 month after LASIK. Near uncorrected visual acuity was significantly better in the combination group than in the artificial tear and diquafosol groups 1 week and 1 month after LASIK. Distance functional visual acuity improved significantly only in the combination group 1 month after LASIK. The Schirmer value in the combination group was significantly higher than that in the hyaluronate group at 1 month after LASIK. Subjective dry eye symptoms in the combination group improved significantly compared with those in the other groups 1 week after surgery.

Conclusions.—Our results suggest that hyaluronate and diquafosol combination therapy is beneficial for early stabilization of visual performance and improvement of subjective dry eye symptoms in patients after LASIK.

▶ The 2 products tested against artificial tears in this study, 3% diquafosol and 0.3% sodium hyaluronate, are not currently commercially available in the United States. Diquafosol went through rigorous Food and Drug Administration (FDA) trials but in the end never received final approval. Although there are artificial tear products available in the United States that have sodium hyaluronate listed as an inactive ingredient, I do not believe they are at concentration levels as high as 0.3%. I selected this article to highlight the fact that it is not only collagen cross-linking that much of the world has that the United States does not.

As far as results, I found it interesting that many of the visual and symptomatic results were better in the eyes that received 1 or both medication drops compared with artificial tears, but there was no difference in the fluorescein staining or tear breakup time scores.

Certainly, the initial decreased vision after laser in situ keratomileusis and subsequent improvement over time is multifactorial (neurotrophic, damage to goblet cells, change in corneal shape, etc), but these medications appear to help, at least in the first month. Perhaps we in the United States will be able to offer these medications to our patients sometime in the future.

C. J. Rapuano, MD

Variation in the effectiveness of refractive surgery during the year: Results from the Hamburg Weather Study

Neuhaus-Richard I, Frings A, Ament F, et al (Univ of Hamburg, Germany)
J Cataract Refract Surg 40:1139-1146, 2014

Purpose.—To examine the impact of seasonality on the refractive and visual outcomes of laser in situ keratomileusis (LASIK) in myopic eyes.

Setting.—Department of Ophthalmology and Care Vision Refractive Centers, University Medical Center Hamburg-Eppendorf, Hamburg, Germany.

Design.—Retrospective cross-sectional data analysis.

Methods.—Two subgroups were defined. The first comprised patients having surgery during meteorological winter and the second, patients having surgery during meteorological summer. The manifest refraction and uncorrected and corrected visual acuities were assessed preoperatively and postoperatively. Robust regression analysis was applied with the efficacy index, safety index, and postoperative SE as dependent variables.

Results.—This study comprised 1052 eyes of 1052 consecutive myopic patients (419 men, 633 women; mean age at surgery 35.0 years ± 9.0 [SD]) with a mean preoperative refractive spherical equivalent (SE) of −3.88 ± 1.85 diopters (D). At the 1-month follow-up (mean 33.0 ± 5.0 days), the mean postoperative SE was −0.18 ± 0.44 D. The efficacy index was 0.023 higher in eyes with refractive surgery during summer than in eyes treated during winter ($P = .032$), indicating less efficacy during winter. The differences in the safety index and postoperative SE between summer and winter were not statistically significant. No eye had a change of more than 1 line on the logMAR scale (corrected distance visual acuity).

Conclusions.—Although the difference in the efficacy index was statistically significant, the difference in the outcomes of LASIK was not clinically relevant, which shows the procedure's highly standardized reliability. Prospective longitudinal studies are warranted to address meteorotropic reactions by evaluating defined meteorological parameters (Fig 2).

▶ Both outdoor and operating room conditions, such as temperature and humidity, have been found to affect post laser in situ keratomileusis (LASIK) results in some studies. This relatively large study found a small difference in

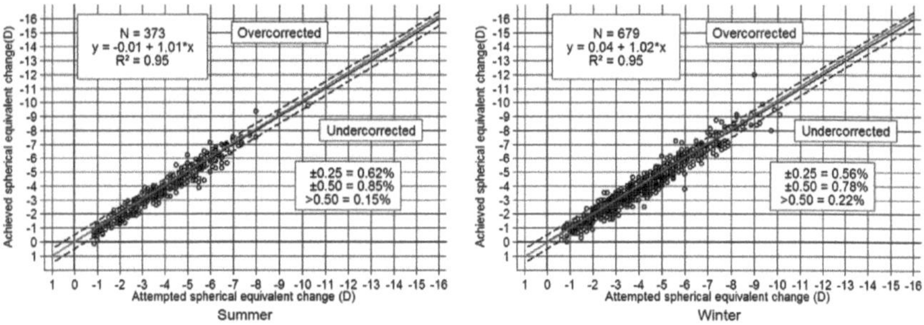

FIGURE 2.—Attempted versus achieved SE correction at 1 month by season. (Reprinted from Journal of Cataract & Refractive Surgery. Neuhaus-Richard I, Frings A, Ament F, et al. Variation in the effectiveness of refractive surgery during the year: results from the Hamburg Weather Study. *J Cataract Refract Surg*. 2014;40:1139-1146, Copyright 2014, with permission from ASCRS and ESCRS.)

LASIK results between the winter and summer months. Although the results were statistically significantly better in the summer, it was such a small difference that the authors felt it was "not clinically relevant" (Fig 2). This is nice to know and confirms many surgeons' clinical impressions, including my own.

Having said that, this study has certain limitations (1) It included only 1052 eyes, which although large, is not huge. (2) It looked at 1-month data, which may not be long enough. (3) It was performed in Germany where the weather in the winter and summer is not as different as it is in many parts of the world. Nonetheless, it is comforting information to learn.

C. J. Rapuano, MD

Association Between the Percent Tissue Altered and Post–Laser In Situ Keratomileusis Ectasia in Eyes With Normal Preoperative Topography

Santhiago MR, Smadja D, Gomes BF, et al (Federal Univ of Rio de Janeiro, Brazil; Univ Ctr Hosp of Bordeaux, France; et al)

Am J Ophthalmol 158:87-95, 2014

Purpose.—To investigate the association of a novel metric, percent tissue altered, with the occurrence of ectasia after laser in situ keratomileusis (LASIK) in eyes with normal corneal topography and to compare this metric with other recognized risk factors.

Design.—Retrospective case-control study.

Methods.—The study included 30 eyes from 16 patients with bilateral normal preoperative Placidobased corneal topography that developed ectasia after LASIK (ectasia group) and 174 eyes from 88 consecutive patients with uncomplicated LASIK and at least 3 years of postoperative follow-up. The following metrics were evaluated: age, preoperative central corneal thickness, residual stromal bed, Ectasia Risk Score System scores, and percent tissue altered, derived from [PTA = (FT + AD)/CCT], where FT = flap thickness, AD = ablation depth, and CCT = preoperative central corneal thickness.

TABLE 4.—Prevalence of Individual Proposed Ectasia Risk Factors in Post-LASIK Ectasia and Control Eyes

Risk Factor	Post-LASIK Ectasia Group	Control Group	*P* Value	Odds Ratio	Confidence Interval	Sensitivity	Specificity	Negative Predictive Value
PTA[a] ≥40%	97%	11%	<.0001[b]	223.3	(28.8–1729.7)	97%	89%	99.4%
RSB ≤300 μm	57%	2%	<.0001[b]	74.5	(19.3–287.7)	57%	98%	92.9%
CCT ≤510 μm	16%	6%	.065	2.9	(0.9–9.2)	16%	93%	86.7%
ERSS ≥4	20%	3%	.001[b]	8.4	(2.4–29.8)	20%	97%	87.5%
ERSS ≥3	43%	12%	.0002[b]	5.3	(2.2–12.3)	43%	87%	89.9%
MRSE ≥8 D	10%	7%	.547	1.5	(0.4–5.7)	10%	93%	85.7%
Age (y) <30	63%	24%	<.0001[b]	5.4	(2.4–12.3)	63%	75%	92.3%

CCT = central corneal thickness; D = diopters; ERSS = Ectasia Risk Score System; MRSE = manifest refractive spherical equivalent; PTA = percent tissue altered; RSB = residual stromal bed.

Ectasia group is composed of ectasia cases after laser in situ keratomileusis with normal preoperative topography and control group is composed of consecutive uneventful laser in situ keratomileusis eyes with at least 3 years follow-up.

[a]Percent Tissue Altered = (Flap Thickness + Ablation Depth)/preoperative Central Corneal Thickness.

[b]Difference statistically significant.

Results.—In the ectasia group, percent tissue altered ≥40 was the most prevalent factor (97%), followed by age <30 years (63%), residual stromal bed ≤300 μm (57%), and ectasia risk score ≥3 (43%) ($P < .001$ for all). Percent tissue altered ≥40 had the highest odds ratio (223), followed by residual stromal bed ≤300 μm (74) and ectasia risk score ≥4 (8). Stepwise logistic regression revealed percent tissue altered ≥40 as the single most significant independent variable ($P < .0001$).

Conclusions.—Percent tissue altered at the time of LASIK was significantly associated with the development of ectasia in eyes with normal preoperative topography and was a more robust indicator of risk than all other variables in this patient population (Table 4).

▶ The concept of percent of tissue ablated or altered as a risk factor for post-laser-assisted in situ keratomileusis (LASIK) ectasia is not new. Many surgeons used to use a "rule of thumb" that the residual stromal bed needed to be > 50% of the preoperative corneal thickness. That was in the earlier days of LASIK when the standard rule was a residual stromal bed of > 250 microns. I must admit, it did not make perfect sense to me that 250-micron residual stromal bed was just as "safe" in a 450-micron cornea as in a 650-micron cornea, so a percent of tissue altered metric seems reasonable.

In this retrospective case-control study, the authors determined that percent of tissue altered was a better predictor of post-LASIK ectasia than other risk factors. They further determined that 40% had the best combination of sensitivity and specificity for predicting the development of post-LASIK ectasia. Forty percent had 97% sensitivity and 89% specificity, combining for a negative predictive value of 99.4%. The negative predictive value is the probability that a negative test really is negative. This is much higher than any of the other commonly used risk factors (Table 4).

Although percent of tissue altered was not a perfect test (11% of the 174 control eyes had a percent tissue altered > 40), it seems as if refractive surgeons should be including some sort of "percent tissue altered" calculation in their preoperative thought process.

C. J. Rapuano, MD

Five-year results of refractive lenticule extraction

Blum M, Flach A, Kunert KS, et al (Univ of Marburg, Germany)

J Cataract Refract Surg 40:1425-1429, 2014

Purpose.—To evaluate the 5-year results of femtosecond laser–assisted refractive lenticule extraction (ReLEx-FLEx) for the treatment of myopia and myopic astigmatism.

Setting.—Departments of Ophthalmology, Helios Klinikum Erfurt, Erfurt, and Phillips Universität Marburg, Marburg, Germany.

Design.—Prospective clinical trial.

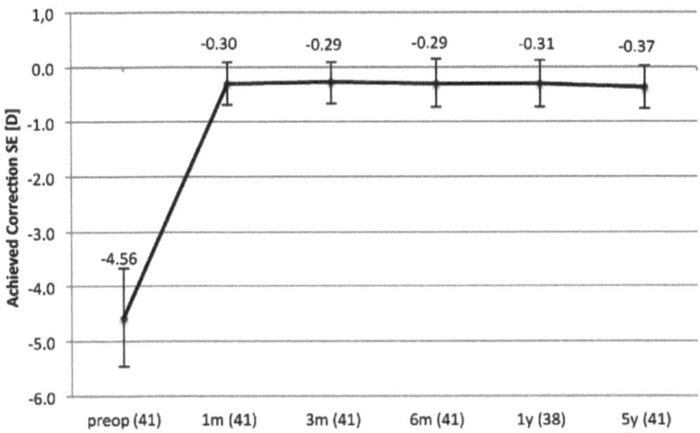

FIGURE 6.—Stability of refractive outcome over the 5-year follow-up (SE = spherical equivalent). (Reprinted from Journal of Cataract & Refractive Surgery. Blum M, Flach A, Kunert KS, et al. Five-year results of refractive lenticule extraction. *J Cataract Refract Surg.* 2014;40:1425-1429, Copyright 2014, with permission from ASCRS and ESCRS.)

Methods.—This was a follow-up of a prospective study that evaluated the first patients treated with refractive lenticule extraction, in which a flap and a refractive lenticule of intrastromal corneal tissue were simultaneously cut using a 200 kHz Visumax femtosecond laser system. Thereafter, the lenticule was manually removed and the flap repositioned. The main outcome measures were the uncorrected and corrected distance visual acuities, objective and manifest refractions, slitlamp examination findings, and side effects after 5 years.

Results.—Forty-one of 108 eyes in the original treatment group were available for a reexamination. Five years postoperatively, 100% of eyes were within ±1.00 diopter (D) of the intended correction and 73% were within ±0.50 D. By 5 years, no eye had lost 2 or more Snellen lines and 1 eye had lost 1 Snellen line. The mean regression was 0.07 D.

Conclusion.—Long-term data indicate that refractive lenticule extraction is an effective and safe procedure for the treatment of myopia and myopic astigmatism and has excellent stability (Fig 6).

► Refractive lenticule extraction was the first of all the femtosecond laser refractive surgery procedures. It uses the femtosecond laser to create a laser-assisted in situ keratomileusis (LASIK)-type flap plus a refractive lenticule. The flap is reflected back as in LASIK, the lenticule is removed manually, and the flap is replaced. This procedure has largely been supplanted by small incision lenticule extraction (SMILE), in which the lenticule is removed through a small 2 to 3 clock-hour opening instead of lifting an entire flap. The importance of this study is that at 5 years, there were no untoward events, but most significantly, the refractions were quite stable (Fig 6). This bodes well for success of the newer SMILE procedure.

C. J. Rapuano, MD

Safety and Complications of More Than 1500 Small-Incision Lenticule Extraction Procedures

Ivarsen A, Asp S, Hjortdal J (Aarhus Univ Hosp, Denmark)
Ophthalmology 121:822-828, 2014

Purpose.—To evaluate the safety and complications of small-incision lenticule extraction (SMILE).

Design.—Clinical control cohort study.

Participants.—A total of 922 healthy patients (1800 eyes) who were treated for myopia or myopic astigmatism between January 2011 and March 2013 at the Department of Ophthalmology, Aarhus, Denmark.

Methods.—Patients received a full preoperative examination and were treated with SMILE in both eyes and followed for 3 months (1574 eyes). Patients with complications, including loss of corrected distance visual acuity (CDVA) or dissatisfaction, were offered a late reexamination.

Main Outcome Measures.—Surgical complications and CDVA.

Results.—Mean preoperative spherical equivalent refraction was −7.25 ± 1.84 diopters (D). Average postoperative refraction was −0.28 ± 0.52 D, and mean error of treatment was −0.15 ± 0.50 D. By 3 months, 86% (1346 eyes) had unchanged or improved CDVA. A loss of 2 or more lines was observed in 1.5% of eyes; however, at a late follow-up visit (average, 18 months), CDVA was within 1 line of the preoperative level in all eyes. Perioperative complications included epithelial abrasions (6%), small tears at the incision (1.8%), and difficult lenticule extraction (1.9%). The cap was perforated in 4 eyes, and a major tear occurred in 1 eye; however, none of these patients had late visual symptoms. In 0.8% (14 eyes), suction was lost during surgery. Re-treatment was successful in 13 eyes, whereas 1 eye had ghost images and was retreated with topography-guided photorefractive keratectomy (PRK). Postoperative complications included trace haze (8%), epithelial dryness on day 1 (5%), interface inflammation secondary to central abrasion (0.3%), and minor interface infiltrates (0.3%); these complications had

TABLE 2.—Preoperative and Postoperative Complications

Preoperative Complications	Postoperative Complications
Abrasion at the incision (114)	Haze, grade 0.5 to 1 (127)
Lenticule extraction difficulties (34)	Dry surface, day 1 (75)
Minor tear at the incision (33)	Epithelial islands at incision (10)
Suction loss (14)	Fiber in interface (6)
Central abrasion (5)	Infiltrates/keratitis (5)
Cap perforation (4)	Monocular ghost images (5)
Major tear (1)	Interface inflammation (4)
Lenticule extraction impossible (1)	

Values in parentheses indicate the number of eyes.

Reprinted from Ivarsen A, Asp S, Hjortdal J. Safety and complications of more than 1500 small-incision lenticule extraction procedures. *Ophthalmology*. 2014;121:822-828.

TABLE 3.—Postoperative Complications: Loss of Corrected Distance Visual Acuity

Eye	Preoperative CDVA	3-Month CDVA	Late CDVA	Notes
1	20/15	20/25	20/15	—
2	20/20	20/30	20/20	Irregular topography
3	20/20	20/30	—	—
4	20/20	20/30	20/20	Decentered ablation
5	20/20	20/30	20/20	Decentered ablation
6	20/20	20/30	—	—
7	20/20	20/40	20/20	—
8	20/20	20/30	20/15	—
9	20/15	20/25	20/20	Slightly irregular topography
10	20/20	20/30	20/15	—
11	20/15	20/25	20/20	Irregular topography
12	20/20	20/30	20/20	Slightly irregular topography
13	20/15	20/25	20/20	—
14	20/20	20/30	20/20	Slightly irregular topography
15	20/20	20/40	20/20	Difficult lenticule extraction, irregular topography, topographic PRK
16	20/30	—	20/30	Major preoperative tear
17	20/20	20/30	20/25	Difficult lenticule extraction, irregular topography
18	20/20	20/40	20/25	Difficult lenticule extraction, irregular topography
19	20/15	20/25	20/15	Irregular topography
20	20/20	20/60	20/15	Grade 1 haze
21	20/15	20/30	20/20	Slightly irregular topography
22	20/15	20/30	20/20	Irregular topography
23	20/15	20/30	20/20	Irregular topography
24	20/15	20/30	—	—

CDVA = corrected distance visual acuity; PRK = photorefractive keratectomy.
Reprinted from Ivarsen A, Asp S, Hjortdal J. Safety and complications of more than 1500 small-incision lenticule extraction procedures. *Ophthalmology.* 2014;121:822-828.

an impact on CDVA at 3 months in only 1 case. Irregular corneal topography occurred in 1.0% of eyes, resulting in reduced 3-month CDVA (12 eyes) or ghost images (6 eyes). Topography-guided PRK was performed in 4 eyes, with improvement in 3 cases. Satisfaction was high, with only 2 patients dissatisfied at their latest visit because of blurred vision or residual astigmatism.

Conclusions.—Overall, SMILE had acceptable safety. Although 1.5% of eyes had reduced CDVA by 3 months, visual acuity was restored in the long term. Likewise, patient satisfaction was high (Tables 2 and 3).

▶ Although not yet Food and Drug Administration approved as of this writing (January 2015), small incision lenticule extraction (SMILE) is gaining traction around the world. This study is the largest I know of that looks at visual results and intraoperative and postoperative complications. This study confirms the excellent clinical results previously reported in smaller studies. There are a few interesting points to glean from this article. Although few and far between, there were several significant intraoperative complications. Four eyes had cap perforations from difficult lenticule extractions. One other eye had a major tear, almost bisecting the cap, and in another eye, the lenticule could not be extracted (Table 2). Twenty-four eyes lost 2 or more Snellen lines of the best corrected visual acuity at 3 months, but all 21 that were examined later (mean of 18 months postoperatively) had improved to within 1 Snellen line of preoperative best corrected vision (Table 3). Patient satisfaction was quite high. At 3 months, 6 patients (9 eyes) were dissatisfied. Topography-guided photorefractive keratectomy (PRK) improved symptoms in 2 of these eyes. One patient (2 eyes) was dissatisfied because of attempted treatment of very high cylinder. At last follow-up, only 2 patients were dissatisfied.

The authors made an interesting observation in the discussion, commenting on the relatively high number of intraoperative complications. They wrote, "Nevertheless, the relatively high frequency of perioperative challenges underlines that SMILE is a technically more demanding procedure then other keratorefractive techniques, including femtosecond LASIK." Aaaahhhhh ... just when I was beginning to think new technology was going to make our lives *easier*.

C. J. Rapuano, MD

Small incision lenticule extraction (SMILE) and femtosecond laser LASIK: comparison of corneal wound healing and inflammation

Dong Z, Zhou X, Wu J, et al (Fudan Univ, Shanghai, PR China; et al)
Br J Ophthalmol 98:263-269, 2014

Aim.—To evaluate and compare early corneal wound healing and inflammatory responses after small incision lenticule extraction (SMILE) versus femtosecond laser laser in situ keratomileusis (LASIK).

Methods.—Thirty-six eyes of 36 rabbits underwent SMILE, while another 36 eyes of 36 rabbits were treated with femtosecond laser LASIK. All the eyes were subjected to the same refractive correction of −6.00 DS/−1.00 DC. Twelve eyes that had no surgery were included for control. After euthanisation, corneal tissue sections were evaluated with terminal deoxyribonucleotidyl transferase-mediated dUTP-digoxigenin nick-end labelling (TUNEL) assay to detect apoptosis at postoperative 4 and 24 h, immunocytochemistry for Ki67 to detect keratocyte proliferation at postoperative day 3, week 1 and month 1, and immunocytochemistry for CD11b to detect inflammation at postoperative day 1, day 3 and week 1, respectively.

Results.—No adverse effects were noted after SMILE or LASIK. Corneal healing postoperatively was uneventful in all cases. There were significantly fewer TUNEL-positive corneal stromal cells after the SMILE procedure at 4 and 24 h postoperatively ($p < 0.01$) compared with the LASIK procedure. In addition, immunocytochemistry showed significantly fewer Ki67-positive cells in the SMILE group than those in the femtosecond laser LASIK group at day 3 and week 1 postoperatively ($p < 0.05$), but there was little expression of Ki67 at month 1 postoperatively in both groups. The CD11b-positive cells were significantly fewer in the SMILE group at day 1, day 3 and week 1 postoperatively ($p < 0.01$).

Conclusions.—SMILE induces less keratocyte apoptosis, proliferation and inflammation compared with femtosecond laser LASIK.

▶ The authors compared SMILE (small incision lenticule extraction, in which a femtosecond laser creates the refractive lenticule and a small superficial incision through which the lenticule is removed) with standard femtosecond laser in situ keratomileusis (LASIK) in rabbits to look at early wound healing and the inflammatory response. Overall, they found less disruption in the SMILE eyes and the LASIK eyes. Although that sounds great—I mean who can argue with less apoptosis and inflammation—what it actually means in real life in human eyes is unknown. If it were to correlate with less regression or less haze or less development of ectasia, *that* would be something. This is a nice beginning for future studies.

C. J. Rapuano, MD

Differences in the Corneal Biomechanical Changes After SMILE and LASIK

Wang D, Liu M, Chen Y, et al (Sun Yatsen Univ, Guangzhou, China; et al)
J Refract Surg 30:702-707, 2014

Purpose.—To compare the corneal biomechanical properties before and after small incision lenticule extraction (SMILE) and femtosecond laser-assisted LASIK in different levels of myopia with the Ocular Response Analyzer (Reichert Ophthalmic Instruments, Depew, NY).

Methods.—A total of 187 and 79 eyes that received SMILE or LASIK, respectively, between January and June 2013 at Zhongshan Ophthalmic Center were enrolled in this study. Patients were grouped according to surgery type (SMILE or LASIK) and −6.00 diopters (D) or less (≤ −6.00 D) or myopia greater than −6.00 D (> −6.00 D). Corneal hysteresis, corneal resistance factor, and 37 waveform parameters were recorded and compared preoperatively and at 1 week and 1 and 3 months postoperatively.

Results.—There was a significant decrease of corneal hysteresis, corneal resistance factor, p1area, and p2area, and an increase of path1 and path2 in both SMILE and LASIK. In myopia −6.00 D or less, the differences between SMILE and LASIK were not significant ($P > .05$), but in myopia greater than −6.00 D, the corneal hysteresis, corneal resistance factor, p1area, and p2area decreased significantly more in LASIK than in SMILE ($P < .05$).

Conclusions.—When comparing SMILE with LASIK, myopia was greater than −6.00 D, and the corneal hysteresis, corneal resistance factor, p1area, and p2area decrease was less after SMILE.

▶ Biomechanical properties of the cornea are difficult to measure in vivo. The Ocular Response Analyzer (ORA) came to market about 8 to 10 years ago with the purpose of measuring corneal "strength." It uses an air puff to analyze deformation and reformation of the corneal curvature. "Weak" corneas, such as those with keratoconus, deform and reform differently from "normal" corneas. One of the main reasons to evaluate corneal strength and weakness is to identify eyes at risk for developing corneal ectasia after refractive surgery. It turns out that this task is not so simple. There was a great degree of overlap in the initial parameters the ORA analyzed between known normal and abnormal eyes. There are now multiple newer parameters that may be better in differentiating normal from abnormal, but more studies are needed.

The authors of this article used the ORA's new parameters to determine whether there were differences in corneal "strength" between the laser-assisted in situ keratomileusis (LASIK) and small incision lenticule extraction (SMILE) procedures for myopia. They did not find differences between the 2 procedures in the lower-myopia treatment group (< −6 D) but did in the higher myopia treatment group (> −6 D). Several parameters consistent with "cornea weakening" were greater in the LASIK eyes than in the SMILE eyes. In their discussion, the authors comment that for myopic errors < 6 D, SMILE removes more corneal tissue than LASIK, whereas the 2 procedures remove similar amounts of tissue when treating eyes with > 6 D of myopia. They state the greater tissue removal in eyes with > 6 D of myopia is compensated for by the lack of a full LASIK flap, which is why the ORA measurements were not different from each other in the 2 lower myopia groups. Although we are not sure exactly what the ORA is actually measuring, these results are additional information supporting the idea that the SMILE technology may have some biomechanical advantages over LASIK.

C. J. Rapuano, MD

Comparison of biomechanical effects of small-incision lenticule extraction and laser in situ keratomileusis: Finite-element analysis

Sinha Roy A, Dupps WJ Jr, Roberts CJ (Case Western Reserve Univ, Cleveland, OH; The Ohio State Univ, Columbus)

J Cataract Refract Surg 40:971-980, 2014

Purpose.—To theoretically compare the corneal stress distribution of laser in situ keratomileusis (LASIK) with the stress distribution of small-incision lenticule extraction.

Setting.—Cleveland Clinic Cole Institute, Cleveland, and The Ohio State University, Columbus, Ohio, USA.

Design.—Computational modeling study.

Methods.—A finite-element anisotropic collagen fiber-dependent model of myopic surgery using patient-specific corneal geometry was constructed for LASIK, small-incision lenticule extraction, and a geometry analog model with unaltered material properties from preoperative but with postoperative geometry including thickness. Surgical parameters, magnitude of myopic correction, LASIK flap thickness, and lenticule depth in small-incision lenticule extraction were varied. Two sets of models, 1 with uniform and 1 with depth-dependent material properties, were constructed.

Results.—Stress distribution between small-incision lenticule extraction simulations and the geometry analog model were similar. In contrast, LASIK consistently reduced stress in the flap and increased stress in the residual stromal bed (RSB) compared with the geometry analog model. An increase in flap thickness or lenticule depth resulted in a greater increase in RSB stress in the LASIK model than in the small-incision lenticule extraction model.

Conclusions.—Small-incision lenticule extraction may present less biomechanical risk to the residual bed of susceptible corneas than comparable corrections involving LASIK flaps. Deeper corrections in the stroma may be possible in small-incision lenticule extraction without added risk for ectasia.

▶ I am not going to even try to pretend that I understood many, if any, of the mathematical formulas in this article. I'm just happy knowing that people much smarter than I am believe that mathematical models are useful predictors of corneal "strength," to use a colloquial term. It makes sense to me that laser-assisted in situ keratomileusis (LASIK), which incises approximately 11 o'clock hours of anterior stroma, would weaken or destabilize the cornea more than small-incision lenticule extraction (SMILE), which only incises approximately 1 to 2 o'clock hours of anterior stroma. I understand that this is a mathematical simulation, but if it turns out to be true, it may be worth considering SMILE over LASIK, especially in eyes with slightly suspicious corneal topographies or where residual stromal bed thickness may be an issue.

C. J. Rapuano, MD

Visual quality comparison of conventional and Hole-Visian implantable collamer lens at different degrees of decentering

Pérez-Vives C, Ferrer-Blasco T, Madrid-Costa D, et al (Univ of Valencia, Spain)

Br J Ophthalmol 98:59-64, 2014

Purpose.—To compare the visual quality of implantable collamer lens (ICL) with and without central hole (Hole ICL and conventional ICL) at different degrees of decentering.

Methods.—An adaptive optics visual simulator (crx1, Imagine Eyes, Orsay, France) was used to simulate the −3, −6 and −12 dioptres (D) conventional and Hole ICLs in three conditions: centred and decentred 0.3 and 0.6 mm. Visual acuity (VA) at high-contrast, medium-contrast and low-contrast and contrast sensitivity (CS) were measured in 15 observers for 3 and 4.5 mm pupils.

Results.—No statistically significant differences in VA and CS were found between conventional and Hole ICLs for any ICL powers and pupil sizes evaluated ($p > 0.05$). Regarding the effect of the ICL decentration on visual performance, we did not find statistically significant differences in VA and CS between centred, 0.3 and 0.6 mm decentred ($p > 0.05$).

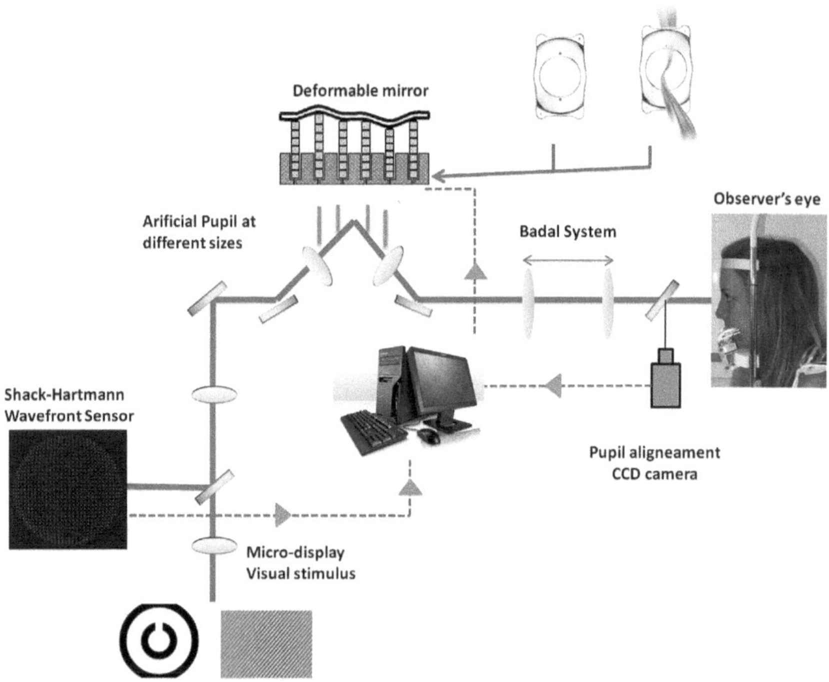

FIGURE 1.—Schematic diagram of the crx1 system (imagine eyes, Orsay, France) used to measure and correct the eye's aberrations. It compromises two basic elements: the Shack–Hartmann wavefront sensor and the correcting device (deformable mirror) conjugated to the pupil plane. The visual test generated on a microdisplay was viewed through the deformable mirror and an artificial pupil. Access the article online to view this figure in colour. (Reprinted from Pérez-Vives C, Ferrer-Blasco T, Madrid-Costa D, et al. Visual quality comparison of conventional and Hole-Visian implantable collamer lens at different degrees of decentering. *Br J Ophthalmol.* 2014;98:59-64.)

Moreover, the ICL decentration affected the same manner on the conventional and Hole ICLs.

Conclusions.—The outcomes showed that conventional and Hole ICLs provided good and comparable visual performance for all powers and pupil sizes evaluated. Besides, ICL decentering affects the same manner both ICL models evaluated. The ICL decentering did not have any effect on the visual performance (Fig 1).

▶ Putting a hole in the middle of a phakic intraocular lens should diminish pupillary block (assuming the hole remains patent) and would consequently eliminate the need for peripheral iridotomies (which have their own complications). Sounds great, but at what (visual) cost? Reports by Shimizu et al in 2012 demonstrated good results with such a lens in a small number of patients.[1,2]

This study used an adaptive optics visual simulator to evaluate the Visian ICL with and without holes at different degrees of decentration and pupil size (Fig 1). They found essentially identical results with the 2 lenses. The authors do acknowledge that surgical effects (eg, induced cylinder), intraocular lens tilt, and other postoperative complications are not taken into account and may affect the results. Assuming such a visual simulator really does mimic real life, this technology should offer a wonderful manner to test new lenses before implantation in patients' eyes.

C. J. Rapuano, MD

References

1. Shimizu K, Kamiya K, Igarashi A, Shiratani T. Early clinical outcomes of implantation of posterior chamber phakic intraocular lens with a central hole (hole ICL) for moderate to high myopia. *Br J Ophthalmol.* 2012;96:409-412.
2. Shimizu K, Kamiya K, Igarashi A, Shiratani T. Intraindividual comparison of visual performance after posterior chamber phakic intraocular lens with and without a central hole implantation for moderate to high myopia. *Am J Ophthalmol.* 2012;154:486-494.

Comparative Study of 2 Types of Implantable Collamer Lenses, 1 With and 1 Without a Central Artificial Hole

Huseynova T, Ozaki S, Ishizuka T, et al (Shinagawa LASIK Ctr, Tokyo, Japan)
Am J Ophthalmol 157:1136-1143, 2014

Purpose.—To compare the outcomes between implantable collamer lenses (ICLs), 1 with and 1 without a central artificial hole.

Design.—Comparative study.

Methods.—We included 65 eyes of 65 patients with refractive error in our study. The mean manifest refraction spherical equivalent (MRSE) was -9.32 ± 4.02 diopters (range, 6.75 to -16.50 diopters). We divided patients into 2 groups based on the type of ICL used, 1 for those without a central artificial hole (Group I, 21 eyes) and 1 for those with a hole (Group II, 44 eyes). The postoperative changes in visual acuity, endothelial cell density, MRSE, higher order aberrations readings, and objective scatter index between the 2 kinds of ICLs were compared. The follow-up period was 3 months.

Results.—There were no statistically significant differences in the postoperative changes in uncorrected distance visual acuity ($P = 0.81$), corrected distance visual acuity ($P = 0.24$), MRSE ($P = 0.18$), and endothelial cell density ($P = 0.76$) between the groups. Also, no difference in objective scatter index was found at 3 months ($P = 0.32$). None of the higher order aberrations readings showed any significant difference between the groups.

Conclusion.—There were no significant differences between the outcomes of these ICLs, either with or without a central artificial hole (Fig 6, Tables 1 and 4).

▶ The implantable collamer lens (ICL) is a phakic posterior-chamber intraocular lens. As noted in the previous comment, there are advantages of placing a hole in the middle of this lens, most notably avoiding the need for a peripheral iridotomy.

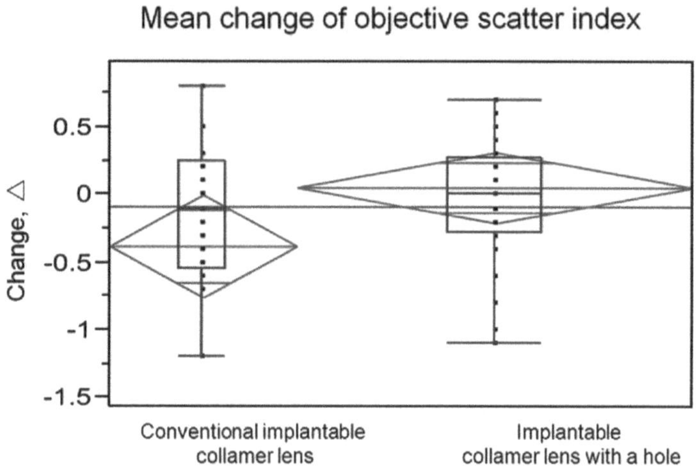

FIGURE 6.—Mean postoperative change of objective scatter index for each group by boxplot. (Reprinted from American Journal of Ophthalmology. Huseynova T, Ozaki S, Ishizuka T, et al. Comparative study of 2 types of implantable collamer lenses, 1 with and 1 without a central artificial hole. *Am J Ophthalmol.* 2014;157:1136-1143, Copyright 2014, with permission from Elsevier.)

TABLE 1.—Preoperative and 3 Months Postoperative Patient Demographics in Eyes Undergoing Implantable Collamer Lens with and Without Central Artificial Hole Implantation

	Groups		
Demographic	Group I (Conventional ICL)	Group II (Hole ICL)	*P* Value
n	21	44	
Age, years	35 ± 5.6 (27 to 44)	35 ± 9.4 (18 to 55)	
MRSE, D			
Preop	−9.51 ± 4.65 (6.75 to −17.00)	−10.05 ± 2.72 (−2.75 to−16.38)	
3 M	1.50 ± 0.20 (0.75 to 1.75)	0.19 ± 0.40 (1.13 to −0.75)	
Δ	11.01 ± 4.80*	10.24 ± 2.76*	0.18
OSI			
Preop	1.24 ± 1.21 (0.30 to 5.30)	1.03 ± 0.66 (0.30 to 3.60)	
3 M	0.86 ± 0.52 (0.20 to 2.10)	1.08 ± 0.80 (0.30 to 3.50)	
Δ	−0.38 ± 1.11	0.05 ± 0.70	0.32
ECD			
Preop	2812 ± 248 (2114 to 3135)	2879 ± 343 (1859 to 3472)	
3 M	2812 ± 303 (2183 to 3344)	2911 ± 318 (2165 to 3497)	
Δ	12.00 ± 253.92	32.35 ± 242.19	0.76
UDVA (logMAR)			
Preop	1.46 ± 0.27 (0.52 to 2.00)	1.49 ± 0.21 (2.00 to 0.01)	
3 M	−0.13 ± 0.10 (0.15 to −0.18)	−0.13 ± 0.08 (0.10 to −0.30)	
Δ	1.32 ± 0.28*	1.35 ± 0.23*	0.82
CDVA (logMAR)			
Preop	−0.12 ± 0.09 (0.15 to −0.18)	−0.12 ± 0.08 (0.22 to −0.18)	
3 M	−0.16 ± 0.07 (0.15 to −0.18)	−0.18 ± 0.04 (−0.30 to −0.08)	
Δ	0.10 ± 0.16*	0.18 ± 0.22*	0.24

CDVA = corrected distance visual acuity; Δ = change; ECD = endothelial cell density; ICL = implantable collamer lens; logMAR = logarithm of the minimal angle of resolution; MRSE = manifest refraction spherical equivalent; n = number of eyes; OSI = objective scatter index; UDVA = uncorrected distance visual acuity.

*Statistical significance of the improvement.

Reprinted from American Journal of Ophthalmology. Huseynova T, Ozaki S, Ishizuka T, et al. Comparative study of 2 types of implantable collamer lenses, 1 with and 1 without a central artificial hole. *Am J Ophthalmol.* 2014;157:1136-1143, Copyright 2014, with permission from Elsevier.

TABLE 4.—Mean Change in Preoperative and 3-Month Postoperative Corneal and Ocular Aberrations for the Implantable Collamer Lens with and Without Central Artificial Hole Implantation

	Groups		
Aberrations	Group I (Conventional ICL)	Group II (Hole ICL)	*P* value
Corneal Aberrations			
4 mm			
ΔS3	0.02	0.02	0.47
ΔS4	0.00	0.02	0.23
ΔTotal	0.02	0.02	0.63
6 mm			
ΔS3	0.09	0.09	0.74
ΔS4	0.01	0.02	0.23
ΔTotal	0.08	0.09	0.78
Ocular aberrations			
4 mm			
ΔS3	0.05	0.13	0.62
ΔS4	0.02	0.06	0.23
ΔTotal	0.05	0.15	0.48
6 mm			
ΔS3	0.18	0.46	0.75
ΔS4	0.16	0.42	0.53
ΔTotal	0.29	0.73	0.68

Δ = change; ICL = implantable collamer lens; RMS = root mean square; S3 = 3rd component of root mean square (coma-like aberration); S4 = 4th component of root mean square (spherical-like aberration).

Reprinted from American Journal of Ophthalmology. Huseynova T, Ozaki S, Ishizuka T, et al. Comparative study of 2 types of implantable collamer lenses, 1 with and 1 without a central artificial hole. *Am J Ophthalmol.* 2014;157:1136-1143, Copyright 2014, with permission from Elsevier.

But at what cost? The previous article[1] found no difference in theoretical results between the ICL with and without a central hole using an adaptive optics visual simulator. In this article, Huseynova et al performed a retrospective clinical study comparing the ICL without a hole to the ICL with a 0.36-mm central hole, looking specifically at higher order aberrations and light scatter.

They found essentially identical results in manifest refraction spherical equivalent, uncorrected distance vision, best corrected distance vision, and endothelial cell density at the 3-month postoperative visit (Table 1). Although the differences were not statistically significant between the 2 lens types, there were more induced ocular aberrations in the ICL with a hole than without a hole for a 4-mm pupil and 6-mm pupil size at 3 months (Table 4). Also, although not statistically significant, there was more light scatter in the ICL with a hole than without a hole (Fig 6). Although I can certainly imagine that a small 0.36-mm hole could clog, there were no episodes of pupillary block in this series (or any reported series that I know of looking at this lens with a central hole).

Although this study is small, it seems to validate that although there may be a slight increase in objective light scatter and ocular aberrations with the addition of a hole in the ICL, they appear to be small and, as per the authors, "had negligible clinical effects." If the holes do in fact stay patent, holes in this lens design may well be worth the trade-off.

C. J. Rapuano, MD

Reference

1. Perez-Vives C, Ferrer-Blasco T, Madrid-Costa D, et al. Visual quality comparison of conventional and Hole-Visian implantable collamer lens at different degrees of decentering. *Br J Ophthalmol.* 2014;98:59-64.

Orthokeratology-Associated Infectious Keratitis in a Tertiary Care Eye Hospital in Hong Kong

Chan TCY, Li EYM, Wong VWY, et al (Hong Kong Eye Hosp, Hong Kong SAR, China; The Chinese Univ of Hong Kong, Hong Kong SAR, China)

Am J Ophthalmol 158:1130-1135, 2014

Purpose.—To analyze cases of orthokeratology-associated infectious keratitis managed in a tertiary care eye hospital in Hong Kong between 2003 and 2013.

Design.—Retrospective study.

Methods.—Case records of patients with infectious keratitis attributable to orthokeratology contact lenses were analyzed. Data analyzed included clinical features, microbiological evaluation, and treatment outcomes.

Results.—A total of 23 patients were included (16 female, 7 male, mean age: 15.0 ± 4.2 years; range: 9—23 years). All patients were using overnight orthokeratology for an average of 2.7 ± 2.8 years (range: 3 months - 10 years) before the onset of infection. Clinical features included corneal infiltrate (n = 14, 60.9%) and corneal perineuritis (n = 12, 52.2%). Fifteen eyes (65.2%) had a positive microbiological culture obtained from corneal scrapings. The most commonly isolated organism was *Pseudomonas aeruginosa* (n = 6), followed by coagulase-negative *Staphylococcus* (n = 5) and *Acanthamoeba* (n = 3). Five cases of *Pseudomonas aeruginosa* and 5 cases of *Acanthamoeba* were identified from contact lenses or contact lens solution. The mean duration from disease onset to remission was 31.9 ± 34.9 days (range: 6—131 days). All patients responded to medical treatment, and no emergency surgical intervention was needed. The best-corrected logMAR visual acuity improved significantly from 0.62 ± 0.51 (20/83 Snellen) to 0.15 ± 0.20 (20/28 Snellen) (Wilcoxon signed rank test, $P < .001$).

Conclusions.—Orthokeratology-associated infectious keratitis continues to be a serious problem, especially in regions with high prevalence of myopia. Early clinical and microbiological diagnosis and intensive treatment can improve final visual outcomes (Table 1).

▶ The fact that orthokeratology lenses (or contact lens wear in general) can cause infectious keratitis is not new. That orthokeratology lens use is concentrated more in children and young adults compared with overall contact lens use may make related corneal infections seem more tragic. This article struck home for me as I have recently cared for 2 children with orthokeratology lens-related corneal ulcers.

TABLE 1.—Year-Wise Trend for Orthokeratology-Related Cases With Keratitis in Comparison to Contact Lens—Related Keratitis Cases and Overall Keratitis Cases Admitted to Hong Kong Eye Hospital Between 2003 and 2013

Year	2003	2004	2005	2006	2007	2008	2009	2010	2011	2012	2013	Total
OrthoK keratitis (cases)	2	3	1	1	1	3	1	1	1	4	5	23
CL keratitis (cases)	6	11	18	20	10	7	5	10	10	9	15	121
Overall keratitis (cases)	37	33	46	62	32	24	22	33	37	39	28	393
Proportion of OrthoK keratitis in CL keratitis (%)	33.3	27.3	5.6	5.0	10.0	42.9	20.0	10.0	10.0	44.4	33.3	19.0
Proportion of OrthoK keratitis in total microbial keratitis (%)	5.4	9.1	2.2	1.6	3.1	12.5	4.5	3.0	2.7	10.3	17.9	5.9
OrthoK *Acanthamoeba* (cases)	0	2	0	1	1	2	0	0	0	3	3	12
CL *Acanthamoeba* (cases)	2	3	5	5	3	5	2	1	0	4	2	32

CL = contact lens—associated; OrthoK = orthokeratology-associated.

Reprinted from American Journal of Ophthalmology. Chan TCY, Li EYM, Wong VWY, et al. Orthokeratology-Associated Infectious Keratitis in a Tertiary Care Eye Hospital in Hong Kong. *Am J Ophthalmol*. 2014;158:1130-1135, Copyright 2014, with permission from Elsevier.

The authors found that *Pseudomonas* and acanthamoeba were the 2 most commonly involved organisms in their patients (Table 1). *Pseudomonas* should not surprise anyone because it is the most common organism associated with soft contact lens-related corneal ulcers. Acanthamoeba, on the other hand, is an uncommon cause of infectious keratitis. Having said that, contact lens use (that is, soft contact lens use, not rigid contact lens use, which is what orthokeratology lenses are) is by far the most common risk factor for acanthamoeba keratitis. I did find it interesting that these authors did not report any cases of fungal keratitis in this series.

Most of the published case series of orthokeratology lens-related corneal ulcers have been from East Asia. That is probably because of the greater use of orthokeratology lenses in that part of the world due to the high prevalence of myopia. Recent studies from Hong Kong and Taiwan showed that 19% to 40% of cases of infectious keratitis in children were related to orthokeratology lenses.[1,2]

The authors recommend that eye care practitioners fully explain the risks of orthokeratology lenses to patients and parents, stressing the early signs and symptoms of infectious keratitis so patients can see an eye doctor promptly when infection is suspected. In Hong Kong, as in the United States, most orthokeratology prescribers are optometrists, whereas those managing most significant cases of infectious keratitis are ophthalmologists. My 2 patients with orthokeratology lens-related infections were fit by optometrists. According to their parents, they were not informed of the increased risk of infection from these lenses compared with other contact lenses or glasses. Both of my patients are currently doing well. One had acanthamoeba keratitis that eventually responded to medical treatment. The other had a fungal keratitis that perforated and required a penetrating graft. Fortunately, there has been no recurrence of fungal keratitis, and the patient's vision has become quite good. Needless to say, that is not always the case with corneal ulcers.

C. J. Rapuano, MD

References

1. Young AL, Leung KS, Tsim N, Hui M, Jhanji V. Risk factors, microbiological profile, and treatment outcomes of pediatric microbial keratitis in a tertiary care hospital in Hong Kong. *Am J Ophthalmol.* 2013;156:1040-1044.
2. Lee YS, Tan HY, Yeh LK, et al. Pediatric microbial keratitis in Taiwan: clinical and microbiological profiles, 1998-2002 versus 2008-2012. *Am J Ophthalmol.* 2014; 157:1090-1096.

3 Cornea

A Comparison of Lamellar and Penetrating Keratoplasty Outcomes: A Registry Study

Coster DJ, for the Australian Corneal Graft Registry Contributors (Flinders Univ, Adelaide, Australia)

Ophthalmology 121:979-987, 2014

Objectives.—To investigate changing patterns of practice of keratoplasty in Australia, graft survival, visual outcomes, the influence of experience, and the surgeon learning curve for endothelial keratoplasty.

Design.—Observational, prospective cohort study.

Participants.—From a long-standing national corneal transplantation register, 13 920 penetrating keratoplasties, 858 deep anterior lamellar keratoplasties (DALKs), and 2287 endokeratoplasties performed between January 1996 and February 2013 were identified.

Methods.—Kaplan-Meier functions were used to assess graft survival and surgeon experience, the Pearson chi-square test was used to compare visual acuities, and linear regression was used to examine learning curves.

Main Outcome Measures.—Graft survival.

Results.—The total number of corneal grafts performed annually is increasing steadily. More DALKs but fewer penetrating grafts are being performed for keratoconus, and more endokeratoplasties but fewer penetrating grafts are being performed for Fuchs' dystrophy and pseudophakic bullous keratopathy. In 2012, 1482 grafts were performed, compared with 955 in 2002, translating to a requirement for 264 extra corneal donors across the country in 2012. Comparing penetrating grafts and DALKs performed for keratoconus over the same era, both graft survival ($P < 0.001$) and visual outcomes ($P < 0.001$) were significantly better for penetrating grafts. Survival of endokeratoplasties performed for Fuchs' dystrophy or pseudophakic bullous keratopathy was poorer than survival of penetrating grafts for the same indications over the same era ($P < 0.001$). Visual outcomes were significantly better for penetrating grafts than for endokeratoplasties performed for Fuchs' dystrophy ($P < 0.001$), but endokeratoplasties achieved better visual outcomes than penetrating grafts for pseudophakic bullous keratopathy ($P < 0.001$). Experienced surgeons (>100 registered keratoplasties) achieved significantly better survival of endokeratoplasties ($P < 0.001$) than surgeons who had performed fewer grafts (<100 registered keratoplasties). In the hands of experienced, high-volume surgeons, endokeratoplasty failures occurred even after 100 grafts had been performed.

Conclusions.—More corneal transplants, especially DALKs and endokeratoplasties, are being performed in Australia than ever before. Survival of DALKs and endokeratoplasties is worse than the survival of penetrating grafts performed for the same indications over the same timeframe. Many endokeratoplasties fail early, but the evidence for a surgeon learning curve is unconvincing.

▶ Over the past 2 decades, corneal transplantation has evolved from penetrating keratoplasty (PK) to various forms of anterior and posterior lamellar keratoplasties. This important registry study presented some surprising outcomes in graft survival and vision of keratoplasties performed in Australia from 1996 to 2013.

Although the number of keratoplasties was stable over the first 10 years in the study, an increase in number of grafts performed annually was noted. Furthermore, changes in practice patterns were noted, such as an increase in deep anterior lamellar keratoplasty (DALK) with fewer PKs for keratoconus and an increase in endokeratoplasties (EK) with fewer PKs for endothelial disease.

The main outcome measure of this study was graft survival, in which unexpected results were found. DALK survival was noted to be worse than PK for keratoconus. No difference in the survival between DALK and PK was noted in nonkeratoconus eyes. Survival of endothelial grafts was worse than PK performed for the same indication over the same period of time.

Visual outcomes were also surprising. Patients who underwent PK had better visual outcomes than those who underwent DALK. In addition, PK was associated with better vision than endothelial keratoplasty for Fuchs' dystrophy, whereas endothelial keratoplasty patients had better visual outcomes than PK for pseudophakic bullous keratopathy.

The authors also evaluated surgeon experience and surgeon learning curves in assessing visual outcomes in endokeratoplasties. Surgeons who performed more than 100 endokeratoplasties had improved graft survival compared with those surgeons who performed fewer than 100 endothelial keratoplasties. Despite improved results, endothelial graft failure was still noted among the more experienced surgeons.

This large study, comprised of more than 17 000 corneal grafts, strongly supports the role of PK when evaluating both visual and graft survival outcomes, even when compared with DALK for keratoconus and EK for Fuchs' dystrophy. Although my experience with DALK and visual outcomes mirror the results of this study, patients undergoing endothelial keratoplasty (specifically Descemet's stripping automated endothelial keratoplasty) for Fuchs' dystrophy do seem to have improved visual outcomes in our practice. Although final visual acuity may be similar, EK patients do have faster visual results with better refractive outcomes, 2 measures that were not evaluated in this study. Furthermore, contrary to the results of this study, there have been other smaller, single-center studies suggesting graft survival was better in EK compared with PK. The authors recognize the difference between small, single-center studies and their broader approach including all corneal surgeons in Australia and the effect this may have on their outcomes.

In conclusion, this is a noteworthy study, based on its high number of corneal grafts, as well as its thought-provoking results. In Australia, despite newer advances in corneal transplantation, penetrating keratoplasty remains superior at this time.

P. K. Nagra, MD

Endophthalmitis After Penetrating Keratoplasty

Chen JY, NHSBT Ocular Tissue Advisory Group and Contributing Ophthalmologists (OTAG Audit Study 18) (Royal Liverpool Univ Hosp, UK; et al)

Ophthalmology 122:25-30, 2015

Purpose.—To determine the incidence of endophthalmitis after penetrating keratoplasty (PK) and patient and donor risk factors.

Design.—Retrospective cohort study using national transplant registry data.

Participants.—All corneal transplant recipients (n = 11 320) registered on the United Kingdom Transplant Registry undergoing their first PK between April 1999 and December 2006.

Methods.—Patients who developed endophthalmitis were identified on the transplant registry. In addition, cases where the fellow cornea from the same donor had been transplanted were included. Clinical information regarding donor and recipient characteristics, surgical details, and postoperative outcomes were collected and analyzed. In cases where endophthalmitis was reported, the diagnosis was verified by a follow-up supplementary questionnaire to the surgeon. Logistic regression was used to investigate differences in the factors associated with the development of endophthalmitis.

Main Outcome Measures.—Incidence of endophthalmitis and graft survival.

Results.—The overall incidence of endophthalmitis occurring after primary PK in the UK was 0.67%. The incidence of endophthalmitis occurring within 6 weeks of surgery was 0.16%. Graft survival after endophthalmitis was 27% (95% confidence interval, 16–38) at 5 years, with a mean best-corrected visual acuity of 1.13 (logarithm of the minimum angle of resolution) for surviving grafts. Factors associated with endophthalmitis were donor cause of death (infection), high-risk cases, and indication for corneal transplantation.

Conclusion.—Endophthalmitis remains a serious issue, with those affected having reduced graft survival and poor visual outcomes. Management of the identified recipient and donor risk factors are important to reduce endophthalmitis risk. In particular, the increased incidence of endophthalmitis when the donor dies of infection requires further explanation and review of current donor eye retrieval and eye bank practices. The delayed presentation of endophthalmitis cases also raises questions regarding possible sequestration of microbes within the corneal tissue and the effect of antimicrobials in storage media.

▶ Endophthalmitis after intraocular surgery remains one of the most concerning postoperative complications, often associated with poor vision and outcome. The authors of this article reviewed the results of 7.5 years of data from the UK national transplant registry to determine the incidence as well as evaluate risk factors for endophthalmitis after penetrating keratoplasty.

An incidence of 0.67% was found, with a much smaller incidence of 0.16% for acute endophthalmitis, occurring in the first 6 weeks after surgery. The rate of endophthalmitis in the fellow donor cornea was 0%, although of 14 fellow donor corneas that were not used, 5 corneas (7%) had antimicrobial growth during organ culture. Risk factors associated with increased endophthalmitis rates were not using a disinfectant at the time of retrieval by the eye bank (which is routinely performed in the United States), increased death to preservation time (mean time in the United Kingdom is 34 hours, compared with 9.25 hours in the United States), and a history of septicemia in the donor (active sepsis at time of death is a contraindication to corneal donation in the United States). Recipient risk factors noted to be associated with increased risk of endophthalmitis included "high-risk" grafts for indications such as infection, injury or ulcerative keratitis, or history of previous ocular surgery, as well as therapeutic corneal transplants.

Because of differences in corneal tissue procurement in the United States compared with the United Kingdom, the donor risks noted in this study may not be relevant to our patients. The recipient risk factors, on the other hand, are more applicable to our patient population. As the authors suggest, the postoperative management of patients undergoing high-risk or therapeutic corneal transplants may warrant "surgeons to be extra vigilant" given the increased risk (compared with low-risk grafts) of endophthalmitis.

P. K. Nagra, MD

Therapeutic and Optical Keratoplasty in the Management of *Acanthamoeba* Keratitis: Risk Factors, Outcomes, and Summary of the Literature

Robaei D, Carnt N, Minassian DC, et al (Moorfields Eye Hosp NHS Foundation Trust, London, UK; EpiVision Ophthalmic Epidemiology Consultants, Bucks, UK)
Ophthalmology 122:17-24, 2015

Objective.—To report the risk factors for and outcomes of therapeutic and optical keratoplasty in the management of *Acanthamoeba* keratitis (AK).

Design.—Retrospective case series.

Participants.—A total of 50 eyes of 196 patients with retrievable medical records, diagnosed with AK at Moorfields Eye Hospital, London, underwent keratoplasty between January 1991 and April 2012.

Methods.—Patient demographics, initial clinical examination findings, and management details were collected. The ophthalmic characteristics of patients who underwent keratoplasty for AK were compared with those who did not. Patients undergoing therapeutic keratoplasty were compared with those undergoing optical keratoplasty for baseline characteristics, management details, and visual outcomes. A multivariate logistic model was used to derive the odds ratios of a poor visual outcome in all keratoplasty patients.

Main Outcome Measures.—Poor visual outcome was defined as final visual acuity of 20/200 or worse. Secondary outcomes of interest included number of clinic visits and the need for additional intraocular surgery.

Results.—Of the 196 AK patients, a total of 50 patients (25.5%) underwent penetrating or anterior lamellar keratoplasty, 10 of whom (20%) underwent repeat procedures. Of these 50 patients, 26 (52%) had therapeutic keratoplasty, predominantly for corneal perforation. The remaining 24 patients (48%) underwent optical keratoplasty for visual rehabilitation. Thirty-seven (80.4%) patients in the keratoplasty group initially were misdiagnosed as having herpes simplex keratitis versus 59 (41.8%) patients who did not require a keratoplasty ($P < 0.001$). Final visual outcomes were significantly better in the optical group compared with the therapeutic group, with 13 (54.2%) achieving visual acuity of 20/30 or better versus 7 (26.9%), respectively. On multivariate analysis, beginning therapy at a hospital other than Moorfields and undergoing a therapeutic, rather than an optical, keratoplasty were associated significantly with a poor visual outcome from keratoplasty.

Conclusions.—The prognosis of keratoplasty differs markedly when performed for therapeutic purposes compared with visual rehabilitation. Where possible, keratoplasty should be delayed until such time as the eye is uninflamed and medically cured of *Acanthamoeba.*

▶ *Acanthamoeba* keratitis (AK) remains one of the more challenging forms of infectious keratitis both to diagnose and treat. Although the rate of this condition has increased over the past decade, it remains uncommon. Several smaller case series have been published, but there are few larger case series in the literature.

The authors of this retrospective review evaluated the risk factors and outcomes for corneal grafts for AK, comparing therapeutic versus optical grafts. Of 196 patients diagnosed at their institution with AK over a 21-year time span, 50 patients went on to have corneal grafts. Of these 50 grafts, 26 patients had therapeutic keratoplasties (TKP), whereas 24 patients underwent optical keratoplasties (OKP). Compared with patients who were treated medically alone, patients who had corneal grafts had a longer delay to treatment (following onset of symptoms) and were more likely to be misdiagnosed as herpes simplex keratitis.

Visually acuity outcomes were much better in the OKP group, with 54.2% of these patients achieving 20/30 or better vision, compared with 26.9% of the TKP group. Conversely, almost 20% of patients undergoing TKP had no light perception vision at their last follow-up. Three patients in the OKP group required more than 1 keratoplasties, compared with 7 patients in the TKP group (1 of these was due to disease recurrence in TKP).

Based on these results, the authors recommend delaying corneal transplantation when possible. Waiting until after completion of antiamebic therapy, when the corneas are stable and uninflamed, before consideration for surgery may lead to the best results. Our approach has been to wait longer than the 1 month the authors describe after discontinuation of antiamebic therapy, typically at least 6 months before consideration for OKP. Unfortunately, corneal perforation for failure of treatment in AK does occur, necessitating the need for TKP. Based on the results of this study, we can counsel patients on the possible poor visual outcomes with possible need for additional surgery following TKP.

P. K. Nagra, MD

Pneumodescemetopexy with perfluoroethane (C_2F_6) for the treatment of acute hydrops secondary to keratoconus

Ting DSJ, Srinivasan S (Univ Hosp Ayr, Scotland, UK; Univ of Glasgow, Scotland, UK)

Eye 28:847-851, 2014

Purpose.—To evaluate the efficacy and safety of pneumodescemetopexy with intracameral perfluoroethane (C_2F_6) gas for the treatment of acute hydrops secondary to keratoconus.

Methods.—Retrospective, non-comparative, interventional case series. Eight eyes of eight patients who presented with acute hydrops secondary to keratoconus between July 2009 and September 2013 were consecutively recruited. All were treated with intracameral 14% isoexpansile concentration of C_2F_6. Preoperative and postoperative best-corrected visual acuities (BCVA), intraoperative and postoperative complications, and time taken for resolution of corneal oedema were assessed.

Results.—All the patients, except for one, were followed up for 1 year. The mean age of the cohort was 29.1 ± 13.5 years. BCVA at presentation was 6/60 or less in all patients. Improvement of BCVA was achieved postoperatively in seven (87.5%) patients, with three (37.5%) patients achieving a BCVA of 6/18. The average time between initial presentation and complete resolution of corneal oedema was 60.0 ± 32.1 days. The C_2F_6 gas persisted in the anterior chamber between 6 and 8 days. All the patients required only one injection during the treatment period. There was no intraoperative or postoperative complication noted during the follow-up period.

Conclusion.—Pneumodescemetopexy with intracameral isoexpansile concentration of C_2F_6 gas serves as a safe and effective treatment modality for patients with acute hydrops secondary to keratoconus.

▶ Corneal hydrops can lead to sudden, marked decline in visual acuity with pain and photophobia. Hydrops is most commonly seen in young patients with keratoconus, can take months to heal, and often leads to a significant corneal scar and need for corneal transplantation. As Fan Gaskin et al elucidate in their article on hydrops, this condition is associated with significant morbidity. They detail conventional treatments (hypertonic solution, topical steroids) as well as newer surgical options (injections of air of gas) but note evidence supporting these treatments is limited.[1]

The authors of the current article present a small, retrospective case series of 8 patients with hydrops who were successfully treated with C_2F_6 injection. C_2F_6 was chosen as a longer acting gas than SF_6, but shorter than C_3F_8. C_3F_8 was avoided because of complications associated with it, specifically pupillary block and cataract formation. All 8 patients in this study were treated within 1 week of presentation, the gas lasted for 6 to 8 days, and no patients developed elevated intraocular pressure. The edema resolved on average of 60 days, and 7 of the 8 patients had a documented improvement in vision. The 1 patient who had no improvement in visual acuity had a history of poor vision due to Leber congenital amaurosis.

Although this is a small, retrospective case series and therefore associated with inherent limitations, it does suggest that there may be a benefit of gas injection to hasten the resolution of hydrops. The gas was well tolerated without any complication, but it does seem reasonable to perform laser or surgical peripheral iridectomies on all patients to prevent pupillary block and acute angle closure glaucoma, a potentially devastating complication. Although smaller case series like this are a start, further prospective studies evaluating the benefit of gas injection compared to conservative treatment in improving visual acuity, hastening resolution, and altering the need for corneal transplantation are warranted.

P. K. Nagra, MD

Reference

1. Fan Gaskin JC, Patel DV, McGhee CHJ. Acute corneal hydrops in keratoconus-new perspectives. *Am J Ophthalmol.* 2014;157:921-928.

Aganirsen Antisense Oligonucleotide Eye Drops Inhibit Keratitis-Induced Corneal Neovascularization and Reduce Need for Transplantation: The I-CAN Study

Cursiefen C, Viaud E, Bock F, et al (Univ of Cologne, Germany; Gene Signal International SA, Boulogne-Billancourt, France; et al)

Ophthalmology 121:1683-1692, 2014

Objective.—Eye drops of aganirsen, an antisense oligonucleotide preventing insulin receptor substrate-1 expression, inhibited corneal neovascularization in a previous dose-finding phase II study. We aimed to confirm these results in a phase III study and investigated a potential clinical benefit on visual acuity (VA), quality of life (QoL), and need for transplantation.

Design.—Multicenter, double-masked, randomized, placebo-controlled phase III study.

Participants.—Analysis of 69 patients with keratitis-related progressive corneal neovascularization randomized to aganirsen (34 patients) or placebo (35 patients). Patients applied aganirsen eye drops (86 mg/day/eye) or placebo twice daily for 90 days and were followed up to day 180.

Main Outcome Measures.—The primary end point was VA. Secondary end points included area of pathologic corneal neovascularization, need for transplantation, risk of graft rejection, and QoL.

Results.—Although no significant differences in VA scores between groups were observed, aganirsen significantly reduced the relative corneal neovascularization area after 90 days by 26.20% ($P = 0.014$). This improvement persisted after 180 days (26.67%, $P = 0.012$). Aganirsen tended to lower the transplantation need in the intent-to-treat (ITT) population at day 180 ($P = 0.087$). In patients with viral keratitis and central neovascularization, a significant reduction in transplantation need was achieved ($P = 0.048$). No significant differences between groups were observed in the risk of graft rejection. However, aganirsen tended to decrease this risk in patients with traumatic/viral keratitis ($P = 0.162$) at day 90. The QoL analyses revealed a significant improvement with aganirsen in composite and near activity subscores ($P = 0.039$ and 0.026, respectively) at day 90 in the per protocol population. Ocular and treatment-related treatment-emergent adverse events (TEAEs) were reported in a lower percentage with aganirsen compared with placebo. Only 3 serious TEAEs (2 with aganirsen and 1 with placebo) were considered treatment-related.

Conclusions.—This first phase III study on a topical inhibitor of corneal angiogenesis showed that aganirsen eye drops significantly inhibited corneal neovascularization in patients with keratitis. The need for transplantation was significantly reduced in patients with viral keratitis and central neovascularization. Topical application of aganirsen was safe and well tolerated.

▶ Aganirsen is a promising antiangiogenic treatment, shown in Phase IIB trials in Europe to decrease corneal neovascularization compared with placebo. This current study detailed the phase III trial, a multicentered, double-masked, randomized, placebo-controlled study evaluating the effect of topical aganirsen taken twice daily for 90 days on corneal neovascularization (NV). The primary end point was visual acuity, with secondary end points, including area of corneal NV, need for transplantation, risk of graft rejection, and quality of life.

There was no statistically significant effect on vision by aganirsen compared with placebo. Aganirsen statistically significantly reduced the relative area of corneal NV by 26.2%, and there was a trend toward decreasing the expected need for corneal transplantation, although this was not significant. Subset analysis suggested a significant decrease in the expected need for transplant when evaluating patients with viral keratitis and corneal NV, although the authors admit that the sample size was small. In addition, there was no significant decrease in the expected risk for graft rejection. Quality-of-life analysis did show a significant improvement in composite scores and near vision subscores at 90 days.

The authors commented that the use of visual acuity as the primary end point may not be appropriate when considering corneal NV. Unlike retinal and especially macular pathology in which pathology often directly affects visual acuity, corneal NV starts peripherally and therefore may not have such a significant effect on visual acuity. Furthermore, corneal NV may be associated with edema, scarring, and lipid deposition, all of which we would not expect to respond to antiangiogenic treatment alone. The most encouraging results are the decrease in relative area of corneal NV. As the authors point out, this novel class of medication may have a role in addition to conventional treatments for certain conditions, such as viral keratitis. The authors term this concept "primary prevention" in that by using both antiangiogenic and antiviral therapy, the need for cornea transplantation may be decreased.

Aganirsen remains a promising treatment for corneal NV. Although a significant improvement with this treatment was not noted for all end points, the results suggest there may be a more beneficial role for this medication for specific conditions, such as viral keratitis. Obviously, additional trials are required before we can determine what the specific role of aganirsen will be in our clinical management of patients.

P. K. Nagra, MD

Topical Cyclosporine in Corneal Transplantation

Ziaei M, Manzouri B (Moorfields Eye Hosp, London, UK)

Cornea 34:110-115, 2015

Purpose.—Corneal transplantation is the most commonly performed tissue transplantation boasting over a century of history, science, and tradition. One of the most promising immunomodulatory substances whose immunosuppressive effect has revolutionized solid organ transplantation is cyclosporine (CsA). We present a literature review on the role of topical cyclosporine in corneal transplantation.

Methods.—A review of the published literature using key databases that include MEDLINE and PubMed was undertaken. Published evidence base for the use of topical cyclosporine in corneal transplantation between 1986 and 2010 was evaluated and summarized.

Results.—There is some scientific evidence to support the use of topical cyclosporine in appropriately selected cases of corneal transplantation. Although some encouraging human case series and case–control studies have been published, to date most randomized controlled trials evaluating the effects of topical cyclosporine in graft rejection prophylaxis and treatment have failed to demonstrate statistically significant improved outcomes.

Conclusions.—Cyclosporine cannot currently be considered as an effective sole agent in prophylaxis and treatment of allograft rejection, and corticosteroids therefore remain the gold standard choice of therapy. Further studies are required to refine the role of cyclosporine in modern corneal transplantation.

▶ Although corneal transplantation has achieved high levels of success in visual rehabilitation, graft rejection remains a major cause of failure. Topical steroids are the standard of care post-operatively, but they are not without complications, including elevated intraocular pressure, steroid-induced glaucoma, and cataract formation. Ideally, an alternative option, for both prevention and treatment of corneal graft rejection, could be used to avoid these complications or provide additional support against rejection in high-risk grafts. Topical cyclosporine has been used in such a role over the past few decades, although with unproven results.

The authors of this article performed a literature review of the use of topical cyclosporine in corneal transplantation over a 25-year period. Not surprisingly, they found topical cyclosporine as monotherapy was not beneficial. However, cyclosporine 1% and 2% used with topical steroids was found to have some encouraging results in some case series, although other series found no statistically significant benefit. Cyclosporine 0.5% and 0.05% with topical steroids were not found to have definitive improvement over topical steroids alone. The authors recognized that one of their main challenges was that negative results are often not published. Therefore, in their review of the published literature, there may have been a bias toward the use of cyclosporine.

The authors conclude that cyclosporine should not be considered monotherapy in the management of patients after corneal transplantation. Further studies are warranted to establish the role of cyclosporine for graft rejection and prevention. In our practice topical steroids remain the gold standard, although possible consideration for cyclosporine 1% or 2% is given in conjunction with topical steroids, especially for high-risk grafts.

P. K. Nagra, MD

Therapeutic effects of 0.1% tacrolimus eye drops for refractory allergic ocular diseases with proliferative lesion or corneal involvement

Fukushima A, Ohashi Y, Ebihara N, et al (Kochi Med School, Japan; Ehime Univ School of Medicine, Japan; Juntendo Univ School of Medicine, Tokyo, et al)

Br J Ophthalmol 98:1023-1027, 2014

Background.—The objective of this study was to investigate the efficacy of topical 0.1% tacrolimus in treating refractory allergic conjunctivitis with proliferative lesions and/or corneal involvement.

Methods.—This prospective observational study included 1436 patients with refractory allergic conjunctivitis whose condition had responded poorly to conventional antiallergic drugs and/or topical steroids and/or topical cyclosporine. All patients received tacrolimus eye drops twice daily during the study period. Ten clinical signs and six clinical symptoms were rated on a four-grade scale. The primary endpoint was the change from baseline in total clinical signs and symptoms score at the last observation or following 6 months of treatment.

Results.—Total signs and symptoms score significantly decreased after 1 month of treatment ($p < 0.001$). Giant papillae and corneal lesions were also reduced by tacrolimus eye drop use ($p < 0.001$). The drug proved effective in patients whose condition did not respond well to topical cyclosporine therapy. About 50% of all patients using topical steroids were weaned. The most common adverse reaction was a transient burning sensation (3.20%).

Conclusions.—Tacrolimus eye drops are highly effective in treating refractory allergic conjunctivitis with proliferative lesions and/or corneal involvement, and may reduce or replace topical steroid use.

Trial Registration Number.—UMIN 000008640 (Table 3).

▶ Treating severe allergic ocular surface disease can be particularly challenging, especially when considering the typically young patient population, as well as the significant, debilitating symptoms often associated with these conditions. These patients often require multiple medical treatments, including antiallergy medications, steroids, and cyclosporine. More than occasionally, patients remain symptomatic despite all these treatment options, which can be especially frustrating for both the clinician and patient alike.

TABLE 3.—Adverse Drug Reactions

Adverse Drug Reactions	Number of Events (%)
Transient burning sensation in eye	46 (3.20)
Eye irritation	34 (2.37)
Eye pain	10 (0.70)
Hordeolum	8 (0.56)
Conjunctival hyperaemia	6 (0.42)
Eye pruritus	4 (0.28)
Foreign body sensation in eye	3 (0.21)
Eye discharge	3 (0.21)
Lacrimation	3 (0.21)
Lid herpes	3 (0.21)
Chalazion	3 (0.21)
Intraocular pressure elevation	3 (0.21)
Photophobia	3 (0.21)
Corneal ulcer	2 (0.14)
Conjunctival oedema	2 (0.14)
Punctate keratitis	2 (0.14)
Bacterial keratitis	2 (0.14)
Corneal erosion	2 (0.14)
Transient blurred vision	2 (0.14)
Herpetic keratitis	2 (0.14)
Other events (one each of 26 cases)	1 (0.07)
Overall: number of patients (%)	117 (8.15)

Reprinted from Fukushima A, Ohashi Y, Ebihara N, et al. Therapeutic effects of 0.1% tacrolimus eye drops for refractory allergic ocular diseases with proliferative lesion or corneal involvement. *Br J Ophthalmol.* 2014;98:1023-1027, with permission from the BMJ Publishing Group Ltd.

The authors of this large, prospective study evaluated the results of 1436 patients with refractory allergic conjunctivitis treated with topical tacrolimus eyedrops. After 1 month of treatment, there was a statistically significant improvement in symptoms and signs (papillae, superficial punctate keratitis, severe keratopathy). In addition, 50% of patients were able to be weaned off steroids, which may help limit complications associated with steroid use such as elevated intraocular pressure, steroid-induced glaucoma, and cataracts. Adverse reactions were noted in 8% of patients (see Table 3), with the most common being burning, noted in 3.2%. Corneal infections (bacterial keratitis, herpetic keratitis, and bacterial corneal ulcer) were noted in 5 of the 1436 patients, all of whom also had atopic dermatitis or asthma.

The results suggest that topical tacrolimus is a highly effective, well-tolerated treatment for refractory allergic conjunctivitis. Furthermore, it may help patients reduce or discontinue the use of topical steroids. Topical tacrolimus is not commercially available in the United States but is available through compounding pharmacies. Although infrequently used in our practice, this study certainly provides motivation to institute use of this drop for our refractory allergic conjunctivitis patients.

P. K. Nagra, MD

Clinical features and management of cytomegalovirus corneal endotheliitis: analysis of 106 cases from the Japan corneal endotheliitis study

Koizumi N, for the Japan Corneal Endotheliitis Study Group (Kyoto Prefectural Univ of Medicine, Japan; et al)

Br J Ophthalmol 99:54-58, 2015

Aims.—The purpose of this study is to elucidate the clinical manifestations and the current treatment status of cytomegalovirus (CMV) endotheliitis via a large case series obtained from a national survey conducted in Japan.

Methods.—The Japan Corneal Endotheliitis Study Group proposed diagnostic criteria for CMV endotheliitis based on a viral examination by PCR of aqueous humour, in combination with clinical manifestations. A national survey was then retrospectively conducted among 1160 members of the Japan Cornea Society. The study reviewed the patient profiles, clinical manifestations, and treatment modalities of individuals who met the diagnostic criteria for CMV endotheliitis.

Results.—The study included 109 eyes of 106 patients. Mean patient age was 66.9 ± 10.9 years (85 males (80.2%), 21 females (19.8%)). Patients were commonly diagnosed with anterior uveitis and ocular hypertension prior to confirmation of CMV endotheliitis. Coin-shaped lesions were observed in 70.6%, and linear keratic precipitates in 8.3% of the patients, respectively. 95% of cases were treated with anti-CMV drugs.

Conclusions.—CMV endotheliitis is most common in middle-aged and elderly men. CMV endotheliitis should be suspected when patients present with corneal endotheliitis involving coin-shaped lesions accompanied by anterior uveitis and ocular hypertension.

▶ Cytomegalovirus corneal endotheliitis is a recently recognized corneal infectious disease for which our current understanding is continuing to evolve. The authors of this study present a large, retrospective series of 109 eyes (of 106 patients) with this condition.

They found a majority of their patients were middle-aged men (80.2% male), of which less than 10% has a history of cancer, and no patients reported HIV infection. Clinically, the most common findings, noted in a majority of patients, were "coin-shaped lesion keratic precipitates (KPs)" (seen in 70.6%) and corneal edema (73.4%), as well as anterior chamber inflammation (67.9%). Fewer patients had linear KPs (8.3%). Elevated intraocular pressure was noted in 38.5% of patients on diagnosis.

Diagnosis was confirmed with positive polymerase chain reaction (PCR) for CMV DNA using aqueous specimens, but negative for herpes simplex virus and herpes zoster virus DNA. Patients were treated with ganciclovir or valganciclovir, either systemically, topically, or both in 104 of 109 eyes. Patients treated both systemically and topically had the best response, although even with both, 5.8% of patients did not respond to treatment. The nonresponding patients were felt to have severe corneal endothelial damage, leading to irreversible corneal edema, requiring corneal transplantation. Recurrence of inflammation was noted in 36% of patients, who were then given another course of anti-CMV treatment.

On the basis of these findings, early diagnosis and management is critical in preserving endothelial cell function. Having a high level of suspicion, especially in middle-aged men with signs of intraocular inflammation and corneal edema, promptly obtaining PCR and starting treatment with oral and topical anti-CMV medications may help avoid the need for corneal transplantation in the future for these patients.

P. K. Nagra, MD

Medically Reversible Limbal Stem Cell Disease: Clinical Features and Management Strategies

Kim BY, Riaz KM, Bakhtiari P, et al (Univ of Illinois Eye and Ear Infirmary, Chicago; Northwestern Univ Feinberg School of Medicine, Chicago, IL; et al)
Ophthalmology 121:2053-2058, 2014

Purpose.—To describe the clinical features and management strategies in patients whose limbal stem cell (LSC) disease reversed with medical therapy.

Design.—Retrospective case series.

Participants.—Twenty-two eyes of 15 patients seen at 3 tertiary referral centers between 2007 and 2011 with 3 months or more of follow-up.

Methods.—Medical records of patients with medically reversible LSC disease were reviewed. Demographic data, causes, location and duration of disease, and medical inventions were analyzed.

Main Outcome Measures.—Primary outcomes assessed included resolution of signs of LSC disease and improvement in visual acuity.

Results.—Causes of the LSC disease included contact lens wear only (13 eyes), contact lens wear in the setting of ocular rosacea (3 eyes), benzalkonium chloride toxicity (2 eyes), and idiopathic (4 eyes). Ophthalmologic findings included loss of limbal architecture, a whorl-like epitheliopathy, or an opaque epithelium arising from the limbus with late fluorescein staining. The superior limbus was the most common site of involvement (95%). The corneal epithelial phenotype returned to normal with only conservative measures, including lubrication and discontinuing contact lens wear in 4 patients (4 eyes), whereas in 11 patients (18 eyes), additional interventions were required after at least 3 months of conservative therapy. Medical interventions included topical corticosteroids, topical cyclosporine, topical vitamin A, oral doxycycline, punctal occlusion, or a combination thereof. All eyes achieved a stable ocular surface over a mean follow-up of 15 months (range, 4–60 months). Visual acuity improved from a mean of 20/42 to 20/26 ($P < 0.0184$).

Conclusions.—Disturbances to the LSC function, niche, or both may be reversible with medical therapy. These cases, which represent a subset of patients with LSC deficiency, may be considered to have LSC niche dysfunction.

▶ Limbal stem cell disease is a condition seen by all corneal specialists and general ophthalmologists. Although many patients may be asymptomatic with a mild variant and can be observed, most patients with advanced limbal stem cell disease are symptomatic. These patients may have more central epithelial changes, leading to decreased vision, irritation, or contact lens intolerance, requiring treatment.

The authors present a case series of 22 eyes (15 patients) that responded to medical treatment for limbal stem cell disease. Conservative measures alone, including discontinuing contact lens wear and lubrication, were successful in 4 eyes, while the remaining 18 eyes required additional treatment following 3 months of conservative measures. Most patients (17 eyes) benefited from anti-inflammatory treatment, specifically topical corticosteroids, and 1 patient had resolution with topical vitamin A ointment at bedtime. Concomitant dry eyes and ocular rosacea was managed as well, and this treatment was maintained after taper of the steroids, including topical cyclosporine, oral doxycycline, punctual occlusion.

The authors distinguish between limbal stem cell deficiency (ie, due to chemical injury), which may not respond to medical treatment, and dysfunction of the limbal stem cells and/or the limbal stem cell microenvironment/niche, which may respond to medical management. The authors theorize that there may be a toxic or traumatic component (contact lens wear, benzalkonium drops) combined with a compromised ocular surface (dry eyes, rosacea) leading to this dysfunction, and treating both components will help the condition resolve.

The authors also present a treatment strategy for patients with presumed limbal stem cell dysfunction, starting with removing any toxic or traumatic factors (ie, discontinue contact lens wear) and optimizing the ocular surface with preservative-free tears and warm compresses. After a few months, if there is no improvement, topical steroids may be considered. As the steroids are tapered, more long-term treatments such as topical cyclosporine could be considered, as well as punctal occlusion and/or oral doxycycline. Autologous serum and/or PROSE lens could be considered for more recalcitrant cases as well.

P. K. Nagra, MD

Collagen Cross-Linking with Photoactivated Riboflavin (PACK-CXL) for the Treatment of Advanced Infectious Keratitis with Corneal Melting

Said DG, Elalfy MS, Gatzioufas Z, et al (Res Inst of Ophthalmology, Cairo, Egypt; Geneva Univ Hosps, Switzerland; et al)

Ophthalmology 121:1377-1382, 2014

Purpose.—To investigate the efficacy and safety of corneal collagen cross-linking (CXL) with photoactivated riboflavin (photoactivated chromophore for infectious keratitis [PACK]–CXL) in the management of infectious keratitis with corneal melting.

Design.—Prospective clinical trial.

Participants.—Forty eyes from 40 patients with advanced infectious keratitis and coexisting corneal melting.

Methods.—Twenty-one patients (21 eyes) underwent PACK-CXL treatment in addition to antimicrobial therapy. The control group consisted of 19 patients (19 eyes) who received only antimicrobial therapy.

Main Outcome Measures.—The slit-lamp characteristics of the corneal ulceration, corrected distance visual acuity, duration until healing, and complications were documented in each group. The Mann–Whitney *U* test was used for statistical analysis. *P* values less than 0.05 were considered statistically significant.

Results.—The average time until healing was 39.76 ± 18.22 days in the PACK-CXL group and 46.05 ± 27.44 days in the control group ($P = 0.68$). After treatment and healing, corrected distance visual acuity was 1.64 ± 0.62 in the PACK-CXL group and 1.67 ± 0.48 in the control group ($P = 0.68$). The corneal ulceration's width and length was significantly bigger in the PACK-CXL group ($P = 0.004$ and $P = 0.007$). Three patients in the control group demonstrated corneal perforation; infection recurred in 1 of them. No serious complications occurred in the PACK-CXL group.

Conclusions.—Corneal CXL with photoactivated riboflavin did not shorten the time to corneal healing; however, the complication rate was 21% in the control group, whereas there was no incidence of corneal perforation or recurrence of the infection in the PACK-CXL group. These results indicate that PACK-CXL may be an effective adjuvant therapy in the management of severe infectious keratitis associated with corneal melting.

▶ Although collagen crosslinking for infectious keratitis is a promising procedure, the only supporting evidence up to this point comprises a few case reports and small case series. This article is a welcome addition to the current body of literature on this topic, representing the largest prospective trial to date. Forty patients with infectious keratitis were included, with 21 undergoing photoactivated chromophore for infectious keratitis (PACK-CXL) in addition to antimicrobial treatment and 19 in a control group who only received antimicrobial therapy.

After initial culture, all patients were started on fortified vancomycin and ceftazidime and oral itraconazole, with changes in this regimen based on culture data or clinical response. Patients in the PACK-CXL group underwent the procedure within 48 hours of initial presentation.

The authors found no significant difference in the time to healing and visual outcomes between the 2 groups. However, 3 patients in the control group developed perforation of their corneal ulcers, and 1 patient in the control group developed a recurrence of the infection. No similar complications were noted among the PACK-CXL treated patients. Transient limbitis was noted in all PACK-CXL-treated patients. In addition, a PACK-CXL-treated patient was noted to have a transient increase in hypopyon size 24 hours after the procedure, which then resolved.

Although no significant improvement in vision or faster recovery was noted in the PACK-CXL-treated patients, the lack of major complications (ie, perforation or recurrence) is encouraging when compared with the control group. Further studies are needed to gain additional understanding of the significance of the posttreatment limbitis noted in all patients, as well as the increased intraocular inflammation noted in 1 patient. Other questions that require additional studies include whether there is a difference in response to PACK-CXL based on the type of organism (bacterial, fungal, etc) and when is the ideal time for treatment (on initial presentation vs 48 hours after antimicrobial treatment vs 1 week after antimicrobial treatment, etc). Although this study suggests PACK-CXL may have a beneficial effect as adjuvant therapy for microbial keratitis, additional studies are needed to further define its role.

P. K. Nagra, MD

Long-term Outcomes of Boston Type 1 Keratoprosthesis Implantation: A Retrospective Multicenter Cohort

Srikumaran D, Munoz B, Aldave AJ, et al (The Johns Hopkins Univ School of Medicine, Baltimore, MD; The Jules Stein Eye Inst, Los Angeles, CA; et al)
Ophthalmology 121:2159-2164, 2014

Purpose.—To study the long-term outcomes of Boston type 1 keratoprosthesis (KPro) surgery.

Design.—Retrospective, multicenter case series.

Participants.—A total of 158 eyes of 150 patients underwent KPro implantation at 5 participating tertiary centers in the United States between January 2003 and December 2006. Of those, 139 eyes of 133 patients were included in the analyses.

Methods.—The medical records of consecutive adult patients who received KPro surgery were reviewed. All patients with at least 1 postoperative visit were retained in the outcomes analyses. In eyes in which a repeat KPro procedure was performed, only the outcomes of the initial surgery were analyzed.

Main Outcome Measures.—Visual acuity (VA) outcomes, postoperative complications, and device retention.

Results.—The mean follow-up was 46.7 ± 26 months with all but 4 eyes having at least 6 months of follow-up. Preoperatively, only 10.8% of the eyes had VA of ≥20/200. Postoperatively, the VA in 70% of eyes improved to ≥20/200. The probability of maintaining VA of ≥20/200 at 7 years was 50%. The device retention rate was estimated at 67% at 7 years. The 7-year cumulative incidence of complications was 49.7%

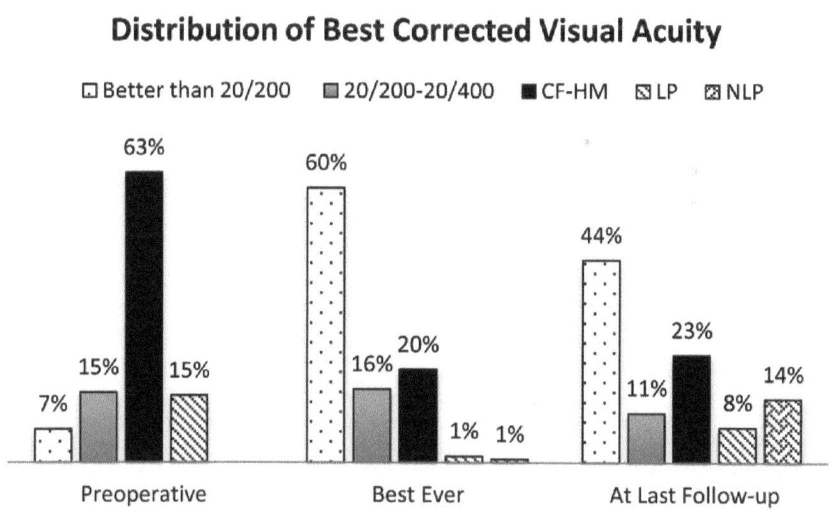

FIGURE 1.—Preoperative visual acuity (VA) in comparison with best-ever vision measured at any time point during follow-up (n = 139) and the vision measured at the last visit (n = 130) in a retrospective cohort of patients who underwent Boston type 1 keratoprosthesis (KPro) surgery before 2007 at 5 tertiary care centers in the United States. The VA at the last follow-up is presented for all eyes in the cohort regardless of retention of the device. One patient with mental retardation could not have vision measured accurately and was excluded from this analysis. Eight eyes with device removal did not have a post-removal acuity recorded and were not included in the distribution for the last visit. The VA was recorded as no light perception if the eye was enucleated during the follow-up. The totals do not add up to exactly 100% because of rounding. CF = counting fingers; HM = hand motions; LP = light perception; NLP = no light perception. (Reprinted from Ophthalmology. Srikumaran D, Munoz B, Aldave AJ, et al. Long-term outcomes of boston type 1 keratoprosthesis implantation: a retrospective multicenter cohort. *Ophthalmology.* 2014;121:2159-2164, Copyright 2014, with permission from the American Academy of Ophthalmology.)

for retroprosthetic membrane formation, 21.6% for glaucoma surgery, 18.6% for retinal detachment, and 15.5% for endophthalmitis.

Conclusions.—Although the risk for complications with longer follow-up seemed to increase, this large multicenter cohort demonstrates favorable outcomes with KPro, with a large number of patients achieving and retaining useful vision over a 7-year period (Fig 1).

▶ This multicenter look at the long-term outcomes of the Boston Keratoprosthesis crystallizes the experience of those who perform this surgery. Analyzing around 150 patients treated at 5 centers, the group reports a significant decline in retention rate of the keratoprosthesis from 2 years postoperatively (82%) to 7 years (67%). Although this is still a relatively high retention rate for this group of high-risk patients, it shows that these patients need ongoing surveillance and follow-up, as problems can surface at any point. Of course, the retention rate is only part of the story. These patients can lose vision, and do lose vision, while still maintaining the device. This is most commonly secondary to glaucoma complications. The visual acuity data of best vision achieved vs final vision shows that the Boston Keratoprosthesis can allow patients to quickly reach the eye's potential vision, but maintaining that may be a struggle (Fig 1). It is very helpful to use the assistance of an interested glaucoma specialist who can aid these patients. All of the patients presented in this report were adults. It is concerning to apply the declining rates of retention and visual acuity to our pediatric population, who have a long road and many years of struggle ahead. For this reason, many, including myself, have less enthusiasm for keratoprosthesis in children over the years. We are appreciative to have the Boston Keratoprosthesis as a tool to care for patients who have limited other options and look forward to advances in the way to care for these patients over the long term.

K. M. Hammersmith, MD

Therapeutic and Optical Keratoplasty in the Management of *Acanthamoeba* Keratitis: Risk Factors, Outcomes, and Summary of the Literature

Robaei D, Carnt N, Minassian DC, et al (Moorfields Eye Hosp NHS Foundation Trust, London, UK; EpiVision Ophthalmic Epidemiology Consultants, Bucks, UK)

Ophthalmology 122:17-24, 2015

Objective.—To report the risk factors for and outcomes of therapeutic and optical keratoplasty in the management of Acanthamoeba keratitis (AK).

Design.—Retrospective case series.

Participants.—A total of 50 eyes of 196 patients with retrievable medical records, diagnosed with AK at Moorfields Eye Hospital, London, underwent keratoplasty between January 1991 and April 2012.

Methods.—Patient demographics, initial clinical examination findings, and management details were collected. The ophthalmic characteristics of patients who underwent keratoplasty for AK were compared with those who did not. Patients undergoing therapeutic keratoplasty were compared with those undergoing optical keratoplasty for baseline characteristics, management details, and visual outcomes. A multivariate logistic model was used to derive the odds ratios of a poor visual outcome in all keratoplasty patients.

Main Outcome Measures.—Poor visual outcome was defined as final visual acuity of 20/200 or worse. Secondary outcomes of interest included number of clinic visits and the need for additional intraocular surgery.

Results.—Of the 196 AK patients, a total of 50 patients (25.5%) underwent penetrating or anterior lamellar keratoplasty, 10 of whom (20%) underwent repeat procedures. Of these 50 patients, 26 (52%) had therapeutic keratoplasty, predominantly for corneal perforation. The remaining 24 patients (48%) underwent optical keratoplasty for visual rehabilitation. Thirty-seven (80.4%) patients in the keratoplasty group initially were misdiagnosed as having herpes simplex keratitis versus 59 (41.8%) patients who did not require a keratoplasty ($P < 0.001$). Final visual outcomes were significantly better in the optical group compared with the therapeutic group, with 13 (54.2%) achieving visual acuity of 20/30 or better versus 7 (26.9%), respectively. On multivariate analysis, beginning therapy at a hospital other than Moorfields and undergoing a therapeutic, rather than an optical, keratoplasty were associated significantly with a poor visual outcome from keratoplasty.

Conclusions.—The prognosis of keratoplasty differs markedly when performed for therapeutic purposes compared with visual rehabilitation. Where possible, keratoplasty should be delayed until such time as the eye is uninflamed and medically cured of Acanthamoeba (Fig 1, Table 3).

▶ This article presents data on keratoplasty for Acanthamoeba keratitis (AK) at Moorefields Eye Hospital over a 20-year period. This group consistently provides insightful and helpful contributions on AK. Twenty-five percent of the nearly 200 cases of AK during this time period required keratoplasty. The authors compare the characteristics of those patients identified over this time who required keratoplasty vs those who did not undergo surgery. Many of the findings here were consistent with previous studies. Patients who required surgery had longer symptom duration before therapy than those who did not (35 days vs 21 days). A significantly larger proportion of patients in the keratoplasty group were misdiagnosed as herpes simplex virus (HSV) vs those who did not require keratoplasty (80% vs 42%). Our group has consistently observed that a large proportion of our patients with AK were misdiagnosed as having herpetic keratitis (usually around 75%). We have not delineated the surgical cases from others, but it remains the most frequent "misdiagnosis" for HSV. Any patient with suspected herpes keratitis and a history of contact lens wear should be treated with caution and watched carefully for rapid resolution to HSV. About half of the grafts were performed as therapeutic ones, mostly for

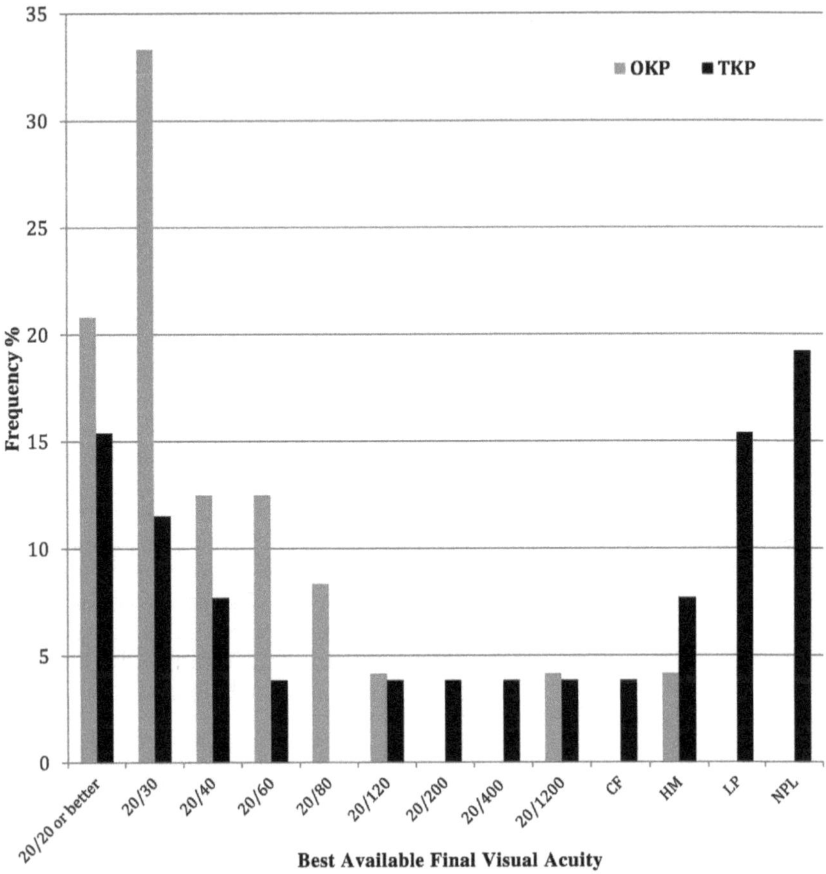

FIGURE 1.—Bar graph showing the distribution of final visual acuity in patients undergoing therapeutic keratoplasty (TKP) and optical keratoplasty (OKP). CF = counting fingers; HM = hand movements; LP = light perception; NLP = no light perception. (Reprinted from Ophthalmology. Robaei D, Carnt N, Minassian DC, et al. Therapeutic and optical keratoplasty in the management of *Acanthamoeba* keratitis: risk factors, outcomes, and summary of the literature. *Ophthalmology.* 2015;122:17-24, Copyright 2015, with permission from the American Academy of Ophthalmology.)

perforation, whereas the other half were performed in quiet eyes, as optical keratoplasty. Not surprisingly, final visual outcomes were significantly better in the optical group, leading the authors to recommend the reservation of keratoplasty for optical indications, except in the cases of perforation or impending perforation. They recommend that optical keratoplasty, either lamellar or penetrating, be performed after all antiamebic and steroid therapy have been discontinued for a minimum of 1 month. We have had a similar experience and, accordingly, delay surgical intervention when possible. Interestingly, the authors do not analyze or comment on glaucoma complications of these patients, which seem

TABLE 3.—Univariate Comparison of Patients Who Underwent Optical Keratoplasty (n = 24) and Those Who Underwent Therapeutic Keratoplasty (n = 26)

	Optical Keratoplasty (n = 24)	Therapeutic Keratoplasty (n = 26)	*P* Value
Mean age (SD), yrs	44.3 (16.6)	43.0 (12.1)	0.826
Male gender, n (%)	12 (50.0)	16 (61.5)	0.569
Initially diagnosed elsewhere, n (%)	11 (45.8)	17 (65.4)	0.254
Topical steroid use before diagnosis, n (%)	21 (91.3)	16 (72.7)	0.135
Unknown	1	4	
Treatment for HSK before diagnosis, n (%)	19 (82.6)	18 (78.3)	>0.999
Unknown	1	3	
Median delay to commencement of antiamebic therapy median (IQR*), days	31 (24.5–91)	39 (27–85)	0.785
Median duration of antiamebic therapy (IQR), mos	11 (6–18)	12 (6–19)	0.627
Median time lag to keratoplasty (IQR), mos	17 (12.5–26)	7 (3.8–13)	<0.001
Patients with multiple keratoplasties, n (%)	3 (12.5)	7 (26.92)	0.294
Final VA, n (%)			
≥20/30	13 (54.2)	7 (26.9)	0.004
20/40–20/60	6 (25.0)	3 (11.5)	
20/80–20/200	3 (12.5)	2 (7.7)	
<20/200	2 (8.3)	14 (53.9)	
Total median no. of clinic visits (IQR)	40 (23–59)	56 (36–68)	0.131
Mean no. of visits/yr (SD)	1.1 (0.75)	1.2 (0.61)	0.332
Patients needing other eye surgery, n (%)	14 (58.3)	23 (88.5)	0.024

HSK = herpes simplex keratitis; IQR = interquartile range; SD = standard deviation; VA = visual acuity.
*A measure of dispersion, presented here as the 25th and 75th percentiles of the data distribution.

paramount in the final outcomes of many of our severe cases, including those who require a keratoplasty.

K. M. Hammersmith, MD

New Therapeutic Modality for Corneal Endothelial Disease Using Rho-Associated Kinase Inhibitor Eye Drops

Koizumi N, Okumura N, Ueno M, et al (Doshisha Univ, Kyotanabe, Japan; Kyoto Prefectural Univ of Medicine, Kyoto, Japan)
Cornea 33:S25-S31, 2014

Corneal endothelial dysfunction accompanied by visual disturbance is a primary indication for corneal endothelial transplantation. However, despite the value and potential of endothelial graft surgery, a strictly pharmacological approach for treating corneal endothelial dysfunction remains

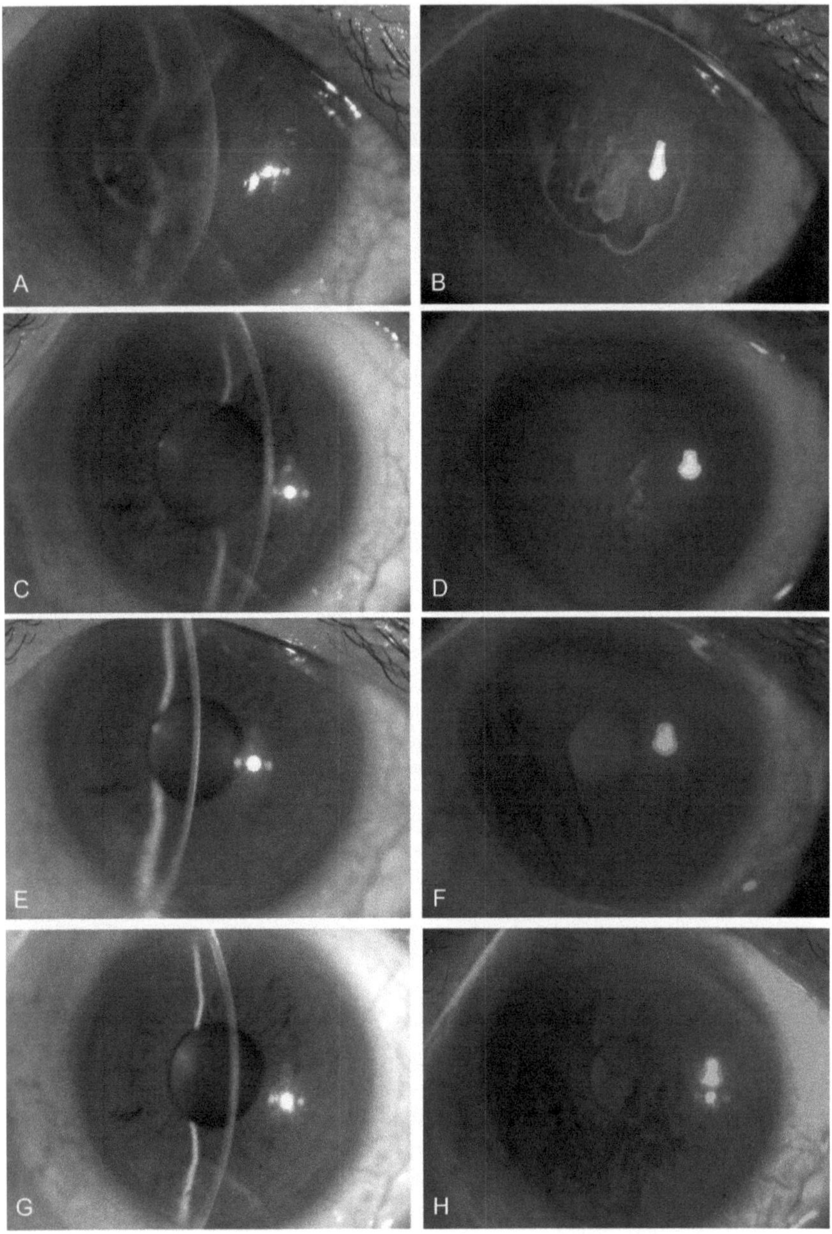

FIGURE 5.—Slit-lamp photographs of a patient with Fuchs corneal dystrophy before and after transcorneal freezing and ROCK inhibitor treatment. Before treatment, a central corneal edema (A) accompanied by a lesion of epithelial bullae (B) was detected. Three days after treatment, the corneal erosion created by the transcorneal freezing had already healed, and mild bullae were detected (C, D). It should be noted that less corneal edema was observed at 2 days than in the pretreatment image. Six months after treatment, the corneal edema was significantly reduced, and the cornea had recovered its clarity (E). No epithelial damage was observed by fluorescein staining (F). Two years after treatment, the patient's cornea remains clear with good (20/16) vision (G, H). Reprinted from Koizumi et al[27] with permission from Lippincott Williams & Wilkins. *Editor's Note*: Please refer to original journal article for full references. (Reprinted from Koizumi N, Okumura N, Ueno M, et al. New therapeutic modality for corneal endothelial disease using rho-associated kinase inhibitor eye drops. *Cornea*. 2014;33:S25-S31, with permission from Lippincott Williams & Wilkins.)

an attractive proposition. Previously, we reported that the selective Rho-associated kinase (ROCK) inhibitor Y-27632 promotes cell adhesion and proliferation, and inhibits the apoptosis of primate corneal endothelial cells in culture. These findings have led us to develop a novel medical treatment for the early phase of corneal endothelial disease using ROCK inhibitor eye drops. In rabbit and monkey models of partial endothelial dysfunction, we showed that corneal endothelial wound healing was accelerated via the topical application of ROCK inhibitor to the ocular surface, resulting in the regeneration of a corneal endothelial monolayer with a high endothelial cell density. Based on these animal studies, we are now attempting to advance the clinical application of ROCK inhibitor eye drops for patients with corneal endothelial dysfunction. A pilot clinical study was performed at the Kyoto Prefectural University of Medicine, and the effects of Y-27632 eye drops after transcorneal freezing were evaluated in 8 patients with corneal endothelial dysfunction. We observed a positive effect of ROCK inhibitor eye drops in treating patients with central edema caused by Fuchs corneal endothelial dystrophy. We believe that our new findings will contribute to the establishment of a new approach for the treatment of corneal endothelial dysfunction (Fig 5).

▶ This article reports on a pilot clinical study using the selective Rho-associated kinase (ROCK) inhibitor in humans with endothelial dysfunction. Previously, this group has demonstrated that the ROCK inhibitor promoted cell adhesion and proliferation and inhibited apoptosis of primate corneal endothelial cells in culture. The authors here continue the journey to identify a pharmacological approach for treating endothelial disease. The authors treated 8 patients, half of whom had bullous keratopathy and the other half with Fuchs dystrophy. All eyes underwent transcorneal freezing followed by the ROCK inhibitory eyedrop 6 times a day for a week. The primary end point was central corneal thickness. There was no improvement in the pseudophakic bullous keratopathy patients, but 3 of the 4 Fuchs patients showed a "decrease in corneal thickness that was maintained with time." The data on the corneal thickness change are not presented. The authors do show impressive clinical photographs of a patient with bullous changes associated with Fuchs dystrophy. After treatment, the patient had complete resolution and attained 20/16 vision at 2 years. The authors admit that it is not clear how much of this effect stems from the ROCK administration and how much may come from the denudation of pathologic endothelial cells. It is exciting work, and we look forward to larger studies, demonstrating sustained effect and safety of this therapy.

K. M. Hammersmith, MD

Ocular and Systemic Morbidity in a Longitudinal Cohort of Sjögren's Syndrome

Akpek EK, Mathews P, Hahn S, et al (The Johns Hopkins Univ School of Medicine, Baltimore, MD; et al)
Ophthalmology 122:56-61, 2015

Purpose.—To report vision-threatening ocular manifestations of primary Sjögren's syndrome (SS).

Design.—Retrospective review.

Participants.—Consecutive patients evaluated at an SS center between January 2007 and May 2011.

Methods.—Data collection was completed in March 2013. The 2002 American-European consensus criteria were used for diagnosis of SS.

Main Outcome Measures.—Frequency of extraglandular ocular findings and timing of their diagnosis relative to that of SS and dry eye were assessed.

Results.—One hundred sixty-three patients were included. Almost all patients (98%) had a history of dry eye for an average of 10.4 years (median, 7.9 years) before presentation. One or more extraglandular ocular manifestations were present in 40 patients (25%), and vision-threatening findings were present in 22 patients (13%). Twelve patients (55%) with a vision-threatening ocular finding did not have a diagnosis of SS at presentation. Sixty-eight patients (42%) had extraglandular systemic manifestations of SS. Patients with vision-threatening ocular findings were 3.9 times more likely to have systemic involvement (95% confidence interval, 1.4-11.0; $P = 0.010$). Peripheral neuropathy, interstitial nephritis, and vasculitis were more common in those with vision-threatening ocular findings compared with patients without ($P < 0.05$ for all).

Conclusions.—These results from a tertiary referral-based cohort demonstrate that primary SS frequently is associated with ocular and systemic complications. Dry eye precedes these findings on average by 1 decade. Therefore, ophthalmologists should consider assessing for SS in patients with clinically significant dry eye.

▶ This is an interesting analysis of patients presenting to a tertiary care center for treatment of Sjögren syndrome (SS) over a 4.5-year period. The authors attempt to assess its relationship to eye disease (and severity of eye disease) and to other systemic manifestations. Not surprisingly, almost all of the patients are women (91%) and had received the diagnosis of SS at a median age of 51 years. Most of them had dry eye symptomatology as their first symptom, preceding systemic ones. Only 63% of these patients, who went on to be identified as having SS, presented with the diagnosis. As ophthalmologists, we have the opportunity to help identify these patients. The group of patients with vision-threatening findings (haze, perforation or impending perforation, etc) also had significantly more systemic issues, such as peripheral neuropathy, vasculitis, and interstitial nephritis. One of the interesting discussions about SS and systemic disease is its relationship with non-Hodgkin lymphoma (NHL). Several studies have shown that SS is an independent risk factor for NHL. In fact, it has been shown to be the autoimmune disease with highest association with malignancy. Akpek et al identified 5 patients with NHL (2.7%) but did not comment on how this compares with expected rates of lymphoma in women older than 50 years. Recently, a new test has become available to detect earlier markers for SS, which is available as the Sjö test (formerly from Nicox Corporation, now Bausch and Lomb). Although the test was originally available only through a physician with an imperfect fingerstick test, it is now becoming more available through commercial laboratories. This will greatly enhance its use. We look forward to the opportunity to reach an earlier diagnosis in younger patients with predominantly dry eye symptomatology with systemic SS so that associated systemic manifestations may be better identified and treated.

K. M. Hammersmith, MD

Treatment of pseudodendrites in herpes zoster ophthalmicus with topical ganciclovir 0.15% gel

Aggarwal S, Cavalcanti BM, Pavan-Langston D (Cornea and Refractive Surgery Service, Boston, MA; Harvard Med School, Boston, MA)

Cornea 33:109-113, 2014

Purpose.—There is no standard of treatment for epithelial pseudodendrites in herpes zoster ophthalmicus (HZO). The purpose of this study is to report the topical antiviral drug, 0.15% ganciclovir for treatment of these lesions.

Methods.—This is a retrospective, interventional case series of 4 patients who were diagnosed with HZO epithelial pseudodendrites despite being given oral antiviral treatment and who underwent 0.15% ganciclovir gel topical treatment. Main outcome measures included epithelial healing time, visual acuity, and corneal sensation.

Results.—All 4 patients were immunocompetent and had epithelial lesions unresponsive to antiviral treatment with oral valacyclovir. Treatment with topical 0.15% ganciclovir gel 5 times a day resulted in the lesions healing successfully within 7 days with improved visual acuity in 3 patients and an increase in corneal sensation in 2 of the 4 patients.

Conclusions.—Topical 0.15% ganciclovir gel, 5 times a day until pseudodendritic lesion healing and tapering to bid for 2 to 4 weeks thereafter, is an effective treatment for pseudodendrites in HZO-affected cases that are often a challenge to manage with other oral or topical antivirals.

► Although it reports a small case series, this article addresses an important clinical question: What is the best way to treat pseudodendrites in patients with varicella zoster keratitis? Over the years, this has been a frustrating problem, with imperfect choices. These include frequent lubrication (often not effective enough), topical trifluridine (too toxic to the already compromised surface), topical vidarabine ointment (only available through compounding pharmacies), and oral antivirals (mixed success). Recently, topical ganciclovir 0.15% ophthalmic gel (Zirgan; Bausch & Lomb, Rochester, NY) has become available in the United States for treatment of herpetic disease. The patients all responded, both with resolution of pseudodendrites and associated epithelial defects, but also with increased corneal sensation in half of the patients. It has been established that the pseudodendrites have viral DNA by polymerase chain reaction. It is reasonable to assume that topical and/or oral antivirals would be helpful. However, there is little consensus about the best way to treat zoster keratitis. We look forward to larger trials assessing the best way to manage these patients, both acutely and chronically. In the meantime, it is reasonable to consider topical ganciclovir gel 0.15% 5 times a day for a week, then 2 to 3 times a day for 1 week to 2 months when faced with pseudodendrites, as the authors suggest.

K. M. Hammersmith, MD

4 Glaucoma

New options for combined cataract and glaucoma surgery

Budenz DL, Gedde SJ (Univ of North Carolina at Chapel Hill; Univ of Miami, FL)

Curr Opin Ophthalmol 25:141-147, 2014

Purpose of Review.—To review the current literature regarding the effectiveness and risks of new surgeries that can be combined with phacoemulsification in the management of cataract and glaucoma.

Recent Findings.—Surgical options for concurrently managing cataract and glaucoma have expanded in recent years. Endoscopic cyclophotocoagulation, trabecular micro-bypass stent, ab interno trabeculectomy, and canaloplasty may be performed in conjunction with cataract extraction to provide additional intraocular pressure (IOP) reduction. Studies evaluating these new glaucoma procedures combined with phacoemulsification generally include retrospective case series without a comparison group. Because cataract surgery alone is associated with IOP reduction, the relative contribution of the glaucoma procedure in lowering IOP cannot be determined in these studies. Randomized clinical trials are needed to better evaluate the efficacy and safety of newer glaucoma procedures in combination with cataract surgery.

Summary.—The newer glaucoma procedures appear less effective than trabeculectomy, but they are associated with a lower risk of surgical complications (Tables 1-3).

▶ New surgical procedures for glaucoma are frequently developed for use in combination with cataract extraction. Although the number of surgeries for glaucoma performed in the United States is not exactly known, it's likely around 80 000 to 100 000 per year.[1] In contrast, estimates of the number of annual cataract surgeries are around 3 million. It's also estimated that about 20% of people undergoing cataract surgery have comorbid glaucoma or ocular hypertension. Therefore, the population of patients who might benefit from a procedure for glaucoma at the time of cataract surgery is 6 times larger than the population who need a glaucoma surgery alone. The process of advancing a surgical device through approval and into clinical use is expensive, so investment in devices that target a broader group seems popular.

Phacoemulsification alone lowers the intraocular pressure. Therefore, separating the benefit of cataract surgery from that of a combined procedure requires careful study. This article is an excellent review of the literature on some of the new glaucoma surgeries when combined with cataract extraction.

TABLE 1.—Studies of Combined Phacoemulsification and Endoscopic Cyclophotocoagulation

Author (Year)	Treatment	Number of Eyes	Follow-Up (Months)	Number (%) Lost to Follow-Up	Change from Baseline Mean IOP (%)	Mean Meds (%)
Clement *et al.* [4■]	PE–ECP	63	12	NR	23.9% Decrease	45.8% Decrease
Lindfield *et al.* [5■]	PE–ECP	58	24	17 (29%)	33.0% Decrease	5.1% Increase
Lima *et al.* [6]	PE–ECP	368	35.2 (Mean)	NR	46.7% Decrease	74.3% Decrease
Kahook *et al.* [7]	PE–ECP (1 site)	15	6	8 (53%)	32.2% Decrease	21.9% Decrease
	PE–ECP (2 sites)	25		12 (48%)	46.9% Decrease	79.7% Decrease
Berke [9]	PE–ECP	626	38.4 (Mean)	NR	17.6% Decrease	57.5% Decrease
	PE	81			4.2% Increase	0%
Gayton *et al.* [10]	PE–ECP	29	23.5 (Mean)	12 (21%)	28.8% Decrease	34.4% Decrease
	PE–trab	29	27.2 (Mean)		31.9% Decrease	29.2% Decrease
Uram [8]	PE–ECP	10	19.2 (Mean)	0 (<1 year)	23.9% Decrease	45.8% Decrease

ECP, endoscopic cyclophotocoagulation; IOP, intraocular pressure; meds, glaucoma medications; NR, not reported; PE, phacoemulsification; trab, trabeculectomy.

Editor's Note: Please refer to original journal article for full references.

Reprinted from Budenz DL, Gedde SJ. New options for combined cataract and glaucoma surgery. *Curr Opin Ophthalmol.* 2014;25:141–147.

TABLE 2.—Studies of Combined Phacoemulsification and iStent

Author (Year)	Treatment	Number of Eyes	Follow-Up (Months)	Number (%) Lost to Follow-Up	Change from Baseline Mean IOP (%)	Mean Meds (%)
Craven *et al.* (2012) [15■■]	PE–1 iStent	117	24	19 (16.2%)	8.1% Decrease	81.3% Decrease
	PE	123		22 (17.9%)	0.6% Decrease	66.7% Decrease
Samuelson *et al.* (2011) [14]	PE–1 iStent	117	12	17 (14.5%)	8.0% Decrease	86.7% Decrease
	PE	123		13 (10.6%)	5.0% Decrease	73.3% Decrease
Fea (2010) [16]	PE–1 iStent	12	15	0	17.3% Decrease	80.0% Decrease
	PE	24		3 (12.5%)	9.2% Decrease	31.6% Decrease
Fernández-Barrientos *et al.* (2010) [17]	PE–2 iStents	17	12	0	27.3% Decrease	100% Decrease
	PE	16		0	16.1% Decrease	41.7% Decrease
Spiegel *et al.* (2009) [18]	PE–1 iStent	48	12	6 (12.5%)	20.3% Decrease	75.0% Decrease

IOP, intraocular pressure; meds, glaucoma medications; PE, phacoemulsification.

Editor's Note: Please refer to original journal article for full references.

Reprinted from Budenz DL, Gedde SJ. New options for combined cataract and glaucoma surgery. *Curr Opin Ophthalmol.* 2014;25:141–147.

It covers procedures for which evidence in peer-reviewed journals exists, including endocyclophotocoagulation (ECP), ab interno trabeculectomy (Trabectome), trabecular micro-bypass stent (iStent), and canaloplasty. Unfortunately, literature on most of these procedures falls short of rigorously controlled randomized clinical trials.

TABLE 3.—Studies of Combined Phacoemulsification and Trabectome

Author (Year)	Treatment	Number of Eyes	Follow-Up (months)	Number (%) Lost to Follow-Up	Change from Baseline Mean IOP (%)	Change from Baseline Mean Meds (%)
Francis (2010) [21]	PE–Trabectome	114	24	47 (41%)	31.1% Decrease	41.7% Decrease
	PE	145		104 (71.7%)	11.7% Decrease	NR
Mosaed *et al.* (2010) [22]	PE–Trabectome	290	12	24 (8%)	22.8% Decrease	33.5% Decrease
Francis and Winarko (2011) [20]	PE–Trabectome	89	12	4 (5%)	30.3% Decrease	43.3% Decrease
Ahuja *et al.* (2013) [23■]	PE–Trabectome	158	24	106 (67%)	22.2% Decrease	31.9% Decrease

IOP, intraocular pressure; meds, glaucoma medications; PE, phacoemulsification; NR, not reported.
Editor's Note: Please refer to original journal article for full references.
Reprinted from Budenz DL, Gedde SJ. New options for combined cataract and glaucoma surgery. *Curr Opin Ophthalmol.* 2014;25:141–147.

Phaco-ECP results show intraocular pressure (IOP) lowering, but studies generally don't include a control group except a trial that was poorly organized (Table 1). Information on phaco-canaloplasty also suffers from lack of rigorous controlled trials. It yields greater IOP lowering but is technically challenging and scars the conjunctiva. Trabectome data are limited by the large number of patients lost to follow-up in the analysis (Table 3).

Phaco-iStent data involve better study design but indicate mild IOP-lowering effect, with most of the device's benefit being in reduction of medication use (Table 2).

If new glaucoma procedures prove effective and safe, better studies may be performed to confirm their benefit as an adjunct to cataract surgery.

S. Fudemberg, MD

Reference

1. Mansouri K, Medeiros FA, Weinreb RN. Global rates of glaucoma surgery. *Graefes Arch Clin Exp Ophthalmol.* 2013;251:2609-2615.

Sustained drug delivery in glaucoma

Knight OJ, Lawrence SD (Univ of North Carolina at Chapel Hill)
Curr Opin Ophthalmol 25:112-117, 2014

Purpose of Review.—This article reviews recently published studies and important clinical trials of novel drug delivery systems for glaucoma and evaluates the potential of these systems to provide sustained therapeutic benefits.

Recent Findings.—The efficacy of topical medications to lower intraocular pressure (IOP) is limited by poor patient adherence, low bioavailability of drug and the potential for local and systemic side effects. Recent studies highlight the potential for sustained drug delivery through innovative delivery platforms. Nanoparticle-based formulations, drug-eluting contact lenses, punctum inserts and bioadhesive matrices placed in the conjunctival sac can enhance drug delivery by increasing precorneal residence time, enhancing corneal permeation and lowering the systemic absorption of drug. Periocular injections and surgically implanted drug reservoirs could offer even greater duration of drug delivery, particularly when the drug is packaged within stable vehicles.

Summary.—Novel platforms for providing sustained drug delivery in glaucoma continue to evolve. The ability to incorporate effective commercially available drugs into more stable compounds is an important element. Although more research is needed to establish their clinical efficacy, novel delivery systems will allow for more targeted medical therapy and for the opportunity to further explore neuroprotective and gene-based therapies.

▶ Minimally invasive glaucoma surgery (MIGS) has captured a tremendous amount of attention in recent years. Sustained-release drug delivery has the potential to provide a similar spark to discussions about glaucoma in the coming years. It's an exciting time for ophthalmologists and glaucoma patients.

We know that glaucoma medications are hugely effective in lowering intraocular pressure (IOP) and preventing blindness from glaucoma. However, their use is limited by expense, side effects, and compliance. Depot medications for glaucoma could be a major breakthrough in reducing the influence of patient compliance on medication efficacy. Furthermore, depending on the location of the depot, the side effect profile of medications may change. For example, the side effect profile of a medication injected inside the eye may differ from topical application (for better or worse). Cost and reimbursement for placement of depot medications will evolve with the possibility of a real impact on the health care system and delivery of glaucoma care.

This article reviews drug delivery in glaucoma. Currently, particular interest is being devoted to injectable systems, medication laden punctal plugs, and devices that fit on the globe and/or in the conjunctival fornices that elute drug.

The pathway for recurring injections of glaucoma medication was paved by the use of anti vascular endothelial growth factor (VEGF) medications for treatment of age-related macular degeneration (ARMD). It is fortuitous that ARMD treatment preceded injectable glaucoma medications. The immediate and profound vision loss characterized by exudative ARMD coupled with the obvious and significant benefit of anti-VEGF agents likely broke down barriers to repeated intraocular injections faster than would have been the case in glaucoma, which is often asymptomatic.

It will take years before many of the products for sustained drug delivery in glaucoma are widely clinically available (if they become available). Patients' response to them will be important. For example, fear of injections could preclude their use. When offered the choice between an eyedrop and an intraocular injection, taking drops may not seem so bad to many patients. Or maybe the opposite will actually be true. Hopefully, the efficacy and tolerability of sustained-release drug delivery systems will be sufficient to drive their adoption.

S. Fudemberg, MD

Intraocular pressure fluctuation and glaucoma progression: what do we know?

Leidl MC, Choi CJ, Syed ZA, et al (Nassau Univ Med Ctr, NY; Harvard Med School, Boston, MA)

Br J Ophthalmol 98:1315-1319, 2014

While mean intraocular pressure (IOP) has long been known to correlate with glaucomatous damage, the role of IOP fluctuation is less clearly defined. There is extensive evidence in the literature for and against the value of short-term and long-term IOP fluctuation in the evaluation and prognosis of patients with glaucoma. We present here the arguments made by both sides, as well as a discussion of the pitfalls of prior research and potential directions for future studies. Until a reliable method is developed that allows for constant IOP monitoring, many variables will continue to hinder us from drawing adequate conclusions regarding the significance of IOP variation.

► Even when following a glaucoma patient closely, one may collect only a handful of intraocular pressure (IOP) measurements over the course of a year. Nonetheless, the IOP measured at follow-up visits plays a significant role in determining the treatment regimen. It is well known that IOP fluctuates in those with and without glaucoma. However, it is not well understood how fluctuation in IOP affects the risk of glaucoma progression. This issue has become more important as increasing data are available from sleep laboratories that record IOP measurements over a period extending beyond typical office hours.[1] Furthermore, advances in technology are yielding new devices for continuous IOP monitoring that will provide a wealth of information about how IOP changes over short and long periods of time.

This article reviews available, and contradictory, studies about IOP fluctuation and glaucoma. There are no standardized time intervals for analysis of short- and long-term IOP fluctuation. Short-term IOP fluctuation may refer to changes over a 24-hour period. Definitions of long-term IOP fluctuation are more variable. The mean IOP, peak IOP, and standard deviation of IOP measurements have all been connected to glaucoma progression in studies. However, findings of other studies call those links into question. No consensus exists.

IOP measurement over a diurnal curve provides many more data points than would otherwise be available for a patient followed for glaucoma on a typical schedule of visits. Continuous IOP monitors provide hugely more information. For example, the Triggerfish telemetric contact lens sensor (Sensimed AG, Lausanne, Switzerland) makes 300 measurements automatically during a 30-second period every 5 minutes and transmits this information to a detector positioned on the orbital rim and then to a recorder worn on the patient's waist. With this information, IOP variation can be recorded over a span of seconds. There are many potential variables that could affect IOP over such short intervals (eye movements, Valsalva maneuver, etc).

Great strides are being made toward gathering data about IOP. Given that IOP is the only known modifiable risk factor for glaucoma, these efforts are fundamentally significant. Unfortunately, data on IOP fluctuation has not coalesced into a clear picture. Enthusiasm for new devices that will deliver exponentially more data about IOP fluctuation is tempered by the fact that we will not immediately know what to do with it.

S. Fudemberg, MD

Reference

1. Holló G, Kóthy P, Vargha P. Evaluation of continuous 24-hour intraocular pressure monitoring for assessment of prostaglandin-induced pressure reduction in glaucoma. *J Glaucoma.* 2014;23:e6-e12.

Nanotechnology and glaucoma: a review of the potential implications of glaucoma nanomedicine

Kim NJ, Harris A, Gerber A, et al (Indiana Univ School of Medicine, Indianapolis)

Br J Ophthalmol 98:427-431, 2014

The purpose of this review is to discuss the evolution of nanotechnology and its potential diagnostic and therapeutic applications in the field of ophthalmology, particularly as it pertains to glaucoma. We reviewed literature using MEDLINE and PubMed databases with the following search terms: glaucoma, nanotechnology, nanomedicine, nanoparticles, ophthalmology and liposomes. We also reviewed pertinent references from articles found in this search. A brief history of nanotechnology and nanomedicine will be covered, followed by a discussion of the advantages and concerns of using this technology in the field of glaucoma. We will look at various studies concerning the development of nanomedicine, its potential applications in ocular drug delivery, diagnostic and imaging modalities and, surgical techniques. In particular, the challenges of assuring safety and efficacy of nanomedicine will be examined. We conclude that nanotechnology offers a novel approach to expanding diagnostic, imaging and surgical modalities in glaucoma and may contribute to the knowledge of disease pathogenesis at a molecular level. However, more research is needed to better elucidate the mechanism of cellular entry, the potential for nanoparticle cytotoxicity and the assurance of clinical efficacy.

▶ The nanoscale ranges from 1 to 100 nanometers, and the authors of this article point out that between 2000 and 2011, governments worldwide invested more than $67 billion in the development of nanotechnology. This review surveys the potential implication of nanotechnology in drug delivery, intraocular pressure

(IOP) measurement, imaging, and treatment of glaucoma. Most projects to date are animal studies and provide a foundation on which nanomedicine at the human level will evolve.

There is tremendous room for improvement in all aspects of glaucoma care. By current standards, drug delivery by topical application to the eye is highly direct, but only a tiny fraction of drug in an eyedrop actually reaches the aqueous humor. Nano-level control over particle size and shape may facilitate major advances in efficiency of drug delivery. For example, experimental nanoparticles loaded with latanoprost have been injected into the subconjunctival space of rabbits to lower IOP. Other nanotechnology concepts help underpin the engineering of small monitors that track biophysical measurements and might ultimately find clinical use in IOP measurement. Nanodevices could be used to aid in aqueous drainage and as adjuncts to transscleral filtration procedures.

Nanotechnology is exciting because the ability to manipulate systems at a molecular level holds broad reaching promise. Although seemingly far from wide clinical application, the significant resources devoted to nanotechnology offer hope for real change.

S. Fudemberg, MD

Teleglaucoma: ready to go?

Strouthidis NG, Chandrasekharan G, Diamond JP, et al (UCL Inst of Ophthalmology, London, UK; Inst of Ophthalmology, London, UK; Bristol Eye Hosp, UK)

Br J Ophthalmol 98:1605-1611, 2014

Telemedicine technologies and services allow today's ophthalmic clinicians to remotely diagnose, manage and monitor several ophthalmic conditions from a distance. But is this the case for glaucomas? There has been a proliferation of telemedicine friendly devices in recent years that improves the capabilities of the clinician in managing glaucomas. The existing instruments still need to align themselves with accepted industry standards. There are successful programmes running in several areas of the world. The safety and efficacy of these programmes needs further exploration. The inability of a single device or test to diagnose glaucomas satisfactorily has also hampered progress in remotely diagnosing these conditions. There is, however, significant potential for telemedicine-friendly devices to remotely monitor the progress of glaucoma, thereby, reduce some of the workload on an overstretched health service.

▶ This article reviews diagnostic information important to identify glaucoma as well as the benefits and limitations of obtaining those data. The essential problem with glaucoma screening is that without a single test, or even a battery of tests, that consistently make the diagnosis, it is difficult to eliminate false negatives (patients with glaucoma who are missed by the screen). Technological advances have increased the range of devices that can collect information remotely and transfer that information for interpretation. Harnessing the power of this technology for glaucoma screening could make a significant public health impact by extending access to underserved populations, but we need to overcome the inherent limitations of screening test for glaucoma.

Intraocular pressure (IOP) measurement is an important part of glaucoma screening. Goldmann applanation remains the gold standard, but it is difficult to use in the field. Noncontact tonometers are improving, and the reliability gap between them and Goldmann applanation has narrowed. Progress on continuous IOP monitoring devices holds promise for providing access to a wealth of data remotely, including in-home monitoring of IOP. Imaging devices are better and easier to use than ever. Nonmydriatic cameras provide high-resolution digital disc photos without dilation, but diagnosis of glaucoma in the absence of extremely normal or abnormal findings is difficult with disc photos alone. Optical coherence tomography (OCT) images could be helpful, especially if serial studies are done over time, but more research is needed to firmly determine the utility of OCT for screening glaucoma patients compared with normals.

At this point, telemedicine lends itself better to stratification of diabetic eye disease by fundus photography than glaucoma screening and diagnosis. The potential of telemedicine is tantalizing given that access to care in the US health care system will be stressed by population dynamics in coming years. Telemedicine would also be a great way to overcome geographic barriers to care. Efforts are underway to pioneer telemedicine networks, but it is still early.

S. Fudemberg, MD

Clinical Outcomes in Cytomegalovirus-Positive Posner-Schlossman Syndrome Patients Treated With Topical Ganciclovir Therapy

Su C-C, Hu F-R, Wang T-H, et al (Natl Taiwan Univ Hosp Hsin-Chu Branch, Taiwan; Natl Taiwan Univ, Taipei)
Am J Ophthalmol 158:1024-1031, 2014

Purpose.—To evaluate the clinical characteristics and therapeutic outcomes of cytomegalovirus (CMV)-positive Posner-Schlossman syndrome patients undergoing topical ganciclovir treatment.

Design.—Retrospective, comparative, and interventional case series.

Methods.—One eye of each of 126 consecutive Posner-Schlossman syndrome patients was investigated using aqueous polymerase chain reaction (PCR) between January 2006 and June 2013. The initial presentations and follow-up data of the CMV-positive patients (68 eyes) and CMV-negative patients (58 eyes) were compared.

Results.—Severe endothelial cell loss ($P < .001$) and a higher number of eyes requiring glaucoma filtering surgery ($P = .017$) were observed in CMV-positive Posner-Schlossman syndrome patients. All CMV-infected eyes treated with continual topical 2% ganciclovir exhibited an undetectable CMV level at the following taps. During follow-up, the average number of antiglaucomatous agents decreased, and a similar frequency of intraocular pressure (IOP) spikes was observed in both groups ($P = .358$).

Patients with CMV-positive eyes with a disease duration over 5 years were likely to require glaucoma surgery (P =.024, log-rank test). All patients receiving surgery exhibited CMV-negative PCR during the IOP attack, but experienced severe peripheral anterior synechiae and pigment clogging. Both groups exhibited a similar endothelial cell decrease (P =.243) and probability of progressive endothelial cell loss (P =.219, log-rank test).

Conclusion.—Ganciclovir treatment was effective for clearing the viral load, assisting the IOP control, and preserving the corneal endothelium of CMV-positive Posner-Schlossman syndrome patients. Early diagnosis and proper treatment could decrease the risk of advanced glaucoma and avoid glaucoma surgery in long-lasting cases.

▶ Posner-Schlossman syndrome (PSS) and Fuchs heterochromic iridocyclitis (FHI) are uncommon causes of anterior uveitis associated with elevated intraocular pressure (IOP). PSS is also known as glaucomatocyclitic crisis and is characterized by unilateral, recurrent episodes of mild, nongranulomatous anterior uveitis with high IOP. FHI also causes mild anterior inflammation that is chronic with formation of posterior subcapsular cataract and significant secondary glaucoma. Unlike PSS, FHI does not respond well to topical steroids. The presence of iris heterochromia in FHI has been overemphasized and is inconsistent, but the lighter colored iris usually indicates the affected eye.

Herpetic anterior uveitis is similar to PSS and FHI in terms of unilaterality, recurrence, small keratic precipitates, iris atrophy, and elevated IOP. Given the similarity, an infectious etiology of PSS and FHI has been sought for years. Relatively recent work with polymerase chain reaction technology indicates that cytomegalovirus may play a significant role in the pathology of PSS and FHI.[1,2]

CMV seems to penetrate and damage the corneal endothelium and trabeculum. This study found that patients with PSS who are also CMV positive tended to have more severe disease with greater endothelial cell loss and worse glaucoma at diagnosis than CMV-negative patients.

Idiopathic uveitis is frustratingly common. Learning of a potentially causal infectious agent is a major breakthrough, but altering the outcome of the disease may still be a challenge. Antiviral therapy could reduce CMV burden and risk of damage to these structures, but recurrence rates are high. This study evaluates topical ganciclovir 2% in CMV-positive patients with PSS. Their findings were positive and indicate that the risk of advanced glaucoma and recurrence of the disease could be decreased by treatment.

S. Fudemberg, MD

References

1. Van Gelder RN. Idiopathic no more: clues to the pathogenesis of Fuchs heterochromic iridocyclitis and glaucomatocyclitic crisis. *Am J Ophthalmol.* 2008;145: 769-771.
2. Chee SP, Jap A. Presumed Fuchs heterochromic iridocyclitis and Posner-Schlossman syndrome: comparison of cytomegalovirus-positive and negative eyes. *Am J Ophthalmol.* 2008;146:883-889.e1.

Three-year Treatment Outcomes in the Ahmed Baerveldt Comparison Study

Barton K, the Ahmed Baerveldt Comparison Study Group (Moorfields Eye Hosp, London, UK; et al)

Ophthalmology 121:1547-1557.e1, 2014

Purpose.—To compare 3-year outcomes and complications of the Ahmed FP7 Glaucoma Valve (AGV) (New World Medical, Cucamonga, CA) and the Baerveldt Glaucoma Implant (BGI) 101-350 (Abbott Medical Optics, Abbott Park, IL) for the treatment of refractory glaucoma.

Design.—Multicenter, randomized, controlled clinical trial.

Participants.—A total of 276 patients: 143 in the AGV group and 133 in the BGI group.

Methods.—Patients aged 18 to 85 years with refractory glaucoma and intraocular pressures (IOPs) ≥18 mmHg in whom an aqueous shunt was planned were randomized to an AGV or a BGI.

Main Outcome Measures.—The IOP, visual acuity (VA), supplemental medical therapy, complications, and failure (IOP >21 mmHg or not reduced by 20% from baseline, IOP <5 mmHg, reoperation for glaucoma or removal of implant, or loss of light perception vision).

Results.—At 3 years, IOP (mean ± standard deviation) was 14.3 ± 4.7 mmHg (AGV group) and 13.1 ± 4.5 mmHg (BGI group)

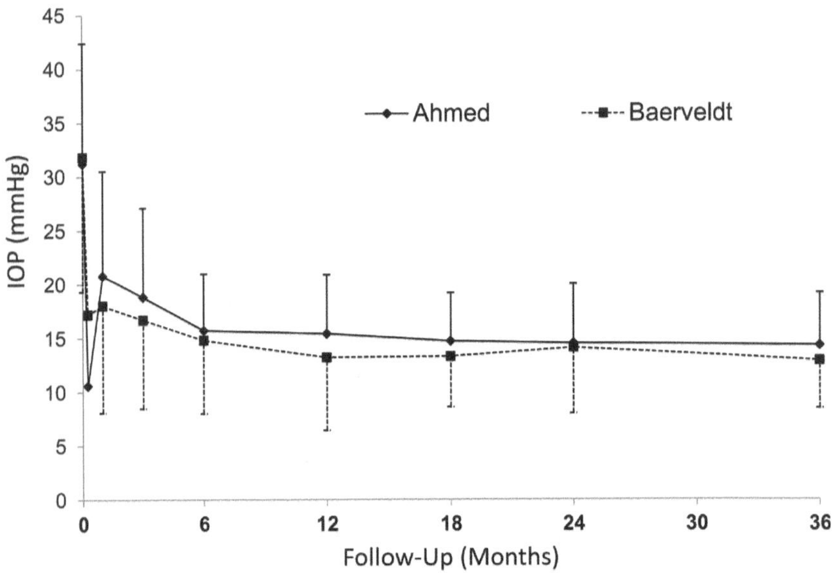

FIGURE 2.—The intraocular pressure (IOP) by randomized treatment group and follow-up visit. Graph of IOP (mmHg) in the Ahmed Baerveldt Comparison Study by randomized study group from preoperative level to last follow-up (mean ± standard deviation). (Reprinted from Ophthalmology. Barton K, the Ahmed Baerveldt Comparison Study Group. Three-year treatment outcomes in the Ahmed Baerveldt comparison study. *Ophthalmology*. 2014;121:1547-1557.e1, Copyright 2014, with permission from the American Academy of Ophthalmology.)

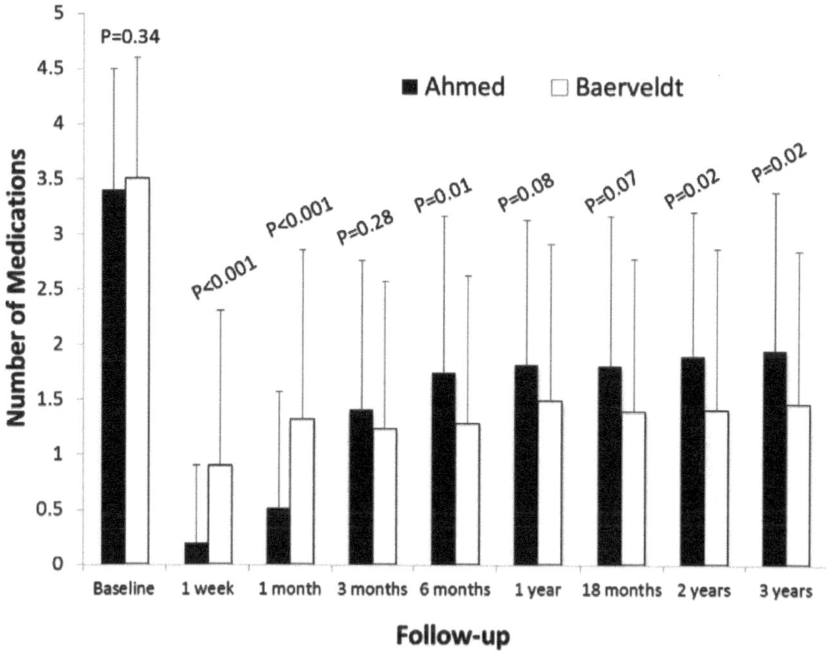

FIGURE 3.—Medication use by randomized treatment group and follow-up visit. Histogram of the number of classes of ocular hypotensive medication used from before surgery to 3-year follow-up visit (mean ± standard deviation). (Reprinted from *Ophthalmology*. Barton K, the Ahmed Baerveldt Comparison Study Group. Three-year treatment outcomes in the Ahmed Baerveldt comparison study. *Ophthalmology*. 2014;121:1547-1557.e1, Copyright 2014, with permission from the American Academy of Ophthalmology.)

($P = 0.086$) on 2.0 ± 1.4 and 1.5 ± 1.4 glaucoma medications, respectively ($P = 0.020$). The cumulative probabilities of failure were 31.3% (standard error [SE], 4.0%) (AGV) and 32.3% (4.2%) (BGI) ($P = 0.99$). Postoperative complications associated with reoperation or vision loss of >2 Snellen lines occurred in 24 patients (22%) (AGV) and 38 patients (36%) (BGI) ($P = 0.035$). The mean change in the logarithm of the minimum angle of resolution VA at 3 years was similar (AGV: 0.21 ± 0.88, BGI: 0.26 ± 0.74) in the 2 treatment groups at 3 years ($P = 0.66$). The cumulative proportion of patients (SE) undergoing reoperation for glaucoma before the 3-year postoperative time point was 14.5% (3.0%) in the AGV group compared with 7.6% (2.4%) in the BGI group ($P = 0.053$, log rank). The relative risk of reoperation for glaucoma in the AGV group was 2.1 times that of the BGI group (95% confidence interval, 1.0–4.8; $P = 0.045$, Cox proportional hazards regression).

Conclusions.—Implantation of the AGV was associated with the need for significantly greater adjunctive medication to achieve equal success relative to implantation of the BGI and resulted in a greater relative risk of

TABLE 2.—Reasons Why Treatment Failure in the Ahmed Baerveldt Comparison Study Were Different by Treatment Group

	Ahmed Group	Baerveldt Group
Inadequate IOP control without additional glaucoma surgery	18 (42)	15 (38)
Reoperation to lower IOP	16 (37)	7 (18)
Explantation for complication	3 (7)	4 (10)
Persistent hypotony*	1 (2)	5 (13)
Loss of light perception	5 (12)	9 (23)
Total	43	40

IOP = intraocular pressure.

Data are presented as number (percentage of the total number of failures in each respective treatment allocation group); $P = 0.109$ (Fisher exact).

There were significantly more failures for IOP elevation and reoperation to lower IOP than other causes of failure ($P = 0.034$).

*IOP ≤5 mm Hg at 2 consecutive visits after 3 months.

Reprinted from *Ophthalmology.* Barton K, the Ahmed Baerveldt Comparison Study Group. Three-year treatment outcomes in the Ahmed Baerveldt comparison study. *Ophthalmology.* 2014;121:1547-1557.e1, Copyright 2014, with permission from the American Academy of Ophthalmology.

reoperation for glaucoma. More subjects experienced serious postoperative complications in the BGI group than in the AGV group (Figs 2 and 3, Table 2).

▶ There are 2 major randomized prospective clinical trials comparing the most commonly used tube shunts, the Ahmed FP7 (AGV) and the Baerveldt BG-101 350 (BGI). The studies are called the Ahmed Baerveldt Comparison study (ABC study) and the Ahmed versus Baerveldt study (AVB study). Both published their 3-year results, the AVB study in 2013[1] and the ABC study in 2014.

Three-year results of the ABC study support the theory that the BGI is more effective but at a greater risk of complications. The failure rates of tube shunts in this study are dramatic. If failure is defined as intraocular pressure (IOP) >17 mm Hg or not reduced by 20%, the cumulative probability of failure is 44% and 37% for the AGV and BGI, respectively. If failure is more strictly defined as IOP >14 or not reduced by 20%, the cumulative probability of failure increases to 67% and 53% for the AGV and BGI, respectively. Patients with AGVs were more likely to fail as a result of inadequate IOP control than those in the BGI group. However, patients in the BGI group were more likely than those in the AGV group to fail as a result of hypotony.

Among those patients who were still defined as successful at 3 years, 80% in the AGV group and 67% in the BGI group required medications to achieve success, and that's with failure defined as IOP >21 mm Hg or not reduced by 20% from baseline. Patients in the AGV were also likely to need more medications at both 2- and 3-year time points.

It is important to note that the case mix in this study was relatively high risk. In comparison, the case mix in the Tube versus Trabeculectomy study was lower risk, and success rates were higher. As well, the AVB study results were similar to the ABC results presented in this article.

Although tubes are an essential part of surgical treatment for glaucoma, in patients with refractory glaucoma, failure is too commonly the outcome.

S. Fudemberg, MD

Reference

1. Christakis PG, Tsai JC, Kalenak JW, et al. The Ahmed versus Baerveldt study: three-year treatment outcomes. *Ophthalmology*. 2013;120:2232-2240.

Increased risk of open-angle glaucoma following chronic rhinosinusitis: a population-based matched-cohort study

Chung S-D, Lin C-C, Ho J-D, et al (Far Eastern Memorial Hosp, Taipei, Taiwan; Taipei Med Univ, Taipei, Taiwan; et al)

Eye 28:225-230, 2014

Purpose.—Anatomically, the eyes and paranasal sinuses are neighboring structures and some studies have mentioned eye disease in conjunction with chronic rhinosinusitis (CRS). However, to the best of our knowledge, no prior research has investigated the risk of developing open-angle glaucoma (OAG) among CRS patients. This study aims to provide an estimated risk of developing OAG among patients with CRS by using a population-based data set in Taiwan.

Methods.—This retrospective cohort study used data sourced from the 'Longitudinal Health Insurance Database 2000'. A total of 15 642 CRS patients were included in the study cohort and 46 926 subjects were randomly extracted as a comparison cohort. A cox proportional-hazards regression analysis was performed to calculate the 5-year risk of subsequently developing OAG following a diagnosis of CRS between the study cohort and the comparison cohort.

Results.—The incidence rate of developing OAG over the 5-year follow-up period was 5.45 (95% CI: 4.95–5.98) per 1000 person-years for the study cohort and 2.80 (95% CI: 2.60–3.03) per 1000 person-years for the comparison cohort. After censoring the cases that died over the 5-year period and adjusting for the factors of monthly income, geographic region, hypertension, diabetes, coronary heart disease, hyperlipidemia, and hypothyroidism the hazard ratio for developing OAG over the 5-year period for subjects with CRS to subjects without CRS was 1.73 (95% CI: 1.53–1.96).

Conclusion.—We found that those subjects with CRS had a significantly higher risk of developing OAG over the 5-year follow-up period as compared with subjects without CRS (Tables 1 and 2).

▶ Patients may ask about a connection between conditions affecting the paranasal sinuses and ocular conditions such as glaucoma, perhaps as a result of the anatomic proximity of the eyes and sinuses and potential to cause discomfort. Although the pathophysiology of chronic rhinosinusitis (CRS) is complex, it

TABLE 1.—Demographic Characteristics of Subjects With Chronic Rhinosinusitis and Comparison Subjects in Taiwan (*n* = 62 568)

Variable	Subjects with Chronic Rhinosinusitis (n = 15 642) Total no.	%	Comparison Subjects (n = 46 26) Total no.	%	*P* Value
Sex					1.000
Male	7247	46.3	21 741	46.3	
Female	8395	53.7	25 185	53.7	
Age (years)					1.000
18–29	3874	24.8	11 622	24.8	
30–39	3862	24.7	11 586	24.7	
40–49	3424	21.9	10 272	21.9	
50–59	2250	14.4	6750	14.4	
60–69	1321	8.4	3963	8.4	
≥70	911	5.8	2733	5.8	
Urbanization level					1.000
1 (Most urbanized)	5288	33.8	15 864	33.8	
2	4571	29.2	13 713	29.2	
3	2648	17.0	7944	17.0	
4	1896	12.1	5688	12.1	
5 (Least urbanized)	1239	7.9	3717	7.9	
Monthly income					0.072
0	4315	27.6	13 224	28.2	
NT$1–15 840	2489	15.9	7468	15.9	
NT$15 841–25 000	5286	33.8	16 035	34.2	
≥NT$25 001	3552	22.7	10 199	21.7	
Geographic region					0.182
Northern	7602	48.6	23 122	49.3	
Central	4183	26.7	12 330	26.3	
Southern	3520	22.5	10 381	22.1	
Eastern	337	2.2	1093	2.3	
Hypertension	3334	21.3	8076	17.2	<0.001
Diabetes	1831	11.7	4238	9.0	<0.001
Hyperlipidemia	2775	17.7	6261	13.3	<0.001
Coronary heart disease	1844	11.8	3737	8.0	<0.001
Hypothyroidism	143	0.9	182	0.4	<0.001

involves hypoxia and inflammation. The pathophysiology of glaucoma is incompletely understood, but there is increasing interest in the role of cardiovascular and circulatory issues in glaucoma.

This study used data from a large national insurance database in Taiwan to compare matched cohorts of people with and without CRS. The authors found that the risk of developing glaucoma was significantly higher among patients with CRS. Information from insurance databases facilitates inclusion of a large number of study subjects but introduces a risk of surveillance bias. The patients with CRS probably engaged with the medical system more frequently than those with fewer health issues, which could affect their likelihood of being diagnosed with glaucoma as well as other diseases. Additionally, patients with CRS may need corticosteroids that could contribute to their higher rate of glaucoma diagnosis. More information is needed to connect

TABLE 2.—Incidence Rate, Crude, and Adjusted Hazard Ratio for Open-Angle Glaucoma Among the Sampled Patients

Presence of Open-Angle Glaucoma	Total (n = 62 568) No.	%	Subjects with Chronic Rhinosinusitis (n = 15 642) No.	%	Comparison Subjects (n = 46 926) No.	%
5-Year follow-up period						
Yes	1111	1.8	426	2.7	658	1.5
Incidence rate per 1000 Person-years (95% CI)	3.82 (3.61–4.04)		5.45 (4.95–5.98)		2.80 (2.60–3.03)	
Adjusted[a,b] HR (95% CI)	—		1.73* (1.53–1.96)		1.00	

*$P < 0.001$.

[a]Hazard ratio was calculated by using stratified Cox proportional regression (stratified on sex, age group, urbanization level, and the year of index date) with cases censored if individuals died during the 5-year follow-up period.

[b]Adjustment for patient's monthly income, geographic region, hypertension, diabetes, coronary heart disease, hyperlipidemia, and hypothyroidism.

glaucoma with sinusitis, but this study indicates that the 2 conditions may be related.

S. Fudemberg, MD

Effect of Early Treatment with Aqueous Suppressants on Ahmed Glaucoma Valve Implantation Outcomes

Pakravan M, Rad SS, Yazdani S, et al (Shahid Beheshti Univ of Med Sciences, Tehran, Iran; et al)

Ophthalmology 121:1693-1698, 2014

Objective.—To evaluate the effect of early aqueous suppressant treatment on Ahmed glaucoma valve (AGV) surgery outcomes.

Design.—Randomized clinical trial.

Participants.—Ninety-four eyes of 94 patients with refractory glaucoma.

Methods.—After AGV implantation, 47 cases (group 1) received topical timolol-dorzolamide fixed-combination drops twice daily when intraocular pressure (IOP) exceeded 10 mmHg, whereas 47 controls (group 2) received conventional stepwise treatment when IOP exceeded target pressure.

Main Outcome Measures.—Main outcome measures included IOP and success rate (6 mmHg < IOP < 15 mmHg and IOP reduction of at least 30% from baseline). Other outcome measures included best-corrected visual acuity, complications, and hypertensive phase frequency.

Results.—Groups 1 and 2 were both followed up for a mean of 45 ± 11.6 and 47.2 ± 7.4 weeks, respectively ($P = 0.74$). Mixed model analysis revealed a significantly greater IOP reduction in group 1 at all intervals ($P < 0.001$). At 1 year, the cases exhibited a significantly higher

TABLE 2.—Intraocular Pressure Changes during the Study Period

Time	Group 1 Mean ± Standard Deviation	Range	Group 2 Mean ± Standard Deviation	Range	*P* Value*
Baseline	30.9±9.3	16–56	31.8±9.3	13–56	0.691
Day1	11.1±8.0	2–50	12.2±6.0	0–34	0.063
Week 1	10.2±6.5	0–38	13.1±7.2	0–46	0.003
Week 2	10.6±6.0	2–24	14.3±7.6	0–46	0.005
Week 3	10.8±5.3	2–23	16.3±7.7	0–46	<0.001
Week 4	12.8±5.3	6–32	17.0±4.9	7–28	0.001
Week 6	14.6±6.1	3–29	18.0±4.2	9–28	0.001
Week 12	14.2±5.4	4–22	18.3±5.1	6–30	<0.001
Week 24	13.1±3.8	2–24	16.9±4.1	8–28	<0.001
Week 54	14.0±4.5	0–22	16.8±4.4	9–28	0.012

Group 1 comprised patients receiving early treatment with timolol plus dorzolamide. Group 2 comprised the controls.
*Mann–Whitney *U* test for baseline and analysis of covariance for follow-up visits.
Reprinted from *Ophthalmology*. Pakravan M, Rad SS, Yazdani S, et al. Effect of Early Treatment with Aqueous Suppressants on Ahmed Glaucoma Valve Implantation Outcomes. *Ophthalmology*. 2014;121:1693-1698, Copyright 2014, with permission from the American Academy of Ophthalmology.

TABLE 3.—Number of Glaucoma Medications* Administered during the Study

Time	Overall Mean ± Standard Deviation	Range	Group 1 Mean ± Standard Deviation	Range	Group 2 Mean ± Standard Deviation	Range	*P* Value†
Baseline	3.6±0.6	3–5	3.7±0.6	3–5	3.6±0.6	3–5	0.650
Day 1	0±0	0–0	0±0	0–0	0±0	0–0	>0.99
Week 1	0±0	0–0	0±0	0–0	0±0	0–0	>0.99
Week 2	0.5±0.8	0–3	0.8±1.0	0–3	0.2±0.5	0–2	<0.001
Week 3	0.6±0.9	0–3	1.2±1.1	0–3	0.3±0.6	0–2	<0.001
Week 4	0.9±1.0	0–3	1.5±1.0	0–3	0.4±0.6	0–2	<0.001
Week 6	1.2±0.9	0–3	1.9±0.8	0–3	0.7±0.7	0–2	<0.001
Week 12	1.4±0.9	0–4	1.8±0.8	0–3	1.1±0.9	0–4	<0.001
Week 24	1.6±1.0	0–4	1.7±1.0	0–3	1.5±1.0	0–4	0.158
Week 54	1.7±1.0	0–4	1.8±1.1	0–4	1.6±1.0	0–4	0.184

Group 1 comprised those who received early treatment with timolol plus dorzolamide. Group 2 comprised the controls.
*We considered the timolol-dorzolamide fixed combination as two medications.
†Mann–Whitney *U* test for baseline and ordinal logistic test for follow-up visits.
Reprinted from *Ophthalmology*. Pakravan M, Rad SS, Yazdani S, et al. Effect of Early Treatment with Aqueous Suppressants on Ahmed Glaucoma Valve Implantation Outcomes. *Ophthalmology*. 2014;121:1693-1698, Copyright 2014, with permission from the American Academy of Ophthalmology.

success rate (63.2% vs. 33.3%; $P = 0.008$) and reduced hypertensive phase frequency (23.4% vs. 66.0%; $P < 0.001$).

Conclusions.—Early aqueous suppressant treatment may improve AGV implantation outcomes in terms of IOP reduction, success rate, and hypertensive phase frequency (Tables 2 and 3).

▶ Ahmed glaucoma valves (AGV) are typically less effective, but with fewer serious complications than the Baerveldt glaucoma implant (BGI) (see review of the ABC Study 3-year data above). The plate of a BGI 350 has a larger surface area than that of an AGV, which may play a role in its greater efficacy. Another theory is that the AGV permits more early flow of aqueous to the plate than a BGI, which is nonvalved and typically occluded in the early postoperative period. There may be something about the effect of aqueous on the conjunctiva and Tenon capsule that causes more inflammation and scarring, which limits the overall success of the AGV. Studies indicate that the contents of glaucomatous aqueous humor trigger an inflammatory response when they come into contact with the conjunctiva and Tenon's capsule. Furthermore, the postoperative course of an AGV is frequently characterized by a hypertensive phase a few weeks after implantation that corresponds with apparent thickening and scarring of the bleb overlying its plate.

This study is a randomized controlled trial to examine the effect of early aqueous suppression on the outcome of the AGV. Not surprisingly, medication use among the intervention group was statistically significantly greater than the control group between weeks 2 and 12. Intraocular pressure (IOP) was statistically significantly lower in the intervention group from week 1 to week 24. By week 54, IOP remained clinically lower but did not achieve statistical significance.

Ultimately, additional information from time points extending beyond 1 year may help elucidate whether minimizing the early flow of aqueous yields better overall success for AGVs. The results of this study indicate that it is at least a possibility.

S. Fudemberg, MD

A Method to Estimate the Amount of Neuroretinal Rim Tissue in Glaucoma: Comparison With Current Methods for Measuring Rim Area

Gardiner SK, Ren R, Yang H, et al (Legacy Res Inst, Portland, OR)

Am J Ophthalmol 157:540-549.e2, 2014

Purpose.—To test whether the minimum rim area assessed by spectral domain optical coherence tomography (SD-OCT), based on the shortest distance from the Bruch membrane opening (BMO) to the inner limiting membrane, corresponds more closely to retinal nerve fiber layer (RNFL) thickness and visual field mean deviation (MD) than current rim measures in early glaucoma.

Design.—Prospective cross-sectional study.

Methods.—We studied 221 participants with non-endstage glaucoma or high-risk ocular hypertension and performed standard automated perimetry. We received SD-OCT and confocal scanning laser ophthalmoscopy (CSLO) scans on the same day. Rim area measured by CSLO was compared with 3 SD-OCT rim measures from radial B-scans: horizontal rim area between BMO and inner limiting membrane within the BMO plane; mean minimum rim width (BMO-MRW); and minimum rim area (BMO-MRA) optimized within sectors and then summed. Correlations

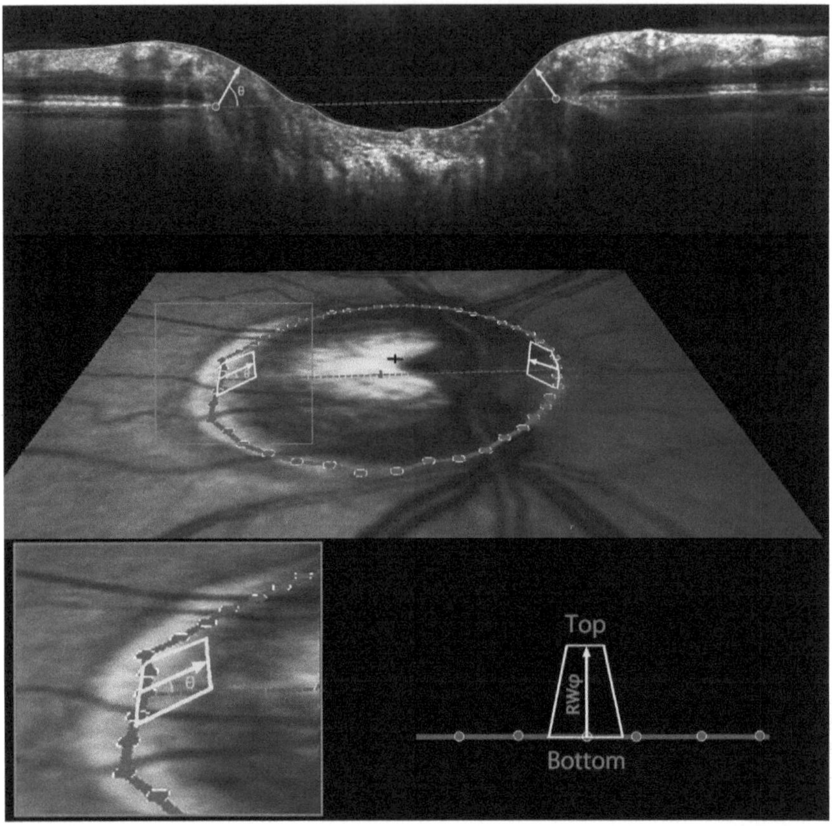

FIGURE 2.—Definition and calculation of the Bruch membrane opening minimum rim width and minimum rim area, as used to estimate the amount of neuroretinal rim tissue in glaucoma (top). Within each of the 24 radial scans, the Bruch membrane opening was delineated (red circles). The minimum rim width within that sector was defined as the shortest distance from this point to the inner limiting membrane (yellow arrow, at angle θ above the Bruch membrane opening plane). These were averaged across sectors to give the global measure of the Bruch membrane opening minimum rim width (middle panel). Within each sector, rim areas (yellow trapezoids) were calculated as the areas of trapezia at varying angles above the Bruch membrane opening plane. The height of each trapezium equals the rim width at this angle, referred to as RW_θ. The base equals the circumference within that sector, $2\pi r/48$, where r represents the distance from the Bruch membrane opening centroid (red cross). The top then has length $2\pi r/48 \times (r - RW_\theta * \cos(\theta))$ (bottom panel). Within each sector, the smallest such area was found, at angle φ, and its area calculated as $(top+bottom) \times RW_\varphi/2$. Note that RWφ will not always be the minimum rim width within this sector, as illustrated in Supplementary Figure S1. The global measure BMO-MRA is generated by summing the areas of these 48 trapeziums. For Interpretation of the references to color in this figure legend, the reader is referred to web version of this article. (Reprinted from *American Journal of Ophthalmology*. Gardiner SK, Ren R, Yang H, et al. A method to estimate the amount of neuroretinal rim tissue in glaucoma: comparison with current methods for measuring rim area. *Am J Ophthalmol.* 2014;157:540-549.e2, Copyright 2014, with permission from Elsevier.)

between these measures and either MD from perimetry or RNFL thickness from SD-OCT were compared using the Steiger test.

Results.—RNFL thickness was better correlated with BMO-MRA ($r = 0.676$) or BMO-MRW ($r = 0.680$) than with either CSLO rim area (r = 0.330, $P < 0.001$) or horizontal rim area (r = 0.482, $P < 0.001$). MD was better correlated with BMO-MRA (r = 0.534) or BMO-MRW (r = 0.546) than with either CSLO rim area (r = 0.321, $P < 0.001$) or horizontal rim area (0.403, $P < 0.001$). The correlation between MD and RNFL thickness was r = 0.646.

Conclusions.—Minimum rim measurements from SD-OCT are significantly better correlated to both RNFL thickness and MD than rim measurements within the BMO plane or based on the clinical disc margin. They provide new structural parameters for both diagnostic and research purposes in glaucoma (Fig 2).

▶ Correlation between structure and function in glaucoma is an exciting prospect but has been difficult in practice. Instruments that measure structure and function are subject to potentially significant inter- and intraindividual variability, which makes structure-function relationships hard to determine. Optical coherence tomography (OCT) testing in glaucoma may provide objective data, but how that data should be applied to guide glaucoma management is not concrete. This study aims to identify parameters that better relate OCT results to functional decline in visual field.

Neuroretinal rim thinning corresponds with glaucoma progression, and sufficient thinning yields vision loss. Quantification of neuroretinal rim loss is predicated on defining the boundaries of the optic disc and also the rim. OCT may provide a better way to consistently set these boundaries than clinical examination because it gives a more detailed view of the anatomy. The area extending from Bruch membrane opening to the inner limiting membrane, as identified by spectral domain OCT, may be a good landmark by which to define the rim. Therefore, the authors provide a way to measure mean minimum rim width and area to create new parameters that could be determined in OCT. They also provide some evidence that these parameters may hold clinical utility. This is an important step toward further utilizing the power of OCT to determine glaucoma progression and guide management.

S. Fudemberg, MD

Ocular hypertension: an approach to assessment and management

Boey PY, Mansberger SL (Devers Eye Inst, Portland, Ore; Singapore Natl Eye Centre)

Can J Ophthalmol 49:489-496, 2014

Ocular hypertension is a common and important problem seen by eye care providers. This review presents a practical approach to individuals with ocular hypertension. It describes the common functional and structural investigations used in evaluation, as well as the advantages and disadvantages of each test. This review also discusses several landmark studies on ocular hypertension and provides a practical guide to the management of this problem.

▶ This article is an excellent review of the pertinent information we use to guide management of glaucoma suspects. Although the factors weighed to determine treatment decisions for these patients are familiar, it is helpful to flesh out the details. As an example, central corneal thickness (CCT) is well known to influence the risk of glaucoma. However, its application may be variable in clinical practice. The clinical definition of thin vs thick CCT is not standardized, and different practitioners may use different thresholds. Although no algorithm has been proven useful for adjusting intraocular pressure measurement for CCT, some doctors still use them. Controversy may be found in the fine points of even broadly accepted tenets of glaucoma care, and looking at a review of the evidence is enlightening. The authors take on risk calculators, disc photography, Heidelberg retinal tomography, optical coherence tomography (including recent and important work regarding new ways to define the optic disc margin using Bruch membrane opening), and perimetry. In a perfect world, specific evidence-based guidelines would make it simple to analyze the risk to an individual patient and the most cost-effective way, on a societal basis, to determine when and whom to treat. We are not there yet.

S. Fudemberg, MD

Effect of Focal Lamina Cribrosa Defect on Glaucomatous Visual Field Progression

Faridi OS, Park SC, Kabadi R, et al (New York Eye and Ear Infirmary of Mount Sinai; New York Med College, Valhalla; et al)
Ophthalmology 121:1524-1530, 2014

Objective.—To evaluate the association between focal, structural defects of the lamina cribrosa (LC) and glaucomatous visual field (VF) progression.

Design.—Retrospective, observational study.

Participants.—A total of 169 patients with glaucoma (169 eyes) with a range of glaucomatous damage.

Methods.—Serial horizontal and vertical enhanced-depth imaging optical coherence tomography (EDI OCT) B-scans of the optic nerve head were obtained from patients with glaucoma with 5 or more prior Humphrey 24-2 VFs (Carl Zeiss Meditec, Inc, Dublin, CA). The EDI OCT scans were reviewed for the presence of focal LC defects (laminar holes or disinsertions with a diameter >100 μm). The VF progression was defined as having ≥2 significantly progressing test points (with a slope calculated using pointwise linear regression [PLR], worse than −1.0 dB/year at $P < 0.01$). Age, intraocular pressure (IOP), baseline VF mean deviation (MD), disc hemorrhage, and central corneal thickness (CCT) were recorded.

Main Outcome Measures.—The relationship between focal LC defects and the rate and risk of VF progression.

Results.—Mean age and VF MD at the time of EDI OCT were 69 ± 12 years and −11.49 ± 6.87 dB, respectively. Sixty eyes (36%) progressed according to PLR criteria. Progression was more common in eyes with, rather than without, focal LC defects (38/81 eyes [47%] vs. 22/88 eyes [25%], $P = 0.003$). Among the evaluated parameters, the presence of focal LC defects, disc hemorrhage, higher mean follow-up IOP, greater number of VFs, and longer follow-up period were significantly associated with VF progression in the multivariable analyses (odds ratios, 2.90, 4.66, 1.22, 1.25, and 1.27, respectively; $P = 0.010$, $P = 0.002$, $P = 0.002$, $P < 0.001$, and $P < 0.001$, respectively). The mean global progression rate was significantly faster in the group with focal LC defect than in the group with no focal LC defect (−0.54 ± 0.99 dB/year vs. −0.28 ± 0.52 dB/year; $P = 0.031$). Among the 60 progressing eyes, despite no significant difference in the mean number of progressing VF points per eye (6.7 ± 7.0 vs. 6.5 ± 4.4; $P = 0.899$), the mean localized progression rate was significantly

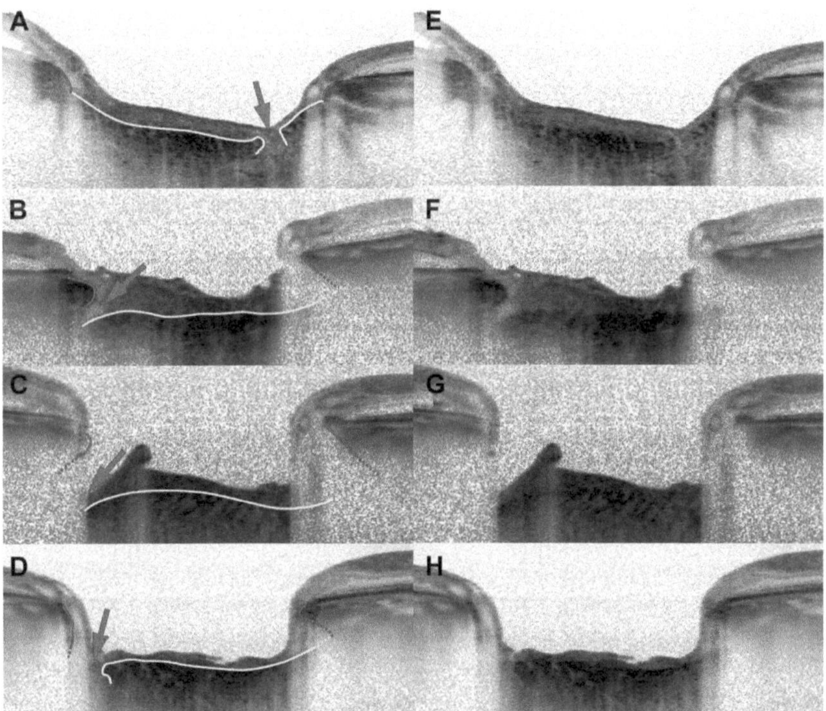

FIGURE 1.—Enhanced-depth imaging optical coherence tomography (OCT) scans of glaucomatous optic discs (**A–D**) and the same images without the labels (**E–H**). A, Laminar hole (*red arrow*). **B** and C, Laminar disinsertions (*red arrows*). **D**, Focal lamina cribrosa (LC) defect with combined features of a laminar hole and a laminar disinsertion (*red arrow*). Red lines indicate the border tissue of Elschnig and scleral canal wall. *Yellow lines* indicate the anterior surface of the LC. *Dotted lines* indicate extrapolation. For Interpretation of the references to color in this figure legend, the reader is referred to web version of this article. (Reprinted from *Ophthalmology.* Faridi OS, Park SC, Kabadi R, et al. Effect of focal lamina cribrosa defect on glaucomatous visual field progression. *Ophthalmology.* 2014;121:1524-1530, Copyright 2014, with permission from American Academy of Ophthalmology.)

TABLE 1.—Number of Eyes with Visual Field Progression in the Group with Focal Lamina Cribrosa Defect and the Group with No Focal Lamina Cribrosa Defect.

	Progression	No Progression	Total
Focal LC defects	38 eyes	43 eyes	81 eyes
No Focal LC defects	22 eyes	66 eyes	88 eyes
Total	60 eyes	109 eyes	169 eyes

LC = lamina cribrosa.

Eyes with VF progression were defined as having at least 2 significantly progressing test points (a progression rate worse than −1.0 dB/yr with $P < 0.01$).

(Reprinted from *Ophthalmology*. Faridi OS, Park SC, Kabadi R, et al. Effect of focal lamina cribrosa defect on glaucomatous visual field progression. *Ophthalmology*. 2014;121:1524-1530, Copyright 2014, with permission from American Academy of Ophthalmology.)

faster in the eyes with focal LC defects than in the eyes with no focal LC defects (−2.85 ± 1.85 dB/year vs. −1.75 ± 0.56 dB/year; $P = 0.009$).

Conclusions.—Focal LC defects are strongly associated with glaucomatous VF progression, and eyes with focal LC defects tend to progress faster than those without (Fig 1; Table 1).

▶ Recently, the lamina cribosa is getting more attention as a potentially important cause and/or marker of glaucoma damage. The lamina cribosa is a conduit for retinal ganglion cells and blood vessels through the scleral canal. Changes in the collagen beams that compose the lamina may be directly related to optic nerve damage in glaucoma. Optical coherence tomography imaging provides a way to examine the lamina, and this study correlated its appearance with visual field progression. Visual field progression was statistically significantly more common among eyes with defects in the lamina cribosa. Additionally, visual field progression among patients with laminar defects occurred at a faster rate. This study evaluated the lamina of patients for whom visual field data were already available. Therefore, one cannot determine if the laminar defects occurred as a result of progression or preceded, and might be a marker for, progression. Ultimately, the identification of visual field progression is not perfectly standardized, and neither is identification of defects in the lamina cribosa. Nonetheless, this article is a compelling demonstration of a relationship between them and an exciting step toward understanding the importance of the lamina cribosa in the pathology of glaucoma.

S. Fudemberg, MD

Effectiveness of Intraocular Pressure–Lowering Medication Determined by Washout

Jampel HD, Chon BH, Stamper R, et al (Johns Hopkins Univ, Baltimore, MD, Duke Univ, Durham, NC; Univ of California, San Francisco; et al)

JAMA Ophthalmol 132:390-395, 2014

Importance.—While medication efficacy is well documented in clinical trials, less is known of medication effectiveness in real-world clinical settings.

Objective.—To assess the effectiveness of intraocular pressure (IOP)–lowering medications in patients with open-angle glaucoma.

Design, Setting, and Participants.—Prospective, multicenter, interventional cohort from the prerandomization phase of a randomized clinical trial at multiple ophthalmology clinics. A total of 603 patients (603 eyes) with primary open-angle glaucoma who were using up to 3 glaucoma medications were included.

Interventions.—One IOP measurement was made while the patient was using his or her usual medications to lower IOP (ON IOP). Eligible participants underwent washout of all IOP-lowering drops, and the diurnal IOP was measured 2 to 4 weeks later (OFF IOP).

Main Outcomes and Measures.—Difference between OFF IOP and ON IOP. The hypothesis was formulated after data collection.

Results.—The mean (SD) ON IOPs for participants using 0 (n = 102), 1 (n = 272), 2 (n = 147), or 3 (n = 82) medications were 24.2 (3.2), 17.5 (3.2), 17.2 (3.1), and 17.2 (3.1) mm Hg, respectively. Patients not using medication had a mean (SD) IOP decrease of 0.2 (2.8) mm Hg at the OFF visit. Patients using 1, 2, and 3 medications had mean (SD) IOP increases of 5.4 (3.0), 6.9 (3.3), and 9.0 (3.8) mm Hg, respectively, at the OFF visit. The percentages of patients with less than a 25% increase in IOP were 38%, 21%, and 13% for those using 1, 2, and 3 medications, respectively.

Conclusions and Relevance.—Discontinuation of 1, 2, and 3 medications was associated with a clinically significant increase in IOP, although with smaller effects for the second and third medications compared with the first medication. A substantial proportion of patients showed only small changes in IOP after medication washout, suggesting either that they were not using the medication effectively or that the medication itself, although used properly, was not lowering the IOP.

Trial Registration.—clinicaltrials.gov Identifier: NCT01085357.

▶ This study provides evidence to support the fundamental concept that glaucoma medications function synergistically to lower intraocular pressure (IOP). Multiple medication use in the treatment of glaucoma is commonplace. Data from the Ocular Hypertension Treatment Study revealed that, even with a relatively modest IOP lowering goal of 20% and IOP ≤24 mm Hg, by 5 years, about 40% of patients required more than 1 medication.[1] The analysis in this article uses data from patients who were washed out of all glaucoma medications in preparation for randomization to treatment with cataract extraction alone or cataract extraction and placement of a CyPass microstent. The CyPass device shunts aqueous into the suprachoroidal space.

When medications were withdrawn, the IOP increased by 33%, 43%, and 55% for patients on 1, 2, or 3 glaucoma drops, respectively. This clearly indicates that adjunctive therapy is more effective at IOP lowering than monotherapy and that the more the medications added, the larger the IOP change. It also shows that the adjunctive agents had less effect than the first medication.

Although these concepts are already widely accepted, the benefit of solid evidence to back clinical practice in glaucoma management has been taken for granted in the past. The information in this study is useful and important.

S. Fudemberg, MD

Reference

1. Kass MA, Heuer DK, Higginbotham EJ, et al. The ocular hypertension treatment study: a randomized trial determines that ocular hypotensive medication delays or prevents the onset of primary open-angle glaucoma. *Arch Ophthalmol.* 2002;120: 701-713.

Glucose-Induced Temporary Visual Recovery in Primary Open-Angle Glaucoma: A Double-Blind, Randomized Study

Casson RJ, Han G, Ebneter A, et al (Univ of Adelaide, South Australia)

Ophthalmology 121:1203-1211, 2014

Purpose.—To investigate the effect of topical glucose on visual parameters in individuals with primary open-angle glaucoma (POAG).

Design.—Double-blind, randomized, crossover study.

Participants.—Nondiabetic pseudophakic patients with definite POAG were recruited; 29 eyes of 16 individuals participated in study 1. A follow-up study (study 2) included 14 eyes of 7 individuals.

Intervention.—Eyes were randomly allocated to receive 50% glucose or saline eye drops every 5 minutes for 60 minutes.

Main Outcome Measures.—The contrast sensitivity and best-corrected logarithm of the minimum angle of resolution (logMAR).

Results.—The 50% glucose reached the vitreous in pseudophakic but not phakic individuals. Glucose significantly improved the mean contrast sensitivity at 12 cycles/degree compared with 0.9% saline by 0.26 log units (95% confidence interval [CI], 0.13–0.38; $P < 0.001$) and 0.40 log units (95% CI, 0.17–0.60; $P < 0.001$) in the follow-up study. The intraocular pressure, refraction, and central corneal thickness were not affected by glucose; age was not a significant predictor of the response.

Conclusions.—Topical glucose temporarily improves psychophysical visual parameters in some individuals with POAG, suggesting that neuronal energy substrate delivery to the vitreous reservoir may recover function of "sick" retinal neurons.

▶ Glaucoma damage is generally considered to be irreversible. It is possible that there is a period after a retinal ganglion cell (RGC) is injured, but before it dies, that it is "sick" and may be saved. This study applies concepts from bench and animal research to test the hypothesis that "sick" RGCs may experience neurorecovery.

The vascular theory of glaucoma, which remains unproven, indicates that ischemic damage to the optic nerve head could be responsible for glaucoma damage in some people. Ocular perfusion pressure (OPP), the relationship between systemic blood pressure and intraocular pressure, may become too low in certain glaucoma patients, resulting in insufficient blood flow to the optic nerve. Especially as cardiologists become increasingly effective at achieving low blood pressure, low OPP may put these patients at risk of glaucoma or worsening glaucoma. Nonetheless, it is important to note that vascular theory of glaucoma is just 1 of the theories receiving attention in the search for the cause of glaucoma. The literature does not conclusively support raising blood pressure in glaucoma patients.

Elevated vitreous glucose levels have been shown to provide neuroprotective benefits in experimental models of retinal ischemia. In the initial phase of this study, a group of patients undergoing vitrectomy for epiretinal membrane peel or macular hole repair were given topical glucose drops before surgery. The authors found that vitreal glucose levels increased in pseudophakic but not phakic patients. Then, in phase 2, they performed a crossover study treating patients with topical glucose drops versus 0.9% saline drops separated by a washout period. Treatment with glucose improved the contrast sensitivity of these patients when compared with saline drops.

This research is particularly interesting because it supports the theory that a population of "sick" RGSs may exist and that an intervention could promote their recovery, which is a step forward in the quest for neuroprotection in glaucoma.

S. Fudemberg, MD

Examining Visual Field Loss in Patients in Glaucoma Clinics During Their Predicted Remaining Lifetime

Saunders LJ, Russell RA, Kirwan JF, et al (City Univ London, UK; Queen Alexandra Hosp, Portsmouth, UK; et al)
Invest Ophthalmol Vis Sci 55:102-109, 2014

Purpose.—To evaluate the proportion of patients in glaucoma clinics progressing at rates that would result in visual disability within their expected lifetime.

Methods.—This retrospective study used visual field (VF) series of at least 3 years' duration from 3790 UK patients in glaucoma clinics calculating rates of loss for each eye using linear regression of mean deviation (MD) over time. Residual life expectancies derived from the UK Office of National Statistics actuarial tables for each patient were combined with these rates to estimate predicted MDs at end of expected lifetime. The proportion of patients projected to progress to visual impairment (MD: −14 dB or worse) or statutory blindness (MD: −22 dB or worse) in both eyes before end of expected lifetime was calculated.

Results.—Only 3.0% (95% confidence interval [CI] 2.7%–3.4%) of patient eyes progressed at faster than −1.5 dB/year (n = 7149 eyes). Of those patients with both eyes followed, 5.2% (CI 4.5%–6.0%) were predicted to progress to statutory blindness, with a further 10.4% (CI 9.4%–11.4%) reaching visual impairment in their lifetime. More than 90% (CI

85.7%–94.3%) of patients predicted to progress to statutory blindness, had an MD worse than −6 dB in at least one eye at presentation.

Conclusions.—This modeling exercise indicates that most patients in glaucoma clinics are not at high risk of progressing to statutory blindness. The likelihood of patients suffering impairment in their lifetimes is linked to VF loss at presentation, which illuminates the importance of reliably detecting significant VF defects in primary care.

▶ Defining progression in glaucoma is one of the most critical problems facing our field. Without an effective and efficient way to identify patients who progress, studying methods to reduce progression is expensive and cumbersome. As long as studying progression is difficult, our ability to evaluate glaucoma management using evidence-based medicine will be limited. Studies have shown that using visual fields to define progression, even with the most basic criteria, may require 6 visual fields.[1] Moreover, the number of fields necessary to identify progression is dependent on assumptions about the rate at which the patients are progressing and the sensitivity with which progression is found. Research on biomarkers for progression and defining progression by changes in structure, rather than functional changes evaluated by visual fields, is fundamentally important.

This study evaluated visual field data from a large group of glaucoma clinic patients in the United Kingdom. The information obtained about the rate of progression is particularly interesting because rate of progression plays a central role in our ability to identify progression. The authors took their analysis a step further. They used actuarial data to determine, based on progression rates, whether the patients would develop sufficient visual field defects to qualify as disabled or blind. Their focus on disability reinforces the concept that visual field damage must reach a threshold before it actually affects an individual's quality of life. For example, a mild nasal step defect may never be noticed by the patient although it appears on our tests.

Treatment for glaucoma does affect quality of life. Medications, lasers, and surgery risk side effects and involve costs—monetary as well as in time and energy. If we strive to minimize glaucoma's negative effect on quality of life, then it would be helpful to know in whom the disease itself would inhibit quality of life as opposed to those who will never reach that degree of glaucoma damage. Unfortunately, actuarial tables work better when applied to a population than an individual. We might be able to approximate when a population will die, but individual life expectancy is harder to predict.

S. Fudemberg, MD

Reference

1. Chauhan BC, Garway-Heath DF, Goñi FJ, et al. Practical recommendations for measuring rates of visual field change in glaucoma. *Br J Ophthalmol.* 2008;92: 569-573.

Is there a link between open-angle glaucoma and dementia? The Three-City–Alienor Cohort

Helmer C, Malet F, Rougier M-B, et al (Inst of Public Health and Development (ISPED), Bordeaux, France; Univ Hospital, Bordeaux, France; et al)
Ann Neurol 74:171-179, 2013

Objective.—Previous research has suggested an association between dementia and glaucoma through common risk factors or mechanisms. Our aim was to evaluate the longitudinal relationship between open-angle glaucoma (OAG) and incident dementia.

Methods.—The Three-City–Bordeaux–Alienor study is a population-based cohort of 812 participants with a 3-year follow-up period. All participants were aged 72 years or older. An eye examination was performed on all subjects. An OAG was determined based on optic nerve damage and visual field loss. Incident dementia was actively screened for and confirmed by a neurologist.

Results.—A total of 41 participants developed dementia over the 3-year follow-up period. Future incident dementia cases had an increased prevalence of OAG (17.5% vs 4.5% for nondemented participants, $p = 0.003$). After adjustment for age, gender, education, family history of glaucoma, vascular comorbidities, and apolipoprotein ϵ4, our results showed that participants with an OAG were four times more likely to develop dementia during the 3-year follow-up period (odds ratio = 3.9, 95% confidence interval = 1.5–10.4, $p = 0.0054$). An increased risk of dementia was also associated with 2 markers of optic nerve degeneration (vertical cup:disk ratio and minimal rim:disk ratio). However, no association was found between a high intraocular pressure and/or the use of intraocular pressure-lowering medications and incident dementia.

Interpretation.—If the association between OAG and dementia is confirmed, direct and noninvasive quantification of the amount of retinal ganglion cell axonal loss may be a useful biomarker of cerebral axonal loss in the future. It may also offer new breakthroughs in understanding the underlying pathophysiological mechanisms of both diseases.

▶ Attention has been drawn to a potential association between glaucoma and dementia. Both are central nervous system disorders for which increasing age is a significant risk factor. Glaucoma may affect the global visual pathway in the brain, and patients with Alzheimer disease may have retinal nerve fiber layer thinning compared with control groups. Although a link between glaucoma and dementia remains unclear, this report provides information that furthers interest in that possibility.

The Three-City study is a prospective, population-based cohort of more than 9000 French adults over the age of 65 living in Bordeaux, Dijon, and Montpellier. It was designed to assess the risk of dementia and cognitive decline as a result of vascular risk factors. At the 7-year follow-up, almost 1000 participants from Bordeaux agreed to join the Alienor study regarding age-related eye disease and nutritional factors. A sample of those patients with 3 years of follow-up was used in this study to examine the relationship between glaucoma and incident dementia.

Ultimately, participants with open-angle glaucoma were 4 times more likely to have subsequent dementia. However, no association was found between elevated intraocular pressure (IOP) or IOP-lowering medications and development of dementia.

This study indicates there is a connection between glaucoma and dementia. Perhaps the results of this study point specifically toward a connection between low-tension glaucoma and dementia. However, the evidence as a whole is mixed. There are other studies that failed to show an increased likelihood of dementia among glaucoma patients using claims databases. Maybe limitations in screening for both conditions affected the outcome of those studies. Hopefully, additional research on this important topic will yield a better understanding of glaucoma and dementia.

S. Fudemberg, MD

5 Retina

Ten-Year Follow-up of Age-Related Macular Degeneration in the Age-Related Eye Disease Study: AREDS Report No. 36

Chew EY, for the Age-Related Eye Disease Study Research Group (Natl Eye Inst, Bethesda, MD; et al)

JAMA Ophthalmol 132:272-277, 2014

Importance.—Providing long-term follow-up of the natural history of age-related macular degeneration (AMD) and associated risk factors will facilitate future epidemiologic studies and clinical trials.

Objective.—To describe 10-year progression rates to intermediate or advanced AMD.

Design, Setting, and Participants.—We observed the Age-Related Eye Disease Study (AREDS) participants for an additional 5 years after a randomized clinical trial of antioxidant vitamins and minerals was completed. Observation occurred at 11 clinical sites of medical retinal practices from academic institutions and community medical centers. Participants aged 55 to 80 years with no AMD or AMD of varying severity (n = 4757) were followed up in the AREDS trial for a median duration of 6.5 years. When the trial ended, 3549 of the 4203 surviving participants were followed for 5 additional years.

Exposure.—Treatment with antioxidant vitamins and minerals.

Main Outcomes and Measures.—Development of varying stages of AMD and changes in visual acuity. The rates of progression to large drusen and advanced AMD (neovascular AMD or central geographic atrophy) were evaluated using annual fundus photographs assessed centrally. Best-corrected visual acuity was measured at annual study visits.

Results.—The risk of progression to advanced AMD increased with increasing age ($P = .01$) and severity of drusen. Women ($P = .005$) and current smokers ($P < .001$) were at increased risk of neovascular AMD. In the oldest participants with the most severe AMD status at baseline, the risks of developing neovascular AMD and central geographic atrophy by 10 years were 48.1%and 26.0%, respectively. Similarly, rates of progression to large drusen increased with increasing severity of drusen at baseline, with 70.9% of participants with bilateral medium drusen progressing to large drusen and 13.8% to advanced AMD in 10 years. Median visual acuity at 10 years in eyes that had large drusen at baseline but never developed advanced AMD was 20/25; eyes that developed advanced AMD had a median visual acuity of 20/200.

Conclusions and Relevance.—The natural history of AMD demonstrates relentless loss of vision in persons who developed advanced AMD. These progression data and the risk factor analyses may be helpful to investigators conducting research in clinic populations.

▶ Despite advancements in the treatment of age-related macular degeneration (AMD), the natural history of this disease process is still overwhelming. It remains the leading cause of blindness in the United States, and the prevalence will double by 2020. This new report presents data approximately 22 years after the original Age-Related Eye Disease Study report in 1992.

The researchers reported progression rates of intermediate and advanced AMD over 10 years. Increasing age, severity of drusen, retinal pigment epithelium abnormalities, and advanced AMD (neovascular AMD or central geographic atrophy) in the fellow eye were all identified as risk factors. Patients with these risk factors need to be followed closely for loss of vision. These patients represent the last cohort of patients that are not addressed by the anti-vascular endothelial growth factor agents. The risk of developing neovascular AMD by 10 years was 48% and central geographic atrophy was 26% in the highest risk cohorts. Multiple reports have provided information on identifying risk factors for progression. One of the biggest challenges is modifying the natural history and improving vision in patients with advanced AMD.

O. P. Gupta, MD

Risk of Geographic Atrophy in the Comparison of Age-related Macular Degeneration Treatments Trials

Grunwald JE, for the CATT Research Group (Univ of Pennsylvania, Philadelphia; et al)

Ophthalmology 121:150-161, 2014

Purpose.—To describe risk factors for geographic atrophy (GA) in the Comparison of Age-related Macular Degeneration Treatments Trials (CATT).

Design.—Cohort within a randomized clinical trial.

Participants.—We analyzed 1024 CATT patients with no GA visible on color fundus photographs (CFPs) and/ or fluorescein angiograms (FAs) at enrollment.

Methods.—Eyes were assigned to ranibizumab (0.5 mg) or bevacizumab (1.25 mg) treatment and to a 2-year monthly or pro re nata (PRN) injection regimen, or monthly injections for 1 year and PRN for 1 year. Demographic, genetic, and baseline ocular characteristics and lesion features of CFP/FA and optical coherence tomography (OCT) were evaluated as risk factors for GA through 2 years of follow-up. Time-dependent Cox proportional hazard models were used to estimate adjusted hazard ratios (aHRs).

Main Outcome Measures.—Development of GA.

Results.—By 2 years, GA developed in 187 of 1024 patients (18.3%). Baseline risk factors for GA development included baseline visual acuity

(VA) ≤20/200 (aHR, 2.65; 95% confidence interval [CI], 1.43–4.93), retinal angiomatous proliferation (RAP; aHR, 1.69; 95% CI, 1.16–2.47), GA in the fellow eye (aHR, 2.07; 95% CI, 1.40–3.08), and intraretinal fluid at the foveal center (aHR, 2.10; 95% CI, 1.34–3.31). Baseline factors associated with lower risk for GA development included blocked fluorescence (aHR, 0.49; 95% CI, 0.29–0.82), OCT measurements of subretinal fluid thickness of >25 μ (aHR, 0.52; 95% CI, 0.35–0.78), subretinal tissue complex thickness of >275 compared with ≤75 μ (aHR, 0.31; 95% CI, 0.19–0.50), and vitreomacular attachment (aHR, 0.55; 95% CI, 0.31–0.97). Ranibizumab compared with bevacizumab had a higher risk (aHR, 1.43; 95% CI, 1.06–1.93), and monthly dosing had a higher risk (aHR, 1.59; 95% CI, 1.17–2.16) than PRN dosing. There were no strong associations between development of GA and the presence of risk alleles for *CFH, ARMS 2, HTRA1*, C3, or *TLR3*.

Conclusions.—Approximately one fifth of CATT patients developed GA within 2 years of treatment. Independent baseline risk factors included poor VA, RAP, foveal intraretinal fluid, monthly dosing, and treatment with ranibizumab. Anti-vascular endothelial growth factor therapy may have a role in the development of GA.

▶ Progression of dry age-related macular degeneration can occur in the setting of neovascular age-related macular degeneration (nAMD). In the treatment of nAMD, often progression of geographic atrophy (GA) can go unnoticed. The authors used a cohort from the Comparison of Age-related Macular Degeneration Treatments Trials (CATT) without GA at enrollment. By 2 years, GA developed in 187 of 1024 patients (18.3%). Baseline risk factors for GA development included baseline visual acuity (VA) ≤20/200, retinal angiomatous proliferation, GA in the fellow eye, and intraretinal fluid at the foveal center. In addition, ranibizumab compared with bevacizumab and monthly dosing compared with as-needed dosing had a higher risk of GA progression. However, there were not strong associations between development of GA and the presence of risk alleles for complement factor H (CFH), age-related maculopathy susceptibility protein 2 (ARMS2), high temperature requirement A1 (HTRA1), complement 3, or toll-like receptor 3 (TLR3). Visual loss in patients with nAMD can occur for a variety of reasons unrelated to the choroidal neovascular membrane. Progression of GA must also be considered part of the disease process as well as related to treatment with intravitreal injections.

O. P. Gupta, MD

The Argus II Retinal Prosthesis: 12-Month Outcomes from a Single-Study Center

Rizzo S, Belting C, Cinelli L, et al (Azienda Ospedaliero-Universitaria Pisana, Pisa, Italy)

Am J Ophthalmol 157:1282-1290, 2014

Purpose.—To study the anatomic and functional outcomes of Argus II Retinal Prosthesis System implantation in patients with retinitis pigmentosa.

Design.—Interventional case series.

Methods.—The study population included 6 patients with visual acuity no better than light perception. After the Argus II Retinal Prosthesis System was implanted, complications and anatomic and functional results were studied. The main outcome measures were mobility, square localization, direction of motion, grating visual acuity, and Goldmann visual field, all of which were assessed. Optical coherence tomography was performed.

Results.—Implantation of the Argus II Retinal Prosthesis System was safely performed in all patients. One patient experienced postoperative elevation in intraocular pressure, which was controlled medically. In 1 patient, moderate detachment of the choroid occurred postoperatively, and it resolved spontaneously. One patient withdrew from the study. Wound dehiscence, endophthalmitis or retinal detachment was not observed. All patients were able to locate a bright light on the ceiling and a dark line on the floor after the surgery. Performance in square localization tests improved in 4 patients, and direction of motion improved in 3 patients. One patient achieved grating visual acuity. Goldmann visual field test results improved in all patients.

Conclusions.—The patients showed improvement in visual tasks after the surgery, and the device was well tolerated and functional over a 1-year follow-up period. A rigorous patient-selection process is necessary to maximize patient compliance with the rigorous follow-up testing schedule. Both patients and medical staff should be prepared for a lengthy, arduous rehabilitation process.

▶ Although the study is small with limited results, the potential future application and improvement of the technology described is attractive. The Argus II Retinal Prosthesis System is used in the setting of retinitis pigmentosa. It is an epiretinal implant consisting of 60 electrodes mounted onto the inner retinal layer. The external system wirelessly communicates with this implant via an eyeglass-mounted camera and a small processor. The camera records real-time images, which are processed and sent wirelessly to the implant, which in turn stimulates the patient's remaining healthy retinal cells.

This was a small study consisting of 6 patients. In all patients, the retinal prosthesis was well tolerated without major safety signals. There was an improvement in the visual tasks postoperatively. Obviously this was a small study with limited follow-up. Although this technology is well beyond a proof of concept, the data are encouraging and indicate that this procedure will continue to evolve. The ultimate question is which retinal prosthesis technology will persevere. The other retinal implants are placed in the subretinal or choroidal space. Each procedure has its own set of advantages and disadvantages.

O. P. Gupta, MD

The Neovascular Age-Related Macular Degeneration Database: Report 2: Incidence, Management, and Visual Outcomes of Second Treated Eyes

Zarranz-Ventura J, for the United Kingdom Age-Related Macular Degeneration Electronic Medical Records Users Group (Moorfields Eye Hosp NHS Trust, London, UK)

Ophthalmology 121:1966-1975, 2014

Purpose.—To study the characteristics of second treated eyes in patients with neovascular age-related macular degeneration (nAMD) treated with ranibizumab in the United Kingdom National Health Service.

Design.—Multicenter national nAMD database study.

Participants.—Twelve thousand nine hundred fifty-one treatment-naïve eyes of 11 135 patients receiving 92 976 ranibizumab injections.

Methods.—Up to 5 years of routinely collected, anonymized data within electronic medical record systems were extracted remotely from 14 centers. Participating centers exclusively used ranibizumab to treat nAMD (loading phase of 3 monthly injections followed by monthly visits and pro re nata re-treatment). The minimum data set included: age, logarithm of the minimum angle of resolution (logMAR) visual acuity (VA) at baseline and at all subsequent visits, and injection episodes.

Main Outcome Measures.—Baseline, change and actual VA over 3 years, and number of treatments and clinic visits.

Results.—During the study, 1816 (16.3%) of the 11 135 patients received treatment to the fellow eye. Mean baseline and final VA were 0.66 (standard deviation, 0.32) and 0.65 (0.40) for first treated eyes and 0.41 (0.34) and 0.56 (0.40) for second treated eyes. The rate of VA loss after the loading phase was similar in first and second treated eyes (0.03 and 0.05 logMAR units/year). When fellow eyes with baseline VA worse than 20/200 were excluded to restrict analyses to eyes at risk of nAMD, the rate of second-eye involvement was 14.0% per year (42%/3 years). Mean number of injections/visits in years 1, 2, and 3 were similar for first and second treated eyes (5.6/8.2, 3.9/8.0, 3.8/8.2 and 5.5/8.7, 3.6/9.4, and 3.8/9.1, respectively).

Conclusions.—Second treated eyes with nAMD commence treatment with better baseline VA, do not show significant vision gain but maintain better VA than first treated eyes at all time points for at least 3 years, making them the more important eye functionally. These data highlight the high burden of second eye involvement, with almost half of all eyes at risk requiring bilateral treatment by 3 years, and the need for regular monitoring of fellow eyes for best visual outcomes which theoretically may reduce the benefits of extended monitoring regimens.

▶ The conversion of dry age-related macular degeneration (AMD) to neovascular AMD can be difficult to detect in patients. Because of the increased frequency with which providers are seeing patients with neovascular AMD, the detection of changes in fellow eye is often identified much earlier. Early detection is critical in the evolution of this disease. Often when exudation is left undetected or untreated, it can lead to irreversible anatomic changes such as subretinal fibrosis. On a histologic level, choroidal neovascularization becomes more resistant to regression due to increased amount of pericytes along the neovascular blood vessels.

The researchers evaluated the visual outcomes and injection requirements in patients who began to need treatment in their fellow eye. The rate of conversion of fellow eyes from nonneovascular to neovascular AMD was 14% per year. However, these eyes maintain a better visual acuity than first-treated eyes. Although this study was performed in the United Kingdom, it has particular importance in the US health care system due to controversy over the value of examining patients who are actively receiving intravitreal injections.

O. P. Gupta, MD

Intravitreal Anti-Vascular Endothelial Growth Factor for Submacular Hemorrhage from Choroidal Neovascularization

Kim JH, Chang YS, Kim JW, et al (Konyang Univ College of Medicine, Seoul, South Korea)

Ophthalmology 121:926-935, 2014

Purpose.—To evaluate the efficacy of intravitreal anti-vascular endothelial growth factor (VEGF) monotherapy for patients diagnosed with exudative age-related macular degeneration (AMD) accompanied by submacular hemorrhage.

Design.—Retrospective, observational case series.

Participants.—Ninety-one eyes of 91 patients who initially presented with submacular hemorrhage associated with exudative AMD from October 2009 to September 2012. Patients were followed up for at least 6 months after treatment.

Methods.—Best-corrected visual acuity (BCVA) was measured at diagnosis and at 1, 3, and 6 months after treatment. The duration of symptoms was estimated. The extent of hemorrhage was estimated using fundus photography, and central foveal thickness was measured using optical coherence tomography. Change in BCVA during 6 months after treatment was estimated. The correlation of BCVA at 6 months with duration of symptoms, extent of hemorrhage, and central foveal thickness was evaluated.

Main Outcome Measures.—The BCVA, duration of symptoms, extent of hemorrhage, and central foveal thickness.

Results.—The mean duration of symptoms was 27.6 ± 39.5 days. The mean extent of hemorrhage was 7.8 ± 5.6 disc areas, and the mean central foveal thickness was 610.1 ± 249.6 mm. All eyes were treated with 3.2 ± 0.8 (range, 1–5) monthly intravitreal anti-VEGF injections during the 6-month follow-up period. The logarithm of the minimum angle of resolution BCVA at diagnosis and at 1, 3, and 6 months after the initial diagnosis was 1.38 ± 0.53 (Snellen equivalent, 20/479), 1.27 ± 0.57, 1.05 ± 0.58, and 0.96 ± 0.65 (Snellen equivalent, 20/182), respectively. The BCVA at 6 months significantly improved from baseline ($P < 0.001$).

Poor BCVA at 6 months correlated with a longer duration of symptoms, greater extent of hemorrhage, and greater central foveal thickness ($P = 0.008$, $P = 0.004$, and $P = 0.014$, respectively).

Conclusions.—Anti-VEGF monotherapy was found to be a useful treatment option for exudative AMD accompanied by submacular hemorrhage. However, the limited efficacy in eyes with large hemorrhage may suggest the need for more aggressive treatment in these cases.

▶ Large submacular hemorrhages secondary to neovascular age-related macular degeneration have traditionally been treated with pars plana vitrectomy with or without tissue plasminogen activator displacement. The visual outcomes have been varied, primarily because of the underlying severity of macular disease. More recently, there have been a number of publications that have evaluated the use of anti-vascular endothelial growth factor (VEGF) agents used in monotherapy regardless of the severity of the submacular hemorrhage.

This retrospective study evaluated outcomes after 6 months of treatment with anti-VEGF monotherapy. The best corrected visual acuity improved by 3 or more lines in 59% of eyes, and the visual acuity was stable in 32% of eyes. Predictors of poor visual acuity at the 6-month time point included longer duration of symptoms, greater extent of hemorrhage, and greater central foveal thickness at time of presentation. There is no clear gold standard in the management of a submacular hemorrhage. All the studies published to date demonstrated that anti-VEGF monotherapy is a viable option that seems to be relatively equivalent to other techniques.

O. P. Gupta, MD

Outer retinal tubulation in the comparison of age-related macular degeneration treatment trails (CATT)

Lee JY, Folgar FA, Maguire MG, et al (Duke Univ Med Ctr, Durham, NC; Univ of Pennsylvania, Philadelphia; et al)

Ophthalmology 121:2423-2431, 2014

Purpose.—To determine the prevalence of, risk factors for, and visual acuity (VA) correlations with outer retinal tubulation (ORT) seen on spectral-domain optical coherence tomography (SD OCT) in eyes with neovascular age-related macular degeneration (AMD) after anti-vascular endothelial growth factor (VEGF) therapy.

Design.—Prospective cohort study within a randomized clinical trial.

Participants.—Patients with SD OCT images at weeks 56 and 104 in the Comparison of AMD Treatments Trials (CATT).

Methods.—Participants in the CATT were assigned randomly to ranibizumab (0.5 mg) or bevacizumab (1.25 mg) treatment and to a monthly or pro re nata (PRN) injection-dosing regimen. A subset of eyes was imaged with SD OCT beginning at week 56. Cirrus 512 × 128 or Spectralis 20° × 20° volume cube scan protocols were used to acquire SD OCT images. Two independent readers at the CATT OCT reading center graded scans, and a senior reader arbitrated discrepant grades. The prevalence of ORT, identified as tubular structures seen on at least 3 consecutive Cirrus B scans or 2 consecutive Spectralis B scans, was determined. The associations of patient-specific and ocular features at baseline and follow-up with ORT were evaluated by univariate and multivariate analyses.

Main Outcome Measures.—Outer retinal tubulations.

Results.—Seven of 69 eyes (10.1%) at 56 weeks and 64 of 368 eyes (17.4%) at week 104 had ORTs. Absence of diabetes, poor VA, blocked fluorescence, geographic atrophy, greater lesion size, and presence of subretinal hyperreflective material at baseline were associated independently with greater risk of ORT at 104 weeks ($P < 0.05$). Neither drug nor dosing regimen were associated significantly with ORT. The mean VA of eyes with ORT at week 104 (58.5 Early Treatment Diabetic Retinopathy Study letters) was worse than the mean VA of eyes without ORT (68.8 letters; $P < 0.0001$).

Conclusion.—At 2 years after initiation of anti-VEGF therapy for neovascular AMD, ORTs are present in a substantial proportion of eyes. We identified baseline features that independently predict ORTs. It is important to identify ORTs because eyes with ORTs have worse VA outcomes than those without this finding.

▶ Outer retinal tubulation (ORT) is the result of degenerating photoreceptors that appear as round or ovoid hyporeflective spaces on optical coherence tomography (OCT). It is typically associated with advanced age-related macular degeneration (AMD) adjacent to areas of retinal pigment endothelium alteration or subretinal fibrosis. It can be misinterpreted for signs of exudation in neovascular AMD.

This current study was a subset analysis of the Comparison of AMD Treatments Trials (CATT) study. Approximately 10% of eyes at 14 months and 17.4% at 26 months demonstrated ORT on OCT. This was not associated with an intravitreal agent but was associated with an absence of diabetes, poor vision, blocked fluorescence, geographic atrophy, greater choroidal neovascularization lesion size, and subretinal hyperreflective material on OCT. These eyes are important to identify because of their poorer visual prognosis and lack of response to anti-vascular endothelial growth factor treatment. Before this anatomic discovery, many "recalcitrant" cases of neovascular AMD were treated unnecessarily.

O. P. Gupta, MD

Treat-and-Extend Bevacizumab for Neovascular Age-Related Macular Degeneration: The Importance of Baseline Characteristics

Rush RB, Simunovic MP, Vandiver L, et al (Southwest Retina Specialists, Amarillo, TX; Sydney Eye Hosp, Australia; Texas Tech Univ Health Science Ctr, Amarillo; et al)

Retina 34:846-852, 2014

Purpose.—To evaluate the factors affecting visual and anatomical outcomes and the number of intravitreal bevacizumab injections required in the treatment of neovascular age-related macular degeneration using a treat-and-extend regimen.

Methods.—Retrospective consecutive case series. The charts of subjects treated with intravitreal bevacizumab for neovascular age-related macular degeneration using a treat-and-extend regimen over a 12-month period were reviewed. The key variables explored were patient age, phakic status, posterior vitreous detachment status, baseline best-corrected visual acuity (BCVA), baseline central macular thickness (CMT), and type of chorodial neovascularization. The primary outcome measures were improvement in BCVA of 3 logMAR lines or more, maintenance of BCVA within 3 logMAR lines of baseline, number of intravitreal injections delivered over a 12-month period, and final CMT on optical coherence tomography.

Results.—A total of 230 eyes met the criteria. Mean presenting BCVA was Snellen 20/55 (0.44 logMAR) and mean final BCVA was Snellen 20/44 (0.35 logMAR) ($P < 0.001$). A total of 23.5% (95% confidence interval [CI], 18.5-29.4%) of the subjects demonstrated an improvement in BCVA of 3 or more logMAR lines, whereas 96.5% (95% CI, 93.3—98.2%) of the subjects lost fewer than 3 logMAR lines. Mean CMT on optical coherence tomography changed from a baseline average of 373.1 μm (95% CI, 360.3—386.1 μm) to a final average of 305.5 μm (95% CI, 290.0—316.0 μm). The average number of injections during the 12-month period was 9.2 (95% CI, 9.0—9.4). Posterior vitreous detachment was associated with fewer injections on univariate and multivariate analysis (8.7 injections in the posterior vitreous detachment group versus 9.8 in the non-posterior vitreous detachment group, $P < 0.001$). Patients with poorer presenting BCVA and greater baseline CMTs were more likely to demonstrate a 3 or more logMAR line improvement in BCVA. Thinner final CMTs were independently associated with thinner presenting CMTs and fewer injections.

Conclusion.—Favorable visual and anatomical outcomes may be achieved with intravitreal bevacizumab in the treatment of neovascular age-related macular degeneration using a treat-and-extend regimen. Our study suggests that posterior vitreous detachment may play a role in the efficacy of intravitreal bevacizumab during the treatment of neovascular age-related macular degeneration.

▶ Modified treatment algorithms for the management of neovascular age-related macular degeneration (AMD) have been reported ever since the pivotal Minimally Classic/Occult Trial of the Anti-Vascular endothelial growth factor (VEGF) Antibody Ranibizumab in the Treatment of Neovascular AMD (MARINA) and the Anti-VEGF Antibody for the Treatment of Predominantly Classic Choroidal Neovascularization in AMD (ANCHOR) trials were published evaluating monthly injections. The treat-and-extend regimen has been by far the most popularly used across the country and worldwide evidenced by numerous formal surveys. More recently, nuances of this regimen have been explored for certain subgroups. In particular, type of anti-VEGF agent, status of a posterior vitreous detachment, and severity of vitreomacular traction are several factors that affect the treat-and-extend protocol.

Baseline characteristics were explored in this study to identify predictors of anatomic and visual outcomes. The anatomic and visual outcomes were similar to those of previous reports evaluating the treat-and-extend regimen. Using regression analysis, the presence of a posterior vitreous detachment was associated with fewer injections. Patients with a poorer presenting best-corrected visual acuity and greater baseline central macular thickness also required more injections.

O. P. Gupta, MD

Polymorphisms in Vascular Endothelial Growth Factor Receptor 2 Are Associated with Better Response Rates to Ranibizumab Treatment in Age-Related Macular Degeneration

Hermann MM, van Asten F, Muether PS, et al (Univ Hosp of Cologne, Germany; Radboud Univ Nijmegen Med Centre, The Netherlands; et al)
Ophthalmology 121:905-910, 2014

Purpose.—Intravitreal anti-vascular endothelial growth factor (VEGF) injections are currently the standard treatment for neovascular age-related macular degeneration (AMD), but a broad range of response rates has been observed. We evaluated the association of single nucleotide polymorphisms (SNPs) in VEGF genes and their receptors (VEGFR) with the response rate to ranibizumab in 366 patients with neovascular AMD.

Design.—Case series study.

Participants.—A total of 366 eyes of 366 patients with neovascular AMD.

Methods.—Visual acuity (VA) was determined at baseline, after 3 monthly ranibizumab injections, and after 1 year of treatment. Genotyping of 126 SNPs in the genes encoding VEGF family members VEGFA, VEGFB, VEGFC, VEGFD (*FIGF*), and placental growth factor (*PGF*); VEGF receptors VEGFR1 (*FLT1*), VEGFR2 (*KDR*), and VEGFR3 (*FLT4*); and the gene encoding pigment epithelium-derived factor (PEDF) (*SERPINF1*) was performed.

Main Outcome Measures.—The changes in VA after 3 injections and after 1 year of treatment and their association with VEGF and VEGFR genotypes.

Results.—Univariate analyses of variance (ANOVAs) revealed a significant effect of SNP rs4576072 in the VEGFR2 gene on VA change after 12 months ($F_{[1,235]} = 14.05$; $P = 0.02$). A stepwise linear regression analysis returned a model ($P = 0.01$) with SNPs rs4576072 and rs6828477 in the *VEGFR2* gene as independent predictors for VA change after 12 months, with a mean increase in VA of 0.26 on the logarithm of the minimum angle of resolution (logMAR) scale in patients with 3 contributing minor alleles compared with a loss of 0.03 logMAR in patients with no minor allele.

Conclusions.—Polymorphisms in the *VEGFR2/KDR* gene significantly influence visual outcome in patients receiving ranibizumab treatment for neovascular AMD. This study shows that genetic variation partially explains the wide range of response to ranibizumab treatment, which in the future might help clinicians tailoring medical interventions to individual needs.

▶ The response to anti-vascular endothelial growth factor (VEGF) agents and visual outcomes can be very different between 2 patients with identical presentations of neovascular age-related macular degeneration (AMD). Although phenotypically they can appear similar, researchers have hypothesized that the genotypes can dictate differences in outcome. Complement factor H, polymorphisms in age-related maculopathy susceptibility 2 (ARMS2), and VEGFA genes have been identified as high-risk alleles and are associated with poor response to ranibizumab and a younger age of onset of neovascular AMD.

This study evaluated polymorphisms of VEGF and VEGF receptors (VEGFR) genes. This evaluation was done using a genotyping technology that identified single nucleotide polymorphisms (SNPs). A linear regression analysis was then performed to establish any association between each SNP and visual outcome. The investigators found that 2 polymorphisms in the VEGFR2 gene were associated with better visual outcomes at 1 year. The goal of this area of research is to help guide clinicians to individualize treatments. It is also interesting and surprising that only two SNPs were identified. Some researchers hypothesized that there is a lot of genetic variability, but this study only identified 2 genes of significance. Further studies with a larger cohort of patients need to be performed to fully understand the genetic variability of this disease.

O. P. Gupta, MD

Intraocular Pressure in Eyes Receiving Monthly Ranibizumab in 2 Pivotal Age-Related Macular Degeneration Clinical Trials

Bakri SJ, Moshfeghi DM, Francom S, et al (Mayo Clinic, Rochester, MN; Stanford Univ School of Medicine, Palo Alto, CA; Genentech, Inc., South San Francisco, CA)

Ophthalmology 121:1102-1108, 2014

Purpose.—To characterize preinjection intraocular pressure (IOP) in eyes receiving monthly ranibizumab versus sham or verteporfin photodynamic therapy (PDT) for age-related macular degeneration (AMD).

Design.—Post hoc analysis of IOP data from 2 phase 3 clinical trials, the Minimally Classic/Occult Trial of the Anti-VEGF Antibody Ranibizumab in the Treatment of Neovascular AMD (MARINA) and the Anti-VEGF Antibody for the Treatment of Predominantly Classic Choroidal Neovascularization in AMD (ANCHOR) trial.

Participants.—All safety-evaluable patients who received 1 or more injections of sham or PDT or of ranibizumab and had 1 or more postbaseline IOP measurements recorded for the study eye.

Methods.—Preinjection IOP measurements for study eyes (n = 1125) and fellow eyes in MARINA and ANCHOR at baseline and at each monthly visit through month 24 were analyzed.

Main Outcome Measures.—End points evaluated were maximum preinjection IOP during the 24-month treatment period; any occurrence of absolute preinjection IOP of 21 mm Hg or more, 25 mm Hg or more, or 30 mm Hg or more; any occurrence of IOP increase of 6 mm Hg or more, 8 mm Hg or more, or 10 mm Hg or more from baseline; any combination of IOP increase of 6 mm Hg or more or 8 mm Hg or more from baseline with concurrent absolute preinjection IOP of 21 mm Hg or more or 25 mm Hg or more; glaucoma-related adverse events; new glaucoma medications used for 45 days or more; and glaucoma filtration or laser surgeries.

Results.—Across treatment groups, 60.1% to 70.9% of study eyes had a maximum preinjection IOP of less than 21 mm Hg. Comparing ranibizumab 0.5 mg versus sham or PTD treatment, respectively: 39.9% versus 29.1% and 10.9% versus 5.1% had maximum preinjection IOPs of 21 mm Hg or more or 25 mm Hg or more, respectively; 44.1% versus 29.9% and 24.2% versus 13.6% had IOP increases from baseline of 6 mm Hg or more or 8 mm Hg or more, respectively; 26.1% versus 13.6% and 16.8% versus 9.0% had 1 or more IOP increase from baseline of 6 mm Hg or more or 8 mm Hg or more, respectively, with a concurrent IOP of 21 mm Hg or more; 9.6% versus 3.7% and 7.5% versus 2.4% had 1 or more IOP increase from baseline of 6 mm Hg or more or 8 mm Hg or more, respectively, with a concurrent IOP of 25 mm Hg or more. No differences were observed in fellow eyes.

Conclusions.—Most ranibizumab-treated eyes did not experience sustained preinjection IOP of 21 mm Hg or more (>2 consecutive visits) over 24 months. When evaluating the combined IOP end point, more ranibizumab-treated eyes had 1 or more IOP increase from baseline of 6 mm Hg or more or 8 mm Hg or more, with concurrent highest IOPs of 21 mm Hg or more and 25 mm Hg or more versus sham or PDT. Intraocular pressure should be monitored in eyes receiving ranibizumab.

▶ Intraocular pressure spikes following intravitreal anti-vascular endothelial growth factor (VEGF) agents have been well described. However, sustained elevated intraocular pressure and glaucomatous progression that may result from routine intravitreal injections is not well understood. Evaluating these data has been difficult because of a lack of controls. In other words, glaucomatous progression may have occurred in some eyes regardless of whether intravitreal injections were performed.

This study examined the intraocular pressure fluctuation in eyes receiving monthly intravitreal injections in 1 eye and used the other eye as a control. The data were from the Minimally Classic/Occult Trial of the Anti-VEGF Antibody Ranibizumab in the Treatment of Neovascular AMD (MARINA) and the Anti-VEGF Antibody for the Treatment of Predominantly Classic Choroidal Neovascularization in AMD (ANCHOR) trials. Participants in these 2 trials received monthly injections of ranibizumab in 1 eye and either photodynamic therapy or a sham injection in the other eye over the course of 24 months. The preinjection and postinjection intraocular pressures were monitored at every visit. Although there are a lot of data presented in this article, the key message is that eyes receiving intravitreal injections can have significant preinjection intraocular elevation compared with control eyes. Some eyes can have sustained elevation for more than 1 visit. Consequently, patients receiving intravitreal injections should be monitored closely for sustained intraocular pressure elevation and glaucomatous progression.

O. P. Gupta, MD

Subfoveal Choroidal Thickness as a Potential Predictor of Visual Outcome and Treatment Response After Intravitreal Ranibizumab Injections for Typical Exudative Age-Related Macular Degeneration

Kang HM, Kwon HJ, Yi JH, et al (Univ College of Medicine, Seoul, South Korea; CHA Univ, Gyunggi-do, South Korea; Jeil Eye Clinic, Gyunggi-do, South Korea; et al)

Am J Ophthalmol 157:1013-1021.e1, 2014

Purpose.—To investigate the prognostic implication of subfoveal choroidal thickness on treatment outcome after intravitreal ranibizumab injections for typical exudative age-related macular degeneration (AMD).

Design.—Retrospective study.

Methods.—A total of 40 eyes of 37 patients who completed 6-month follow-up were analyzed. Patients' data were retrieved from medical records including best corrected visual acuity (BCVA). Subfoveal choroidal thickness at baseline, 3 months, and 6 months was measured by enhanced depth imaging optical coherence tomography and adjusted for age and sex before statistical analysis. Treatment response was after 3 monthly intravitreal ranibizumab injections. Responders (responder group) were defined as a 100 μm or more decrease or complete resolution of subretinal fluid, whereas nonresponders (nonresponder group) were defined as changes less than 100 μm or more than 100 μm increase of subretinal fluid by optical coherence tomography.

Results.—Mean age at diagnosis was 72.1 ± 8.1 years, and 22 eyes (55.0%) were responders. The responder group had thicker subfoveal choroid (257.2 ± 108.3 μm) and smaller lesions (1.3 ± 0.8 μm) at baseline than the nonresponder group (167.1 ± 62.4 μm, $P = .003$; and 2.0 ± 1.0 μm, $P = .008$). The responder group showed significantly better BCVA and thicker subfoveal choroid than the nonresponder group at 3 months ($P = .002$ and $P = .023$) and 6 months ($P = .004$ and $P = .031$). Stepwise and binary regression analysis demonstrated that subfoveal choroidal thickness was significantly correlated with visual outcome ($B = -0.002$, $P = .003$) and treatment response ($B = 8.136$, $P = .018$).

Conclusion.—Subfoveal choroidal thickness may be a predictive factor for visual outcome and treatment response in typical exudative AMD after intravitreal ranibizumab injections.

▶ With advancements in optical coherence tomography technology, researchers are gaining a better understanding of pathophysiology and guide treatment options. Subfoveal choroidal thickness has been an important feature in several retinal diseases such as central serous chorioretinopathy. In addition, the treatment response to anti-vascular endothelial growth factor agents has been varied across all patients with neovascular age-related macular degeneration (AMD). Although some of the varied outcomes can be explained by some clinical features, such as subretinal fibrosis or size of choroidal neovascular membrane, the authors report that choroidal thickness as measured on enhanced depth imaging optical coherence tomography may also predict treatment response.

Patients with a thinner subfoveal choroid showed a worse response to intravitreal ranibizumab and poorer visual outcomes compared with patients with a thicker choroid. This research adds to the growing body of work that may help providers individualize treatment to patients with neovascular AMD.

O. P. Gupta, MD

Exacerbation of choroidal and retinal pigment epithelial atrophy after anti-vascular endothelial growth factor treatment in neovascular age-related macular degeneration

Young M, Chui L, Fallah N, et al (Univ of British Columbia, Vancouver, Canada; Rick Hansen Inst, Vancouver, British Columbia, Canada)

Retina 34:1308-1315, 2014

Purpose.—To study the progression of retinal pigment epithelium (RPE) and choroidal atrophy in patients with neovascular age-related macular degeneration (AMD) and to assess for a possible association with the number and type of anti-vascular endothelial growth factor treatments.

Methods.—Patients with neovascular AMD and a minimum of 1-year follow-up were reviewed. Fellow eyes with nonneovascular AMD were used as control eyes. Retinal pigment epithelial atrophy area and choroidal thickness were determined using spectral-domain optical coherence tomography. Multivariable regression models were used for statistical analyses.

Results.—A total of 415 eyes were included in the study, with a mean follow-up of 2.2 years. Eyes with neovascular AMD had greater progression of RPE atrophy and choroidal atrophy compared with those with nonneovascular AMD ($P < 0.001$). Progression of RPE atrophy and choroidal atrophy was independently associated with the total number of injections of bevacizumab and ranibizumab (all P values ≤ 0.001). In the subgroup of 84 eyes with neovascular AMD and without RPE atrophy at baseline, only bevacizumab was associated with the progression of RPE atrophy ($P = 0.003$). This study likely lacked statistical power to detect an association with ranibizumab in this subgroup.

Conclusion.—Retinal pigment epithelial atrophy and choroidal atrophy in neovascular AMD seem to be exacerbated by anti-vascular endothelial growth factor treatment. Possible differences between bevacizumab and ranibizumab require further investigation.

▶ Anti-vascular endothelial growth factor (VEGF) agents have made an extraordinary impact on the management of neovascular age-related macular degeneration (AMD). Initial analyses primarily focused on the impressive visual acuity gains that were achieved with this treatment. Recently, more attention is being paid to the progression of geographic atrophy in patients receiving this treatment. This important research may help guide treatment by bringing attention to other etiologies of visual loss in the setting of neovascular AMD.

The current study evaluated progression of retinal pigment epithelium and choroidal atrophy in patients receiving anti-VEGF therapy. The fellow nonneovascular eye was used as the control. The researchers reported that the neovascular eye showed a greater progression of retinal pigment epithelium and choroidal atrophy compared with the fellow eye. This finding was independent of the total number of injections. The authors noted some differences between ranibizumab and bevacizumab, but unfortunately this study lacked statistical power to detect differences between these subgroups. These findings add to the growing body of literature and should give providers pause when injecting anti-VEGF agents. Vision loss can occur in the setting of neovascular AMD that is not related to any sign of exudation.

O. P. Gupta, MD

Safety of Intravitreal Ocriplasmin for Focal Vitreomacular Adhesion in Patients with Exudative Age-Related Macular Degeneration

Novack RL, Staurenghi G, Girach A, et al (Retina Vitreous Associates, Los Angeles, CA; Luigi Sacco Hosp, Milan, Italy; NightstaRx Ltd, London, UK; et al)

Ophthalmology 122:796-802, 2015

Purpose.—The evaluation of the safety and preliminary efficacy of 125 μg ocriplasmin intravitreal injection in patients with focal vitreomacular adhesion (VMA) and exudative age-related macular degeneration (AMD).

Design.—Randomized, sham-injection controlled, double-masked, multicenter, phase II trial.

Participants.—A total of 100 patients with VMA and wet AMD were randomized 3:1 to receive 125 μg ocriplasmin intravitreal injection or sham injection.

Methods.—Study treatment was administered in the mid-vitreous cavity by injection. Post-treatment safety and efficacy assessments were made at baseline and on days 7, 14, and 28 and months 3, 6, and 12 after injection. Secondary efficacy end points were exploratory in nature.

Main Outcome Measures.—The safety and tolerability of ocriplasmin were evaluated. The primary efficacy end point was the proportion of patients with VMA release at day 28 after injection. Secondary end points reported included VMA release over time, total posterior vitreous detachment (PVD), change in visual acuity from baseline, and number of anti–vascular endothelial growth factor (VEGF) injections.

Results.—The safety of ocriplasmin in patients with VMA and wet AMD was shown to be comparable to the known safety profile, with the majority of adverse events in the study eye occurring in the first 7 days after study treatment. A greater proportion of patients achieved VMA resolution and total PVD at month 12 with ocriplasmin compared with sham treatment. There was a decrease in the number of anti-VEGF injections with ocriplasmin at month 12 compared with the sham group, although no differences in visual acuity were observed.

Conclusions.—Ocriplasmin treatment in this population seems to be generally safe and well tolerated and resulted in more patients achieving VMA resolution and PVD with less anti-VEGF use compared with sham treatment.

▶ The relationship between neovascular age-related macular degeneration (AMD) and other concurrent macular diseases is not well understood. Vitreomacular traction and vitreomacular adhesion (VMA) in the setting of neovascular AMD are reported to be a common confounding factors. In particular, traction at the vitreoretinal interface can cause progression of both nonneovascular and neovascular AMD. Signs of exudation in patients with neovascular AMD can be more difficult to treat given the tractional component to the macular edema. Ocriplasmin is found to be effective at pharmacologically releasing vitreomacular traction.

The researchers of this study randomly assigned 100 patients to receive ocriplasmin or sham injection along with concurrent anti-vascular endothelial growth factor (VEGF) treatment. Although it was expected that more patients would achieve resolution of VMA and a posterior vitreous attachment in the intervention arm compared with sham injection, the interesting results are related to the anti-VEGF frequency. The study reported that in the ocriplasmin arm, almost 2 fewer injections of anti-VEGF were required over the course of 1 year compared with the sham group. Ocriplasmin is a potentially better option compared with vitrectomy because of the preservation of a reservoir for anti-VEGF. Some have proposed that anti-VEGF agents may have a longer duration of action in eyes with vitreous compared with eyes after vitrectomy.

O. P. Gupta, MD

Baseline Choroidal Thickness as a Predictor for Response to Anti–Vascular Endothelial Growth Factor Therapy in Diabetic Macular Edema

Rayess N, Rahimy E, Ying G-S, et al (Retina Service of Wills Eye Hosp, Philadelphia, PA; Univ of Pennsylvania, Philadelphia)

Am J Ophthalmol 159:85-91.e1-3, 2015

Purpose.—To determine the association between baseline subfoveal choroidal thickness and short-term response to intravitreal anti–vascular endothelial growth factor (anti-VEGF) therapy in diabetic macular edema (DME).

Design.—Retrospective, consecutive case series.

Methods.—Fifty-three eyes from 42 patients diagnosed with treatment-naïve DME were treated with 3 monthly intravitreal injections of ranibizumab or bevacizumab. Serial enhanced depth imaging optical coherence tomography scans were used to measure subfoveal choroidal thickness and central macular thickness (CMT). Anatomic response (CMT decrease ≥50 μm) and functional response (best-corrected visual acuity gain ≥1 line) were assessed at 3 months follow-up using univariate and multivariate analyses.

Results.—After 3 monthly anti-VEGF treatments, subfoveal choroidal thickness decreased significantly (225 μm at baseline, 201 μm at 3 months, $P < .0001$). The anatomic responder group (32 eyes) had a greater baseline choroidal thickness (243 ± 15 μm) than the nonresponder group (21 eyes, 198 ± 13 μm, $P = .03$). Similarly, the functional responder group (28 eyes) tended to have a greater baseline subfoveal choroidal thickness (239 ± 12 μm) than the nonresponder group (25 eyes, 211 ± 16 μm, $P = .08$). Multivariate analyses revealed that a greater baseline subfoveal choroidal thickness was associated with a better anatomic (odds ratio = 1.12 for every 10 μm increase, $P = .03$) and functional response (odds ratio = 8.45 for >200 μm vs ≤200 μm, $P = .008$).

Conclusion.—Baseline subfoveal choroidal thickness may help predict which patients with DME will respond more favorably in the short term to intravitreal anti-VEGF pharmacotherapy. In this study, eyes with a thicker baseline subfoveal choroidal thickness had better short-term anatomic and functional responses.

▶ Enhanced depth-imaging optical coherence tomography has provided additional anatomic information in the analysis of macular disease. As mentioned previously, it is a risk factor for development in central serous chorioretinopathy. Researchers are also using this technology to predict response to anti-vascular endothelial growth factor (VEGF) treatments. Evidence suggests that patients with a thicker choroid have been visual outcomes in the setting of neovascular age-related macular degeneration.

This study evaluated choroidal thickness in the setting of diabetic macular edema. This was a retrospective study that looked at anatomic and functional response after three monthly injections. Better anatomic and functional responses were associated with a greater baseline choroidal thickness. This has been hypothesized owing to retinal hypoxia, higher VEGF levels, and breakdown of the blood-retinal barrier in patients with a thinner choroid.

O. P. Gupta, MD

Intravitreal Aflibercept for Diabetic Macular Edema

Korobelnik J-F, Do DV, Schmidt-Erfurth U, et al (Hôpital Pellegrind—CHU de Bordeaux, France; Univ of Nebraska Med Ctr, Omaha; Med Univ of Vienna, Austria; et al)

Ophthalmology 121:2247-2254, 2014

Purpose.—A head-to-head comparison was performed between vascular endothelial growth factor blockade and laser for treatment of diabetic macular edema (DME).

Design.—Two similarly designed, double-masked, randomized, phase 3 trials, $VISTA^{DME}$ and $VIVID^{DME}$.

Participants.—We included 872 patients (eyes) with type 1 or 2 diabetes mellitus who presented with DME with central involvement.

Methods.—Eyes received either intravitreal aflibercept injection (IAI) 2 mg every 4 weeks (2q4), IAI 2 mg every 8 weeks after 5 initial monthly doses (2q8), or macular laser photocoagulation.

Main Outcome Measures.—The primary efficacy endpoint was the change from baseline in best-corrected visual acuity (BCVA) in Early Treatment Diabetic Retinopathy Study (ETDRS) letters at week 52. Secondary efficacy endpoints at week 52 included the proportion of eyes that gained ≥15 letters from baseline and the mean change from baseline in central retinal thickness as determined by optical coherence tomography.

Results.—Mean BCVA gains from baseline to week 52 in the IAI 2q4 and 2q8 groups versus the laser group were 12.5 and 10.7 versus 0.2 letters ($P < 0.0001$) in VISTA, and 10.5 and 10.7 versus 1.2 letters ($P < 0.0001$) in VIVID. The corresponding proportions of eyes gaining ≥15 letters were 41.6% and 31.1% versus 7.8% ($P < 0.0001$) in VISTA, and 32.4% and 33.3% versus 9.1% ($P < 0.0001$) in VIVID. Similarly, mean reductions in central retinal thickness were 185.9 and 183.1 versus 73.3 μm ($P < 0.0001$) in VISTA, and 195.0 and 192.4 versus 66.2 μm ($P < 0.0001$) in VIVID. Overall incidences of ocular and nonocular adverse events and serious adverse events, including the Anti-Platelet Trialists' Collaboration–defined arterial thromboembolic events and vascular deaths, were similar across treatment groups.

Conclusions.—At week 52, IAI demonstrated significant superiority in functional and anatomic endpoints over laser, with similar efficacy in the 2q4 and 2q8 groups despite the extended dosing interval in the 2q8 group. In general, IAI was well-tolerated.

▶ Intravitreal ranibizumab was the first US Food and Drug Administration-approved anti-vascular endothelial growth factor (VEGF) agent in the treatment of diabetic macular edema. Intravitreal aflibercept was studied in the VISTA and

VIVID trials for this indication. Four-week and 8-week dose administration was compared with laser photocoagulation. The visual acuity gains and 3-line gainers were substantially better compared with those of focal laser. The efficacy of 4- and 8-week dosing was similar.

This study reaffirms the complete revolution in treatment that has occurred in the treatment of diabetic macular edema. Focal laser was the mainstay in treatment. Intravitreal anti-VEGF injections have radically improved outcomes. Although these results were encouraging, further studies need to explore the sustainability of this treatment. In particular, maintaining these visual acuity gains without frequent injections would be ideal. Likely, combination treatment will be further explored.

O. P. Gupta, MD

Effect of combined cataract surgery and ranibizumab injection in postoperative macular edema in nonproliferative diabetic retinopathy

Chae JB, Joe SG, Yang SJ, et al (Chungbuk Natl Univ, Cheongju, Korea; Univ of Ulsan, Seoul, Korea; Univ of Ulsan, Gangneung, Korea)

Retina 34:149-156, 2014

Purpose.—To evaluate whether intravitreal ranibizumab injection at cataract surgery prevents postoperative diabetic macular edema (PME) in patients with stable diabetic retinopathy without significant macular edema.

Methods.—Eighty patients with cataract, stable diabetic retinopathy, and no significant macular edema were randomized to a sham group (cataract surgery only) or a group undergoing cataract surgery plus intraoperative ranibizumab injection. Best-corrected visual acuities, central subfield thickness, and total macular volume were assessed at baseline and 1 week, 1, 3, and 6 months postoperatively by spectral domain optical coherence tomography. Clinically meaningful PME (central subfield thickness increase >60 μm relative to baseline) was computed.

Results.—The groups did not differ in baseline best-corrected visual acuity, central subfield thickness, and total macular volume. Compared with the ranibizumab injection group, the sham group had significantly larger central subfield thickness increases relative to baseline at 1 week and 1 month; larger total macular volume increases at all time points ($P = 0.012$, $P = 0.005$, $P < 0.001$, $P < 0.001$, $P = 0.005$, $P = 0.017$, respectively); higher PME frequency at 1 month ($P = 0.019$); and poorer best-corrected visual acuity improvement from baseline to 6 months after surgery ($P = 0.046$).

Conclusion.—In patients with stable diabetic retinopathy without significant macular edema, intravitreal ranibizumab injection at cataract surgery may prevent the postoperative worsening of macular edema and may improve the final visual outcome without affecting safety.

▶ Increased risk of postoperative diabetic macular edema or progression of diabetic retinopathy after cataract surgery has been well studied. In addition, preexisting diabetic macular edema is not a prerequisite to postoperative macular edema. Subsequently, these patients are often difficult to treat, given the mixed mechanism. The current study randomized patients with stable retinopathy and no significant macular edema to an injection arm that received an intraoperative ranibizumab injection compared with a sham arm that underwent cataract surgery alone. The sham arm was reported to have a greater central subfield thickness, higher frequency of clinically meaningful diabetic macular edema (> 60 μm increase from baseline), and worse visual acuity from baseline at 6 months postoperatively. In the absence of preoperative macular edema, this compelling evidence indicates that an intravitreal ranibizumab injection may prevent postoperative worsening of macular edema and improve the final visual outcome.

O. P. Gupta, MD

Intravitreal Aflibercept Injection for Macular Edema Due to Central Retinal Vein Occlusion: Two-Year Results from the COPERNICUS Study

Heier JS, Clark WL, Boyer DS, et al (Ophthalmic Consultants of Boston, MA; Palmetto Retina Ctr, West Columbia, SC; Retina-Vitreous Associates Med Group, Beverly Hills, CA; et al)

Ophthalmology 121:1414-1420.e1, 2014

Purpose.—To evaluate the efficacy and safety of intravitreal aflibercept injection (IAI) for the treatment of macular edema secondary to central retinal vein occlusion (CRVO).

Design.—Randomized, double-masked, phase 3 trial.

Participants.—A total of 188 patients with macular edema secondary to CRVO.

Methods.—Patients received IAI 2 mg (IAI 2Q4) (n = 114) or sham injections (n = 74) every 4 weeks up to week 24. During weeks 24 to 52, patients from both arms were evaluated monthly and received IAI as needed, or pro re nata (PRN) (IAI 2Q4 + PRN and sham + IAI PRN). During weeks 52 to 100, patients were evaluated at least quarterly and received IAI PRN.

Main Outcome Measures.—The primary efficacy end point was the proportion of patients who gained ≥15 letters in best-corrected visual acuity (BCVA) from baseline to week 24. This study reports week 100 results.

Results.—The proportion of patients gaining ≥15 letters was 56.1% versus 12.3% ($P < 0.001$) at week 24, 55.3% versus 30.1% ($P < 0.001$) at week 52, and 49.1% versus 23.3% ($P < 0.001$) at week 100 in the IAI 2Q4 + PRN and sham + IAI PRN groups, respectively. The mean change from baseline BCVA was also significantly higher in the IAI 2Q4 + PRN group compared with the sham + IAI PRN group at week 24 (+17.3 vs. −4.0 letters; $P < 0.001$), week 52 (+16.2 vs. +3.8 letters; $P < 0.001$), and week 100 (+13.0 vs. +1.5 letters; $P < 0.0001$). The mean reduction from baseline in central retinal thickness was 457.2 versus 144.8 μm ($P < 0.001$) at week 24, 413.0 versus 381.8 μm at week 52 ($P = 0.546$), and 390.0 versus 343.3 μm at week 100 ($P = 0.366$) in the IAI 2Q4 + PRN and sham + IAI PRN groups, respectively. The mean number (standard deviation) of PRN injections in the IAI 2Q4 + PRN and sham + IAI PRN groups was 2.7 ± 1.7 versus 3.9 ± 2.0 during weeks 24 to 52 and 3.3 ± 2.1 versus 2.9 ± 2.0 during weeks 52 to 100, respectively. The most frequent ocular serious adverse event from baseline to week 100 was vitreous hemorrhage (0.9% vs. 6.8% in the IAI 2Q4 + PRN and sham + IAI PRN groups, respectively).

Conclusions.—The visual and anatomic improvements after fixed dosing through week 24 and PRN dosing with monthly monitoring from weeks 24 to 52 were diminished after continued PRN dosing, with a reduced monitoring frequency from weeks 52 to 100.

▶ Macular edema secondary to central retinal vein occlusion continues to result in significant visual loss even in those eyes receiving intravitreal injections. The COPERNICUS study randomly assigned patients to either monthly intravitreal aflibercept or sham injections for the first 6 months, then all patients were eligible to receive intravitreal aflibercept on an as-needed basis until the 1-year endpoint.

At each time point, the aflibercept group achieved a higher percentage of patients that gained 15 letters or more and improved central retinal thickness. The significant functional and anatomic benefits were maintained from the 6-month to 1-year time point. However, at the 1-year time point, monthly injections were discontinued, and all patients received quarterly examinations with as-needed injections. In both arms, the percentage of patients that maintained 15 letters or more improvement over baseline was significantly reduced.

This study shows the improvement in vision that can be achieved with intravitreal aflibercept for macular edema secondary to central retinal vein occlusion but also reinforces that some patients require injections long term. Identifying risk factors for poor visual outcome and long-term treatment will be very helpful for management.

O. P. Gupta, MD

Vitrectomy for Floaters: Prospective Efficacy Analyses and Retrospective Safety Profile

Sebag J, Yee KMP, Wa CA, et al (VMR Inst, Huntington Beach, CA; et al)

Retina 34:1062-1068, 2014

Purpose.—Floaters impact vision but the mechanism is unknown. We hypothesize that floaters reduce contrast sensitivity function, which can be normalized by vitrectomy, and that minimally invasive vitrectomy will have lower incidences of retinal tears (reported at 30%) and cataracts (50–76%).

Methods.—Seventy-six eyes (34 phakic) with floaters were evaluated in 2 separate studies. Floater etiologies were primarily posterior vitreous detachment in 61 of 76 eyes (80%) and myopic vitreopathy in 24 of 76 eyes (32%). Minimally invasive 25G vitrectomy was performed without posterior vitreous detachment induction, leaving anterior vitreous, and using nonhollow probes for cannula extraction. Efficacy was studied prospectively (up to 9 months) in 16 floater cases with Freiburg Acuity Contrast Testing (Weber index [%W] reproducibility = 92.1%) and the National Eye Institute Visual Function Questionnaire. Safety was separately evaluated in 60 other cases followed up on an average of 17.5 months (range, 3–51 months).

Results.—Floater eyes had 67% contrast sensitivity function attenuation (4.0 ± 2.3%W; control subjects = 2.4 ± 0.9%W, $P < 0.013$). After vitrectomy, contrast sensitivity function normalized in each case at 1 week (2.0 ± 1.4%W, $P < 0.01$) and remained normal at 1 month (2.0 ± 1.0%W, $P < 0.003$) and 3 months to 9 months (2.2 ± 1.5%W, $P < 0.018$). Visual Function Questionnaire was 28.3% lower in floater patients (73.2 ± 15.6, N = 16) than in age-matched control subjects (93.9 ± 8.0, N = 12, $P < 0.001$), and postoperatively improved by 29.2% ($P < 0.001$). In the safety study of 60 floater cases treated with vitrectomy, none developed retinal breaks, infection, or glaucoma after a mean follow-up of 17.5 months. Only 8 of 34 cases (23.5%) required cataract surgery (none younger than 53 years) at an average of 15 months postvitrectomy.

Conclusion.—Floaters lower contrast sensitivity function, which normalizes after vitrectomy. Visual Function Questionnaire quantified improvement in satisfaction. Not inducing posterior vitreous detachment reduced retinal tear incidence from 30% to 0% ($P < 0.007$). Postvitrectomy cataract incidence was reduced from 50% to 23.5% ($P < 0.02$). This approach thus seems effective and safe in alleviating the visual dysfunction induced by floaters.

▶ Pars plana vitrectomy for floaters, or floaterectomy, has been a relatively controversial topic. Much of the controversy is based on the value of the procedure weighed against the inherent risks of the surgery. Because of the advancements of vitreoretinal surgical instrumentation, small-gauge vitrectomy has approached the complication rate of standard cataract surgery. Surgeons and patients appreciate the high degree of satisfaction that can be achieved with this surgery.

This study explores the mechanism that causes floaters to result in decreased vision. The safety profile of this procedure is also reported. Contrast sensitivity was attenuated 67% compared with that in control eyes. The Visual Function Questionnaire results were approximately 28% lower as well. Postoperatively, the contrast sensitivity normalized in all cases and the Visual Function

Questionnaire results improved by more than 29%. The safety profile was favorable, and 23.5% of cases required cataract surgery 15 months postoperatively.

O. P. Gupta, MD

6 Uveitis

The Future of Uveitis Treatment

Lin P, Suhler EB, Rosenbaum JT, et al (Oregon Health & Science Univ, Portland; et al)

Ophthalmology 121:365-376, 2014

Uveitis is a heterogeneous collection of diseases with polygenic and environmental influences. This heterogeneity presents challenges in trial design and selection of end points. Despite the multitude of causes, therapeutics targeting common inflammatory pathways are effective in treating diverse forms of uveitis. These treatments, including corticosteroids and immunomodulatory agents, although often effective, can have untoward side effects, limiting their utility. The search for drugs with equal or improved efficacy that are safe is therefore paramount. A mechanism-based approach is most likely to yield the future breakthroughs in the treatment of uveitis. We review the literature and provide examples of the nuances of immune regulation and dysregulation that can be targeted for therapeutic benefit. As our understanding of the causes of uveitis grows we will learn how to better apply antibodies designed to block interaction between inflammatory cytokines and their receptors. T-lymphocyte activation can be targeted by blocking costimulatory pathways or inhibiting major histocompatibility complex protein interactions. Furthermore, intracellular downstream molecules from cytokine or other pathways can be inhibited using small molecule inhibitors, which have the benefit of being orally bioavailable. An emerging field is the lipid-mediated inflammatory and regulatory pathways. Alternatively, anti-inflammatory cytokines can be provided by administering recombinant protein, and intracellular "brakes" of inflammatory pathways can be introduced potentially by gene therapy. Novel approaches of delivering a therapeutic substance include, but are not limited to, the use of small interfering RNA, viral and nonviral gene therapy, and microparticle or viscous gel sustained-release drug-delivery platforms.

► In this Translational Science Review directed toward uveitis specialists, the authors summarize the current understanding of the pathophysiology of uveitis, the drugs available to treat the disease, and the challenges in trial design and selection of end points in evaluating their efficacy. The authors summarize the current state of uveitic therapy as "too toxic, too nonspecific, [and] too few choices." An improved understanding of the cytokines involved in uveitis should allow development of more specific drugs. For example, the pro-inflammatory mediators include T-helper (Th)1 and Th17 lymphocytes and the cytokines interleukin (IL)-1β, IL-6, IL-17, IL-23, and tumor necrosis factor (TNF)-α; the TNF antagonists adalimumab and infliximab, although not approved by the US Food and Drug Administration (FDA) for uveitis, are widely used off label when conventional therapy has failed and may be considered as first-line therapy in patients with severe ocular Behcet's disease. Gevokizumab, an IL-1β antagonist, is in clinical trials for treatment of Behcet's disease. Conversely, anti-inflammatory mediators such as IL-10, IL-27, IL-35, and transforming growth factor (TGF)-β might be used to treat uveitis. However, the authors note that some cytokines, such as interferon (IFN)-γ, can be protective or inflammatory and that systemically administered IL-17 has actually been found to be protective against the development of uveitis in several animal models of uveitis. Furthermore, despite a good therapeutic rationale, several clinical trials of the anti-IL-17A monoclonal antibody secukinumab were discontinued because of the failure to meet the primary efficacy endpoints. Finally, different forms of biologic agents appear to act differently in different parts of the body. Etanercept, which blocks the interaction of TNF with cell surface TNF receptors, is very effective in rheumatoid arthritis but less effective than the anti-TNF agents, infliximab and adalimumab, which are monoclonal antibodies directed against TNF-α. Etanercept may, in fact, exacerbate or even induce ocular inflammation.

Targeted drug therapy (eg, intravitreal injections)[1,2] offers the hope of greater efficacy and reduced toxicity. The authors emphasize the difficulty in creating viable clinical trials for which there are ideal endpoints for a relatively rare and heterogenous disease.[3] Reduction in vitreous haze, for example, is a reasonable outcome to measure in eyes with a significant intermediate uveitis component but is meaningless in eyes with purely posterior uveitis. At the same time, using the same drug to treat 2 or more different types of uveitis (say, birdshot chorioretinopathy and sarcoid-associated panuveitis) may yield conflicting results. A critical issue limiting drug development that is not addressed by the authors is cost.[4] Biologic and other drugs targeted against a single pathway or cytokine are extraordinarily expensive. Without FDA approval for use in uveitis, insurance companies are increasingly likely to deny coverage for these drugs.

J. P. Dunn, MD

References

1. Hamam RN, Barikian AW, Antonios RS, et al. Intravitreal adalimumab in active noninfectious uveitis: a pilot study. *Ocul Immunol Inflamm.* 2014:1-8 [Epub ahead of print].
2. Reddy AK, Cabrera M, Yeh S, Davis JL, Albini TA. Optical coherence tomography-guided ranibizumab injection for cystoid macular edema in well-controlled uveitis: twelve-month outcomes. *Retina.* 2014;34:2431-2438.
3. Mesquida M, Molins B, Llorenç V, Sainz de la Maza M, Adán A. Long-term effects of tocilizumab therapy for refractory uveitis-related macular edema. *Ophthalmology.* 2014;121:2380-2386.
4. Multicenter Uveitis Steroid Treatment (MUST) Trial Research Group, Sugar EA, Holbrook JT, Kempen JH, et al. Cost-effectiveness of fluocinolone acetonide implant versus systemic therapy for noninfectious intermediate, posterior, and panuveitis. *Ophthalmology.* 2014;121:1855-1862.

Expert Panel Recommendations for the Use of Anti–Tumor Necrosis Factor Biologic Agents in Patients with Ocular Inflammatory Disorders

Levy-Clarke G, Jabs DA, Read RW, et al (St. Luke's Cataract and Laser Inst, Tarpon Springs, FL; the Mount Sinai Med School, NY; Univ of Alabama at Birmingham School of Medicine; et al)

Ophthalmology 121:785-796.e3, 2014

Topic.—To provide recommendations for the use of anti-tumor necrosis factor α (TNF-α) biologic agents in patients with ocular inflammatory disorders.

Clinical Relevance.—Ocular inflammatory diseases remain a leading cause of vision loss worldwide. Anti–TNF-α agents are used widely in treatment of rheumatologic diseases. A committee of the American Uveitis Society performed a systematic review of literature to generate guidelines for use of these agents in ocular inflammatory conditions.

Methods.—A systematic review of published studies was performed. Recommendations were generated using the Grading of Recommendations Assessment, Development, and Evaluation group criteria.

Results.—Numerous studies including controlled clinical trials have demonstrated that anti–TNF-α biologic agents (in particular infliximab and adalimumab) are effective in the treatment of severe ocular inflammatory disease. Based on these studies, the expert panel makes the following recommendations.

Conclusions.—Infliximab and adalimumab can be considered as first-line immunomodulatory agents for the treatment of ocular manifestations of Behçet's disease. Infliximab and adalimumab can be considered as secondline immunomodulatory agents for the treatment of uveitis associated with juvenile arthritis. Infliximab and adalimumab can be considered as potential second-line immunomodulatory agents for the treatment of severe ocular inflammatory conditions including posterior uveitis, panuveitis, severe uveitis associated with seronegative spondyloarthropathy, and scleritis in patients requiring immunomodulation in patients who have failed or who are not candidates for antimetabolite or calcineurin inhibitor immunomodulation. Infliximab and adalimumab can be considered in these patients in preference to etanercept, which seems to be associated with lower rates of treatment success.

► A subcommittee of the American Uveitis Society reviewed roughly 400 articles describing the use of antitumor necrosis factor (anti-TNF) agents in the treatment of uveitis and scleritis. Similar to a 2000 study including many of the same authors that evaluated the use of corticosteroids for ocular inflammatory disease, recommendations for clinicians regarding the use of anti-TNF drugs were based on the Scottish Intercollegiate Guideline Network (SIGN) for individual studies. The panel reviewed the potential adverse effects common to all anti-TNF drugs, including infection, sepsis, reactivation of granulomatous disease such as tuberculosis (TB) and invasive fungal infections, exacerbation of heart failure, and development of autoimmune disorders such as lupuslike disease (even with the fully humanized monoclonal antibody adalimumab). Anecdotal evidence (SIGN Level III) suggested that etanercept is associated with a significantly greater number of new uveitis cases than adalimumab or infliximab.[1] The authors recommended that patients taking etanercept with incompletely controlled uveitis or new ocular disease should consider switching to infliximab or adalimumab. The Food and Drug Administration (FDA) has mandated a black box warning about an increased risk of lymphoma in children taking any anti-TNF drug. However, 2 large observational databases of uveitis patients have shown no increased risk of malignancy except for nonmelanoma skin cancer (odds ratio 1.5) in one of the studies. The authors noted that reports of an increased risk of lymphoma in patients treated for rheumatoid arthritis (RA) with anti-TNF drugs have not established a causal relationship; they emphasized that RA alone may increase the risk of lymphoma. Based on the overall analysis, clinicians should incorporate the following recommendations:

Before treatment:

1. All patients should be tested for TB and appropriate anti-TB therapy begun for patients with latent TB. Anti-TNF therapy may be started 1 month after anti-TB therapy has been initiated.
2. Before initiation of anti-TB therapy, patients should have received pneumococcal, killed influenza virus, and hepatitis B vaccinations.
3. Patients should not receive live virus vaccinations such as measles, varicella zoster, oral polio, or live influenza.
4. In patients with intermediate uveitis, magnetic resonance imaging of the brain should be performed to exclude multiple sclerosis.

Treatment of noninfectious ocular inflammatory disease:

1. Infliximab or adalimumab may be considered as first- or second-line corticosteroid-sparing therapy for ocular Behcet disease; infliximab may be considered first- or second-line corticosteroid-sparing therapy for acute exacerbations of the disease.
2. Infliximab and adalimumab may be considered as second-line corticosteroid-sparing therapy for the following:
   - Severe uveitis associated with juvenile idiopathic arthritis or seronegative spondyloarthropathy;
   - Other forms of noninfectious uveitis (eg, birdshot chorioretinitis) in patients with corticosteroid-dependent disease who have failed first-line immunomodulatory therapy, such as antimetabolites or calcineurin inhibitors; and
   - Chronic or severe scleritis.

No doubt the indications for anti-TNF agents and other biologic agents will change as new drugs come to the market, clinicians have greater experience in the use of these drugs in patients with uveitis,[2-4] clinical trials are completed, and the FDA approves the drugs for ophthalmic use.

J. P. Dunn, MD

References

1. Wendling D, Joshi A, Reilly P, Jalundhwala YJ, Mittal M, Bao Y. Comparing the risk of developing uveitis in patients initiating anti-tumor necrosis factor therapy for ankylosing spondylitis: an analysis of a large US claims database. *Curr Med Res Opin.* 2014;30:2515-2521.
2. Cordero-Coma M, Yilmaz T, Onal S. Systematic review of anti-tumor necrosis factor-alpha therapy for treatment of immune-mediated uveitis. *Ocul Immunol Inflamm.* 2013;21:19-27.
3. Schaap-Fogler M, Amer R, Friling R, Priel E, Kramer M. Anti-TNF-α agents for refractory cystoid macular edema associated with noninfectious uveitis. *Graefes Arch Clin Exp Ophthalmol.* 2014;252:633-640.
4. Simonini G, Druce K, Cimaz R, Macfarlane GJ, Jones GT. Current evidence of anti-tumor necrosis factor α treatment efficacy in childhood chronic uveitis: a systematic review and meta-analysis approach of individual drugs. *Arthritis Care Res (Hoboken).* 2014;66:1073-1084.

Incidence of Visual Improvement in Uveitis Cases with Visual Impairment Caused by Macular Edema

Levin MH, for the Systemic Immunosuppressive Therapy for Eye Diseases Cohort Study (Univ of Pennsylvania, Philadelphia; et al)

Ophthalmology 121:588-595.e1, 2014

Purpose.—Among cases of visually significant uveitic macular edema (ME), to estimate the incidence of visual improvement and identify predictive factors.

Design.—Retrospective cohort study.

Participants.—Eyes with uveitis, seen at 5 academic ocular inflammation centers in the United States, for which ME was documented to be currently present and the principal cause of reduced visual acuity (<20/40).

Methods.—Data were obtained by standardized chart review.

Main Outcome Measures.—Decrease of ≥0.2 base 10 logarithm of visual acuity decimal fraction-equivalent; risk factors for such visual improvement.

Results.—We identified 1510 eyes (of 1077 patients) with visual impairment to a level <20/40 attributed to ME. Most patients were female (67%) and white (76%), and had bilateral uveitis (82%). The estimated 6-month incidence of ≥2 lines of visual acuity improvement in affected eyes was 52% (95% confidence interval [CI], 49%–55%). Vision reduced by ME was more likely to improve by 2 lines in eyes initially with poor visual acuity (≤20/200; adjusted hazard ratio [HR] 1.5; 95% CI, 1.3–1.7), active uveitis (HR, 1.3; 95% CI, 1.1–1.5), and anterior uveitis as opposed to intermediate (HR, 1.2), posterior (HR, 1.3), or panuveitis (HR, 1.4; overall $P = 0.02$). During follow-up, reductions in anterior chamber or vitreous cellular activity or in vitreous haze each led to significant improvements in visual outcome ($P < 0.001$ for each). Conversely, snowbanking (HR, 0.7; 95% CI, 0.4–0.99), posterior synechiae (HR, 0.8; 95% CI, 0.6–0.9), and hypotony (HR, 0.2; 95% CI, 0.06–0.5) each were associated with lower incidence of visual improvement with respect to eyes lacking each of these attributes at a given visit.

Conclusions.—These results suggest that many, but not all, patients with ME causing low vision in a tertiary care setting will enjoy meaningful visual recovery in response to treatment. Evidence of significant ocular damage from inflammation (posterior synechiae and hypotony) portends a lower incidence of visual recovery. Better control of anterior chamber or vitreous activity is associated with a greater incidence of visual improvement, supporting an aggressive anti-inflammatory treatment approach for ME cases with active inflammation.

▶ Macular edema (ME) is the leading cause of visual loss in patients with uveitis, but the factors affecting visual recovery in these patients have not been well elucidated.[1,2] In this study, the authors performed a retrospective cohort study from 5 uveitis tertiary care referral centers in the United States of 1510 eyes in 1077 patients with uveitic ME causing reduced visual acuity of < 20/40. The majority of patients were female, white, and had bilateral uveitis. Overall, 52% of eyes had improvement in vision of > 2 lines, with the rate of improvement tending to be higher in the first few months of therapy. Factors associated with visual improvement included initially poor visual acuity (< 20/200), active uveitis, and anterior (as opposed to other anatomic locations) uveitis. Reduction in anterior chamber cells and vitreous cells and haze also correlated with visual improvement. Eyes with snowbanking (but not snowballs), posterior synechiae, and especially hypotony (intraocular pressure < 5 mm Hg) had worse visual outcomes compared with eyes without these findings. A history of cataract, glaucoma, or vitreoretinal surgery was not associated with improvement of ME-induced visual decline. A history of vitreoretinal, cataract, or glaucoma before the diagnosis of ME was not associated with visual improvement, nor was a trend toward improved vision identified in the small number of eyes undergoing such surgeries during follow-up. Of particular note was the fact that visually significant ME was diagnosed in 29% of eyes with inactive uveitis at baseline, confirming that ME might evolve or persist despite control or remission of inflammation. Age and the presence of systemic autoimmune disease did not influence visual outcomes. Active cigarette smoking (which has been shown to increase the risk of both ME in uveitic eyes and relapse of uveitis) was not associated with worse visual outcomes; the authors suggested that smoking might affect the risk of ME more than degree to which it affected the prognosis of established ME.

The study was not designed to assess the cost-effectiveness or relative efficacy of different forms of medical therapy or surgical interventions such as pars plana vitrectomy. Nonetheless, the authors recommended aggressive anti-inflammatory therapy early in the course of disease and emphasized that treatment specifically for ME rather than just uveitis should be evaluated in future studies. One limitation to the study was the fact that ME was diagnosed by clinical examination alone in 77% of patients, compared with optical coherence tomography (OCT; 18%) and fluorescein angiography (FA; 5%), reducing the certainty by which ME rather than epiretinal membrane or vitreomacular traction was the principal cause of visual impairment. In the subset of eyes with ME diagnosed by OCT or FA, however, the results were similar except that intermediate uveitis was associated with a similar rather than less favorable outcome than anterior uveitis, and a history of pars plana vitrectomy was associated with a reduced incidence of visual improvement. The study is strengthened by the large number of patients but does not make specific treatment recommendations. Clinicians should be aware of the potential for visual acuity improvement despite macular edema and that macular edema may persist despite control of the uveitis.

J. P. Dunn, MD

References

1. Lozano López V, Serrano García M, Mantolán Sarmiento C, et al. A cost-effectiveness study of dexamethasone implants in macular edema. *Arch Soc Esp Oftalmol.* 2015;90:14-21.
2. Tomkins-Netzer O, Talat L, Bar A, et al. Long-term clinical outcome and causes of vision loss in patients with uveitis. *Ophthalmology.* 2014;121:2387-2392.

Risk for Uveitis With Oral Moxifloxacin: A Comparative Safety Study

Eadie B, Etminan M, Mikelberg FS (Univ of British Columbia, Vancouver, Canada)

JAMA Ophthalmol 133:81-84, 2015

Importance.—Numerous case reports have suggested that the recent use of moxifloxacin may lead to uveitis. This epidemiologic study is, to our knowledge, the first to explore the relationship between oral moxifloxacin hydrochloride use and uveitis.

Observations.—We conducted a case-control study within a cohort of men aged 40 to 85 years followed up from January 2001 through December 2011. All cases with a new diagnosis of uveitis were identified. For each case, 10 control subjects were matched by age, cohort entry date, and follow-up duration. For identified uveitis cases, current use of moxifloxacin, levofloxacin, or ciprofloxacin hydrochloride was compared with nonuse. Rate ratios were adjusted for potential confounding variables. We identified 13 313 uveitis cases and 133 130 corresponding controls. Compared with nonusers of fluoroquinolones, current first-time users of moxifloxacin demonstrated the highest risk for uveitis (adjusted rate ratio, 2.98 [95% CI, 1.80-4.94]). Current first-time users of ciprofloxacin (adjusted rate ratio, 1.96 [95% CI, 1.56-2.47]) showed an increased risk for uveitis, while current first-time users of levofloxacin (adjusted rate ratio, 1.26 [95% CI, 0.90-1.77]) did not show a significant association with uveitis.

Conclusion and Relevance.—Current use of moxifloxacin or ciprofloxacin appears to increase the risk for uveitis. A statistically significant association of current first-time use of levofloxacin with uveitis could not be

identified. Levofloxacin may pose the least risk for uveitis compared with moxifloxacin and ciprofloxacin.

▶ Drug-induced uveitis accounts for only a small percentage of all uveitis cases but may be underreported. Anecdotal reports suggest that oral (but not topical) fluoroquinolones (FQs) may precipitate acute bilateral anterior uveitis and pigmentary dispersion with atonic pupils.[1–4] However, the incidence of uveitis and drugs in causing uveitis has not been reported. In addition, most reports describe uveitis associated with moxifloxacin, but because this drug is prescribed much more commonly than other FQs, the relative risk of different FQs is unknown. Using a comprehensive database in British Columbia, Eadie and colleagues undertook a time-matched, case-control study of 1 million men aged 40 to 85 years (mean 67.2). For each study patient (defined by the development of acute anterior uveitis within 15 days of the diagnosis of uveitis after receiving a prescription for an oral FQ), 10 age-matched controls were also studied, allowing for assessment of the rate ratio (RR). The RR was adjusted for potential causes of uveitis such as inflammatory bowel disease and ankylosing spondylitis. A group of patients treated with finasteride (a drug not associated with the development of uveitis) also served as controls. First-time users of moxifloxacin had the highest risk of uveitis (adjusted RR 2.98), followed by ciprofloxacin (adjusted RR 1.96); levofloxacin (RR 1.26, 95% confidence interval 0.90-1.77) and finasteride were not associated with uveitis. The risk of uveitis with repeated use of moxifloxacin and ciprofloxacin was lower compared with first-time users. FQ-induced uveitis has been attributed to direct toxic effects on the iris and ciliary body. The authors postulated that oral moxifloxacin has a higher tissue-binding affinity than other FQs, thus explaining its higher association with uveitis. It is not clear why only older men were studied, and the study could not determine whether prescriptions given were actually used. Characteristics of FQ-induced uveitis (laterality, granulomatous vs nongranulomatous, and ocular complications) and treatment were not evaluated. Nonetheless, FQ-induced uveitis should be considered in the differential diagnosis of acute anterior uveitis. Interestingly, an earlier nested case-control study using the same database and with at least 1 of the same authors also found an association between onset of uveitis and antecedent macrolide or beta-lactam use, raising the possibility that the uveitis might be secondary to the underlying infection and not the drug itself. Additional studies are needed to confirm the risk and determine the most effective therapy.

J. P. Dunn, MD

References

1. Wefers Bettink-Remeijer M, Brouwers K, van Langenhove L, et al. Uveitis-like syndrome and iris transillumination after the use of oral moxifloxacin. *Eye (Lond).* 2009;23:2260-2262.
2. Knape RM, Sayyad FE, Davis JL. Moxifloxacin and bilateral acute iris transillumination. *J Ophthalmic Inflamm Infect.* 2013;3:10.

3. Forooghian F, Maberley D, Albiani DA, Kirker AW, Merkur AB, Etminan M. Uveitis risk following oral fluoroquinolone therapy: a nested case-control study. *Ocul Immunol Inflamm*. 2013;21:390-393.
4. Hinkle DM, Dacey MS, Mandelcorn E, et al. Bilateral uveitis associated with fluoroquinolone therapy. *Cutan Ocul Toxicol*. 2012;31:111-116.

Tatto-Associated Uveitis

Ostheimer TA, Burkholder BM, Leung TG, et al (Johns Hopkins Univ School of Medicine, Baltimore, MD)
Am J Ophthalmol 158:637-643.e1, 2014

Purpose.—To describe the clinical presentation of uveitis with coincident onset of raised and indurated tattooed skin.

Design.—Case series.

Methods.—Seven consecutive patients were evaluated at a tertiary ophthalmologic facility with coincident uveitis and cutaneous tattoo induration over an 18-month period. All subjects underwent complete ophthalmic examination and a focused systemic medical evaluation including serologic testing and imaging studies. Two participants underwent biopsy of their tattoos. The patients' clinical courses and responses to treatment over a followup period of 1–20 months are reported (mean followup = 9 months). Main outcome measures included degree of intraocular inflammation, ocular complications, visual acuity, clinically observable tattooed skin changes, and biopsy results.

Results.—Five of 7 patients had bilateral nongranulomatous anterior uveitis: 4 with chronic and 1 with recurrent disease. The remaining 2 patients had bilateral chronic granulomatous panuveitis. Biopsies of raised and indurated tattoos were performed in 2 patients and demonstrated noncaseating granulomatous inflammation surrounding tattoo ink in the dermis. The skin changes resolved in all patients, with a faster response noted in those treated with high-dose oral prednisone for intraocular inflammation. Five patients subsequently experienced recurrent flares of intraocular inflammation in conjunction with the recurrence of raised and indurated tattoos.

Conclusions.—These cases represent a subset of patients in whom skin tattooing may have incited an immune response leading to simultaneous inflammation of the eyes and tattooed skin.

▶ In this single-center case series, the authors identified a series of 7 patients over a 20-month period whose uveitis appeared to be associated with a hypersensitivity reaction to tattoo ink, including induration and inflammation of pigmented skin but not adjacent nonpigmented skin. Six patients were black and 5 were male. Five patients had bilateral nongranulomatous anterior uveitis (4 chronic and 1 recurrent), and 2 patients had bilateral chronic granulomatous panuveitis. Biopsies of the skin lesions in 2 patients revealed noncaseating granulomata surrounding tattoo ink in the dermis. Although corticosteroid therapy resulted in resolution of the skin changes in all cases, 5 patients had recurrent uveitis in conjunction with tattoo induration, and 4 patients required immunomodulatory therapy to control the uveitis. All patients tested negatively for syphilis (fluorescent treponemal antibody absorption and rapid plasma reagin) and sarcoidosis (chest x-ray and/or computed chest tomography and serum angiotensin-converting enzyme and/or serum lysozyme), and no other infectious or autoimmune causes of uveitis were identified. Ocular complications include glaucoma, posterior synechiae, pupillary membranes, optic nerve swelling and hyperemia, cystoid macular edema, papillomacular exudates, epiretinal membranes, and retinal pigment endothelium detachment. The indurated skin did not occur at the time of the tattoo and developed subsequently only in areas of black tattoo pigment, ranging from focal nodular elevation to uniform elevation. The authors noted that the association of tattoos and uveitis is likely underreported[1,2] and that, given the 24% prevalence of tattoos among adults aged 18 to 50 in the United States, a history of tattoos be sought in the workup of the patient with uveitis. The histopathologic findings in the 2 patients who underwent biopsy could have been caused by a delayed-type hypersensitivity reaction to specific components of tattoo pigment, or a manifestation of systemic sarcoidosis may be the end result of immune responses in genetically susceptible individuals to a large variety of environmental triggers.

J. P. Dunn, MD

References

1. Saliba N, Owen ME, Beare N. Tattoo-associated uveitis. *Eye (Lond)*. 2010;24:1406.
2. Mansour AM, Chan CC. Recurrent uveitis preceded by swelling of skin tattoos. *Am J Ophthalmol*. 1991;111:515-516.

The Value of Measuring Urinary β2-Microglobulin and Serum Creatinine for Detecting Tubulointerstitial Nephritis and Uveitis Syndrome in Young Patients With Uveitis

Hettinga YM, Scheerlinck LME, Lilien MR, et al (Univ Medical Ctr Utrecht, the Netherlands; et al)
JAMA Ophthalmol 133:140-145, 2015

Importance.—Tubulointerstitial nephritis and uveitis (TINU) syndrome is characterized by tubulointerstitial and ocular inflammation. Thus far, the value of noninvasive diagnostic tests is not known.

Objective.—To determine whether urinary β2-microglobulin (β2M), urinary protein, and serum creatinine have predictive value for detecting TINU syndrome in young patients with uveitis.

Design, Setting, and Participants.—This prospective cohort study was conducted July 2010 through February 2013 at a tertiary care referral center in Utrecht, the Netherlands. Forty-five consecutive new patients with uveitis aged 22 years or younger were enrolled.

Exposures.—Urinary β2M, urinary protein, and serum creatinine were measured prospectively, and the estimated glomerular filtration rate was calculated.

Main Outcomes and Measures.—A post hoc analysis was performed to determine whether urinary β2M, urinary protein, serum creatinine, estimated glomerular filtration rate, and/or pyuria were correlated with definitive and probable cases of TINU syndrome.

Results.—Eighteen of the 45 patients (40%) in our cohort had elevated urinary β2M levels, and 10 patients (22%) had elevated serum creatinine levels. Twenty of 43 patients (47%) had proteinuria. Eight of the 45 patients were diagnosed by a pediatric nephrologist as having renal dysfunction that suggested acute interstitial nephritis. Of these 8 patients, 2 were definitively diagnosed as having TINU syndrome (confirmed by renal biopsy). After excluding other causes of renal dysfunction, the remaining 6 patients with uveitis and renal dysfunction fulfilled the criteria of probable TINU syndrome. The 8 patients with definitive or probable TINU syndrome had higher urinary β2M levels than patients with normal renal function (median β2M, 1.95 mg/L; 95% CI, 1.26-5.16 mg/L vs 0.20 mg/L; 95% CI, 0.19-0.21 mg/L; $P < .001$; Mann-Whitney *U* test). Our analysis revealed that the positive predictive value of increased β2M combined with increased serum creatinine was 100% for detecting definitive and/or probable TINU syndrome.

Conclusions and Relevance.—These data suggest that urinary β2M and serum creatinine levels are sensitive and relatively simple diagnostic screening tools for detecting renal dysfunction to diagnose TINU syndrome in young patients with uveitis similar to those evaluated in this study.

▶ Tubulointerstitial nephritis and uveitis (TINU) syndrome has usually been considered an uncommon cause of uveitis in children and young adults, peaking in incidence at age 14.[1,2] It is characterized by the sudden onset of bilateral anterior uveitis with mild to moderate vitreous inflammation and, occasionally, chorioretinal scars. Systemic symptoms include malaise, fever, and joint pain. The acute tubulointerstitial nephritis (AIN) component typically precedes the uveitis and is often asymptomatic but can lead to chronic kidney disease. Renal biopsy is necessary to make a definitive diagnosis but is usually not performed because of the risks. Furthermore, AIN is often self-limited, but oral corticosteroids will hasten resolution. Hence, Hettinga et al suggest that the nephritis is "grossly underestimated" as a cause of uveitis, compared with published estimates of 1% to 2%. They performed a retrospective study at a large uveitis tertiary care referral center in the Netherlands to assess the predictive positive value of urinary β2-microglobulin, urinalysis including protein, serum creatinine, and age-adjusted estimated glomerular filtration rate in diagnosing TINU in young patients with uveitis. β2-microglobulin is a 120-kDa protein that is usually excreted by the glomeruli and then reabsorbed by the tubules; in AIN, reabsorption is diminished, resulting in elevated urinary levels. Forty-five patients aged 4 to 22 were included, of whom 8 (18%, 5 male and 3 female) were diagnosed by a pediatric nephrologist as having probable or definitive TINU based on renal biopsy and/or laboratory testing. Seven of these patients had elevated urinary β2-microglobulin (> 1.0 mg/L) with a statistically higher mean (1.95 mg/L) vs those patients with uveitis of other causes (0.20 mg/L). The positive predictive value (PPV) and negative predictive value (NPV) of urinary β2-microglobulin > 1.0 mg/L were 88% and 97%, respectively. For age-adjusted serum creatinine, the PPV and NPV were 80% and 100%, respectively. Combining the 2 tests resulted in PPV of 100% and NPV 97%. It appears that TINU is an underdiagnosed cause of uveitis in young patients and clinicians should strongly consider this in the differential diagnosis. In fact, because elevated urinary β2-microglobulin is transient and affected patients may not be seen promptly by a nephrologist or ophthalmologist, their estimate of the number of patients with TINU may actually be low. By providing useful statistical guidelines for the diagnosis of this disease, the authors have helped to reduce the numbers of patients with the frustrating diagnosis of "idiopathic uveitis." The sample size is small, however, and confirmation of the authors' findings by other centers is necessary.

J. P. Dunn, MD

References

1. Rosenbaum JT. Nibbling away at the diagnosis of idiopathic uveitis. *JAMA Ophthalmol.* 2015;133:146-147.
2. Mackensen F, Smith JR, Rosenbaum JT. Enhanced recognition, treatment, and prognosis of tubulointerstitial nephritis and uveitis syndrome. *Ophthalmology.* 2007;114:995-999.

Differential diagnosis of macular edema of different pathophysiologic origins by spectral domain optical coherence tomography

Munk MR, Sacu S, Huf W, et al (Med Univ of Vienna, Austria)
Retina 34:2218-2232, 2014

Purpose.—To develop a classification approach based solely on spectral domain optical coherence tomography to differentiate macular edema (ME) of different disease entities and to determine underlying pathology.

Methods.—A cross-sectional study including 153 participants: 27 with Irvine–Gass, 31 with uveitic ME, 24 with ME after branch retinal vein occlusion, 13 with central retinal vein occlusion, 44 with diabetic ME, and 14 controls. Spectral domain optical coherence tomography was graded according to a standardized reading protocol. Grading characteristics were: ME pattern in the central line (horizontal/vertical) and in volume scans, distribution of cysts in Early Treatment Diabetic Retinopathy Study grid, morphologic features, and quantitative parameters such as individual layer thickness. The parameters in a best-fitting multivariate model were evaluated for reliability to predict the underlying pathology using a leave-one-out crossover-validation analysis. To evaluate clinical reliability, two masked clinicians graded spectral domain optical coherence tomography images according to the assessed parameters.

Results.—The best-fitting multivariate model revealed that microfoci, ME pattern in vertical line scan, and foveal retinal nerve fiber layer thickness are the best indicators of the underlying pathology of ME. Classification accuracy of this model was 96%, mean cross-validated test classification accuracy was 84% ($r^2 = 0.95$, $P < 0.0001$). Clinical relevance was examined with 2 independent readers, yielding classification accuracies of 86% in both cases.

Conclusion.—Macular edema demonstrates characteristic patterns, morphologic features, and layer thicknesses dependent on the underlying disease process. Diagnostic recognition of these features may allow clinical and automated disease identification based primarily on spectral domain optical coherence tomography analysis.

▶ The pathophysiology of macular edema (ME) includes such factors as proinflammatory mediators, oxidative stress, hypoxia, and increased hydrostatic pressure, each of which can be more or less prominent depending on the underlying disease. However, correlation of morphologic features and patterns of ME with the underlying disease process has not previously been reported. Spectral domain optical coherence tomography (SD-OCT) is superior to fluorescein angiography (FA) for quantitative and qualitative analysis of retinal structures, including macular thickening, but FA has been found to detect macular leakage better than OCT; the 2 tests offer only moderate agreement in assessing the status of ME in eyes with uveitis. Both tests are more sensitive in detecting ME than biomicroscopy. Detection of the cause of ME may have important therapeutic implications. For example, persistent ME in eyes with quiet uveitis may respond best to anti-vascular endothelial growth factor therapy, whereas true uveitic ME may require more aggressive corticosteroid or immunosuppressive therapy.

In this masked, controlled, cross-sectional study, the authors examined 44 eyes that had diabetic ME, 24 with branch retinal vein occlusion, 13 with central retinal vein occlusion, 31 with uveitic macular edema, and 13 control eyes to see if macular edema of different causes could be distinguished using SD-OCT. Macular edema was defined as central retinal thickness greater than 300 μ with either expanded areas of reduced intraretinal reflectivity or the presence of intraretinal cystoid-like spaces. Definitions of ME patterns in horizontal and vertical scans were created (eg, diffuse and focal retinal thickening, generalized ME, central ME). Morphologic features such as epiretinal membrane, microaneurysms, cotton-wool spots, retinal nerve fiber layer (RNFL) thickness, and microfoci-hard exudates were assessed. Patients with vitreomacular traction were excluded. A best-fitting multivariate model was evaluated for reliability to predict the underlying pathology using a leave-one-out crossover-validation analysis. Clinical reliability was assessed using 2 masked graders of the OCT images. The authors found that microfoci, ME pattern in vertical line scans, and foveal retinal nerve fiber layer thickness best predicted the underlying pathology of the ME. Uveitic ME was characterized by absence of intraretinal microfoci, a vertical symmetric ME pattern, and foveal RNFL thickness similar to that of controls. Diabetic ME was characterized by the presence of microfoci with a foveal RNFL thickness similar to that of controls. Branch retinal vein occlusion-associated

ME showed a combination of vertical inferior or superior ME (depending on the location of the vein occlusion) and a foveal RNFL thickness almost double that of controls. Central retinal vein occlusion-associated ME showed a symmetric ME pattern on vertical scans, microfoci, and a foveal RNFL thickness greater than 4 times that of controls. Irvine-Gass syndrome showed absence of intraretinal microfoci and a symmetric ME pattern in vertical line scans with foveal RNFL thickness roughly 3 times that of controls. Given that OCT is less costly and safer than FA, this study confirms earlier work recommending that OCT be the first test used to evaluate macular edema.[1,2]

J. P. Dunn, MD

References

1. Kempen JH, Sugar EA, Jaffe GJ, et al; Multicenter uveitis steroid treatment (MUST) trial research group. Fluorescein angiography versus optical coherence tomography for diagnosis of uveitic macular edema. *Ophthalmology.* 2013;120: 1852-1859.
2. Onal S, Tugal-Tutkun I, Neri P, P Herbort C. Optical coherence tomography imaging in uveitis. *Int Ophthalmol.* 2014;34:401-435.

Viral Retinitis following Intraocular or Periocular Corticosteroid Administration: A Case Series and Comprehensive Review of the Literature

Takakura A, Tessler HH, Goldstein DA, et al (California Pacific Med Ctr, San Francisco; Univ of Illinois at Chicago; Northwestern Univ Feinberg School of Medicine, Chicago, IL; et al)

Ocul Immunol Inflamm 22:175-182, 2014

Purpose.—To describe viral retinitis following intravitreal and periocular corticosteroid administration.

Methods.—Retrospective case series and comprehensive literature review.

Results.—We analyzed 5 unreported and 25 previously published cases of viral retinitis following local corticosteroid administration. Causes of retinitis included 23 CMV (76.7%), 5 HSV (16.7%), and 1 each VZV and unspecified (3.3%). Two of 22 tested patients (9.1%) were HIV positive. Twenty-one of 30 (70.0%) cases followed one or more intravitreal injections of triamcinolone acetonide (TA), 4 (13.3%) after one or more posterior sub- Tenon injections of TA, 3 (10.0%) after placement of a 0.59-mg fluocinolone acetonide implant (Retisert), and 1 (3.3%) each after an anterior subconjunctival injection of TA (together with IVTA), an anterior chamber injection, and an anterior sub-Tenon injection. Mean time from most recent corticosteroid administration to development of retinitis was 4.2 months (median 3.8; range 0.25–13.0). Twelve patients (40.0%) had type II diabetes mellitus. Treatments used included systemic antiviral agents (26/30, 86.7%), intravitreal antiviral injections (20/30, 66.7%), and ganciclovir intravitreal implants (4/30, 13.3%).

Conclusions.—Viral retinitis may develop or reactivate following intraocular or periocular corticosteroid administration. Average time to development of retinitis was 4 months, and CMV was the most frequently observed agent. Diabetes was a frequent co-morbidity and several patients with uveitis who developed retinitis were also receiving systemic immunosuppressive therapy.

▶ Periocular and intravitreal corticosteroid injections and implants have been shown to help control uveitis and to reduce uveitic macular edema.[1-4] Cataract causing vision of <20/40 and glaucoma (intraocular pressure >24 mm Hg) were reported in 34% and 20% of patients within 1 year of receiving a periocular corticosteroid injection in 1 study. The development of Cushingoid features has been described in children. Takakura et al analyzed 25 previously published and 5 unreported cases of unilateral viral retinitis after periocular or intraocular corticosteroid injections and undertook a comprehensive review of the literature. Of the 30 cases, 23 (77%) were caused by cytomegalovirus (CMV), 5 (17%) by herpes simplex virus, and 1 (3%) by varicella zoster virus; the cause of the remaining case was not identified, but acute retinal necrosis was diagnosed clinically. The mean age was 63 years, and 63% of patients were male. Retinitis occurred after 1 or more injections of intravitreal triamcinolone acetonide (TA) in 21 eyes (70%), 1 or more posterior sub-Tenon's TA injections in 4 eyes (13%), after a fluocinolone acetonide 0.59 mg implant in 3 eyes (10%), and in 1 case (3%) each after subconjunctival and intravitreal TA, anterior sub-Tenon's TA, and anterior chamber TA. Reasons for the corticosteroid injections included macular edema associated with retinal vein occlusion, epiretinal membrane, diabetes, or uveitis, choroidal neovascularization, and immune recovery uveitis. The mean time from the most recent corticosteroid injection was 4.2 months. Twelve patients (40%) had concurrent type II diabetes mellitus. The authors suggested that diabetic vasculopathy might facilitate entry of CMV into the retina and noted published data showing the circulating CMV levels tend to be higher in patients with diabetes. Nine patients (30%) were receiving immunosuppressive therapy for underlying disease. Treatments included systemic antivirals in 26 patients (87%), intravitreal antiviral injections in 20 eyes (67%), and the ganciclovir implant in 4 eyes (13%). Retinitis was controlled in all patients, and no eyes with a fluocinolone implant required removal. However, visual outcomes were poor, with final acuity of <20/200 in 58% of eyes due to macular scarring or retinal detachment. Although the study was not designed to determine the incidence of viral retinitis after corticosteroid injections or to assess treatment options, the authors cautioned clinicians about the risks of such injections (not to mention cataract and glaucoma) and emphasized the importance of aggressive antiviral therapy for retinitis. The role of immunosuppressive therapy and the relative risk of periocular vs intraocular corticosteroid injections or implants in precipitating viral retinitis remain unclear. No cases of infectious retinitis were described in the largest reported series of patients undergoing periocular corticosteroid injections (1192 eyes of 914 patients), so the risk appears to be low.

J. P. Dunn, MD

References

1. Sen HN, Vitale S, Gangaputra SS, et al. Periocular corticosteroid injections in uveitis: effects and complications. *Ophthalmology.* 2014;121:2275-2286.
2. Salek SS, Leder HA, Butler NJ, Gan TJ, Dunn JP, Thorne JE. Periocular triamcinolone acetonide injections for control of intraocular inflammation associated with uveitis. *Ocul Immunol Inflamm.* 2013;21:257-263.
3. Leder HA, Jabs DA, Galor A, Dunn JP, Thorne JE. Periocular triamcinolone acetonide injections for cystoid macular edema complicating noninfectious uveitis. *Am J Ophthalmol.* 2011;152:441-448.
4. Habot-Wilner Z, Sallam A, Roufas A, et al. Periocular corticosteroid injection in the management of uveitis in children. *Acta Ophthalmol.* 2010;88:e299-e304.

British Ocular Syphilis Study (BOSS): 2-Year National Surveillance Study of Intraocular Inflammation Secondary to Ocular Syphilis

Mathew RG, Goh BT, Westcott MC (Moorfields Eye Hosp, London, United Kingdom; et al)

Invest Ophthalmol Vis Sci 55:5394-5400, 2014

Purpose.—The British Ocular Syphilis Study (BOSS) is the first national prospective epidemiological study of intraocular syphilis (IOS) in light of the global increase in early syphilis (ES). The aims were to ascertain the UK incidence, demographics, clinical features, laboratory data, and post-treatment visual outcomes of patients with IOS.

Methods.—Prospective study of IOS, reported through the national reporting system (British Ocular Surveillance Unit) from 2009 to 2011. Case definition was any adult presenting with intraocular inflammation in ES.

Results.—A total of 41 new cases (63 eyes) of IOS were reported, giving an annual incidence of 0.3 per million UK adult population. Mean age was 48.7 years (range, 20.6–75.1); 90.2% were male. All had RPR/VDRL titers of ≥1:16. Bilateral ocular involvement occurred in 56%; in unilateral cases, the left eye was more commonly affected ($P = 0.009$). Mean presenting logMAR visual acuity was 0.52 (20/63 Snellen; range, −0.2 to 2.30 logMAR). Panuveitis was the commonest diagnosis, seen in 41.3%, and isolated anterior uveitis was uncommon (9.5%). Subgroup analysis between HIV-positive and -negative patients found no significant differences in terms of proportion of bilateral disease, presenting or post treatment acuity. HIV-positive patients had higher rates of panuveitis. At final follow-up, 92.1% had visual acuity ≥0.3 logMAR (20/40 Snellen) after antibiotic therapy.

Conclusions.—This study is the largest prospective series of ocular syphilis in the post-penicillin era. It confirms good visual outcomes for treated IOS, irrespective of HIV status or time to presentation. The study identified an unexpected preponderance for left eye involvement in uniocular cases; which is unexplained.

▶ Syphilis, in the eye and elsewhere in the body, is one of the "great mimickers" and should be considered in virtually any case of uveitis in adults.[1,2] Most uveitis surveillance studies have reported that syphilis accounts for 1% to 2% of all uveitis.[1] Because syphilis has been increasing in frequency in recent years (including a 1032% increase in the United Kingdom between 1999 and 2008), there is a concern that the incidence of syphilitic uveitis will similarly increase. Mathew and colleagues undertook the first national prospective epidemiologic study of intraocular syphilis in the United Kingdom from 2009 to 2011. Sixty-three eyes of 41 patients were reported, giving an annual incidence of 0.3 per million adults, or roughly 0.6% of all patients infected with syphilis. The mean age was 48.7 years; 90% of patients were male. Bilateral inflammation occurred in 56%; interestingly, the left eye was much more commonly affected than the right eye in unilateral cases; the authors postulated that this might reflect the more direct blood flow to the left side of the head than to the right side. The mean Snellen visual acuity was 20/63. The most common presentation was panuveitis, seen in 41% of eyes; isolated anterior uveitis (9.5%) was the least common clinical presentations. Anterior uveitis and vitritis were the most common presenting signs. Coinfection with human immunodeficiency virus (HIV) was found in 32% of patients, all of whom were male and significantly younger (mean age 39 years) compared with the HIV-negative patients. At follow-up, 92% of patients had visual acuity of >20/40 after treatment. There was no difference in bilaterality, presenting acuity, or posttreatment acuity between HIV-positive and HIV-negative patients. The study did not find the expected increase in the incidence of intraocular syphilis; the authors postulated that perhaps increased awareness of syphilis and earlier treatment of systemic disease might keep the risk of intraocular involvement low. Finally, the study looked only at patients with early syphilis and specifically excluded patients with late latent or tertiary syphilis. The authors emphasized the need to consider syphilis in any adult-onset uveitis and the importance of early treatment in maximizing visual outcomes. All patients with ocular syphilis should be tested for HIV and vice versa.[3]

J. P. Dunn, MD

References

1. Moradi A, Salek S, Daniel E, et al. Clinical features and incidence rates of ocular complications in patients with ocular syphilis. *Am J Ophthalmol.* 2015;159:334-343.
2. Davis JL. Ocular syphilis. *Curr Opin Ophthalmol.* 2014;25:513-518.
3. Fonollosa A, Martinez-Indart L, Artaraz J, et al. Clinical manifestations and outcomes of syphilis-associated uveitis in Northern Spain. *Ocul Immunol Inflamm.* 2014:1-6 [Epub ahead of print].

Characterisation of uveitis in association with multiple sclerosis

Messenger W, Hildebrandt L, Mackensen F, et al (Oregon Health & Science Univ, Portland; Univ of Heidelberg, Germany; et al)

Br J Ophthalmol 99:205-209, 2015

Purpose.—To characterise uveitis in association with multiple sclerosis (MS).

Methods.—We conducted a retrospective chart review of patients with uveitis and MS at two uveitis centres (Portland, Oregon, USA and Heidelberg, Germany). Baseline characteristics and ophthalmic data were collected at the patient's first and last visits. Additionally, neurological records were obtained when possible.

Results.—We identified 113 patients (196 eyes) with uveitis and MS. Of these, 53 had a diagnosis of MS confirmed by review of neurological records, 50 additional patients fulfilled the Poser criteria for MS and 10 with MS were referred by an outside neurologist. Among them, 83 (73%) were women and the mean age of presentation was 40.6 years (range 13-64 years). The average visual acuity in affected eyes at presentation was 20/39. There were 90 patients (80%) who presented with intermediate uveitis and 24 patients (15%) with anterior uveitis. Posterior and panuveitis were found in four patients (3%) and two patients (2%), respectively. During a median follow-up of 3.2 years (range 0.04-21 years), visual acuity improved -0.09 logMar/year. Compared with our location-matched controls with idiopathic intermediate uveitis ($n = 16$), patients with MS and intermediate uveitis were significantly older when diagnosed with uveitis ($p = 0.027$) and more likely to be female ($p = 0.01$). There was no statistical difference in visual acuity or rate of vision change between our cases and controls ($p = 0.58$ and $p = 0.36$, respectively).

Conclusions.—Uveitis with MS generally presents as intermediate uveitis with a minority presenting with anterior uveitis. Patients are significantly older and more likely to be women than patients with idiopathic intermediate uveitis. The visual prognosis is generally favourable.

▶ Multiple sclerosis (MS) is one of the best-known causes of optic neuritis, and the diagnosis, ocular and systemic manifestations, and treatments are well described. The association between MS and uveitis is less well described, with most reports emphasizing the findings of intermediate uveitis and peripheral retinal phlebitis.[1,2] The authors conducted a retrospective review of 196 eyes of 113 patients with uveitis and MS at 2 tertiary care referral centers to characterize the clinical course of disease, time of presentation of uveitis with respect to MS, and visual prognosis. A control group of 16 patients with non-MS-related intermediate uveitis was also studied. Ninety patients (80%) with MS/uveitis had intermediate uveitis, 24 (15%) had anterior uveitis, 4 (3%) had posterior uveitis, and 2 (2%) had panuveitis. Roughly three-fourths of patients had bilateral uveitis. The MS was diagnosed before uveitis in 29% of patients, simultaneously in 15%, and after uveitis in 56%. When recorded, the uveitis was chronic in 74% of patients, recurrent in 19%, and acute in 7%. Visual acuity improved on average by -0.09 logMar/y over a median follow-up of 3.2 years, although 28% of eyes lost vision. Compared with the control group with idiopathic uveitis, patients with MS/uveitis were significantly more likely to be female and older (31 vs 18 years) at the time of diagnosis of uveitis. There was no significant difference between the 2 groups in terms of visual acuity or rate of vision change. Thirty-nine patients (35%) presented with or had self-reported history of optic neuritis. The authors estimated that MS is roughly 20 times more likely in patients with uveitis than in the general population. Key points of this study, by far the largest of all published studies on MS and uveitis, include the unexpectedly high prevalence of anterior uveitis, the high incidence of patients whose MS was diagnosed after uveitis (including 22% of patients with an interval of more than 5 years), the fairly stable visual prognosis, and the older age and female predilection in patients with MS and intermediate uveitis compared with those with idiopathic intermediate uveitis. The report did not address the efficacy of different treatment options, nor did the authors give an opinion on whether patients with intermediate uveitis should routinely undergo MRI of the brain.

J. P. Dunn, MD

References

1. Burkholder BM, Dunn JP. Multiple sclerosis-associated uveitis. *Expert Rev Ophthalmol.* 2012;7:587-594.
2. Towler HM, Lightman S. Symptomatic intraocular inflammation in multiple sclerosis. *Clin Experiment Ophthalmol.* 2000;28:97-102.

7 Oculoplastic Surgery

Reduced Risk of Compressive Optic Neuropathy Using Orbital Radiotherapy in Patients With Active Thyroid Eye Disease

Shams PN, Ma R, Pickles T, et al (Univ of British Columbia, Vancouver)

Am J Ophthalmol 157:1299-1305, 2014

Purpose.—To compare the risk of developing compressive optic neuropathy in patients with active thyroid eye disease (TED) treated with corticosteroids with or without orbital radiotherapy.

Design.—Retrospective single-center case-control study

Methods.—The clinical charts of 351 patients with active TED who received corticosteroids with or without orbital radiotherapy between 1999 and 2010 were reviewed. Patients with compressive optic neuropathy at the time of presentation were excluded. Group 1 received corticosteroids only and Group 2 received corticosteroids as well as orbital radiotherapy. The primary outcome measure was the development of compressive optic neuropathy. Secondary outcome measures were changes in other parameters indicating the activity of TED, including soft tissue inflammation, diplopia, ocular motility restriction, and appearance.

Results.—There were 144 cases in Group 1 and 105 in Group 2. Both groups were matched for age, sex, and stability of thyroid function. The 2 groups differed only in the modality of treatment for active TED. The main indication for treatment in both groups was soft tissue inflammation. Corticosteroids were initiated an average of 2.6 months following symptom onset in Group 1 and 2.5 months in Group 2. Group 2 received orbital radiotherapy on average 4.2 months following the initiation of corticosteroid therapy and 8% (9/105) were intolerant to corticosteroids. At an average of 3.2 years follow-up, compressive optic neuropathy had developed in 17% (25/144) of Group 1 and 0% of Group 2 ($P < .0001$), on average 5.5 months following the initiation of corticosteroid therapy. Although both groups experienced a significant reduction in periocular inflammation, the radiotherapy-treated group demonstrated a significantly greater improvement in ocular motility.

Conclusion.—The rate of compressive optic neuropathy was significantly lower and improvement in ocular motility greater in patients receiving orbital radiotherapy in addition to corticosteroids. Patients with active TED appear to have an effective and sustained response to orbital radiotherapy combined with corticosteroids that is protective against disease progression and the development of compressive optic neuropathy.

▶ The controversy over radiotherapy for thyroid eye disease (TED) has been present since the Mayo Clinic Study[1] in 2001 suggested that orbital radiation was not effective in the treatment of TED. A number of smaller studies since that time have suggested possible value of orbital radiotherapy but nothing conclusive.

This is a retrospective study that looked at active TED patients who received corticosteroids. They were then divided into 2 groups. One group received orbital radiation, and the other group did not. The study conclusion was that 17% of the nonirradiated patients developed compressive optic neuropathy versus 0% in the irradiated group. Both groups, over time, had improvement in the inflammation. The other benefit of orbital irradiation was improvement in diplopia and restriction of motility in the radiated group. No side effects were found from the radiation in this study.

We have looked at 100 patients recently at Wills in an as yet unpublished study and found similar results. No progression to compressive optic neuropathy in the radiated orbits and also shorter time period for stabilization of motility in the radiated group were found.

This is a significant study in that it shows the value of orbital radiation in patients with active TED. Orbital radiotherapy appears to protect them from compressive optic neuropathy and also stabilizes motility faster in some and allows for earlier muscle surgery in those requiring surgery. From these results, any patient with active TED who develops dysmotility and is progressing should be considered for treatment with orbital radiation.

R. B. Penne, MD

Reference

1. Gorman CA, Garrity JA, Fatourechi V, et al. A prospective, randomized, double-blind, placebo-controlled study of orbital radiotherapy for Graves' ophthalmopathy. *Ophthalmology*. 2001;108:1523-1534.

Orbital Fractures and Ocular Injury: Is a Postoperative Ophthalmology Examination Necessary?

Peacock ZS, Boulos T, Miller JB, et al (Massachusetts General Hosp, Boston; Massachusetts Eye and Ear Infirmary, Boston; et al)

J Oral Maxillofac Surg 72:1533-1540, 2014

Purpose.—To determine whether formal ophthalmology evaluation is necessary after operative repair of orbital fractures and the association of an ocular injury to the severity of facial injury.

Patients and Methods.—This was a retrospective cohort study of patients with orbital fractures undergoing operative repair from 2005 to 2013. Subjects were included if they had undergone reconstruction of orbital floor

TABLE 4.—Ocular Findings

Pt. No.	Fractures (n)	Ocular Findings by Ophthalmology* Preoperative	Postoperative	New Postoperative Finding	Change in Management Because of Ocular Findings	Notes
1	2	Ø	Ø	Ø	Ø	
2	6	OD: IRH OS: IRH, EOMD[†]	OD: IRH OS: IRH, EOMD	Ø	Ø	EOMD resolved 4 wk postop
3	3	EOMD[†]	Ø	Ø	Ø	
4	3	Ø	EOMD	EOMD	Ø	EOMD resolved 1 wk postop
5	3	ON	ON	Ø	Ø	Neuro-ophthalmology referral postop; improved monocular diplopia 6 wk postop
6	1	CA	CA	Ø	Ø	
7	4	OHT	Ø	Ø	Ø	
8	8	OD: NLP[†] (fixed dilated pupil), EOMD[†] OS: Ø	OD: NLP[†] (fixed dilated pupil), EOMD[†] OS: Ø	Ø	OD: Ø OS: orbital defect not treated because of loss of vision in OD	ORIF delayed 12 days because of intracranial injury
9	3	EOMD,[†] CR	EOMD[†]	Ø	Additional ophthalmology follow-up	EOMD resolved 4 wk postop
10	2	EOMD[†]	EOMD[†]	Ø	Ø	EOMD resolved 4 wk postop
11	1	OD: OHT OS: ↓VA,[†] OHT, SRH, CR, CA, MH	OD: Ø OS: OHT, CR	Ø	ORIF delayed 1 week due to MH	
12	3	CA, DR, VH	CA, DR, VH	Ø	Ø	
13	2	Ø	Ø	Ø	Ø	
14	7	OD: ↓VA,[†] IRH, SRH, PRH, ON, ME OS: Ø	OD: IRH, SRH, PRH, ON, ME OS: Ø	Ø	Ø	
15	4	CA, PRH, IRH, MH, EOMD[†] (IR entrapment[†])	CA, PRH, IRH, MH	Ø	Ø	Repaired emergently due to muscle entrapment
16	2	Ø	Ø	Ø	Ø	
17	2	Ø	Ø	Ø	Ø	

(Continued)

TABLE 4.—(*Continued*)

		Ocular Findings by Ophthalmology*				
Pt. No.	Fractures (n)	Preoperative	Postoperative	New Postoperative Finding	Change in Management Because of Ocular Findings	Notes
18	2	Ø	Ø	Ø	Ø	
19	1	Ø	Ø	Ø	Ø	
20	8	TI, H, EOMD†	TI, EOMD	Ø	ORIF delayed 11 days due to H	TI resolved at 2 wk follow-up
21	3	Ø	Ø	Ø	Ø	
22	2	Ø	Ø	Ø	Ø	
23	2	I, MH, CA	CA	Ø	MH resolved after 4 days	
24	2	Ø	Ø	Ø	Ø	
25	2	Ø	Ø	Ø	Additional ophthalmology follow-up for asymmetric IOP preoperatively	
26	7	OD: ↑IOP OS: ↑IOP	OD: ↑IOP OS: ↑IOP	Ø	Brimodidine for ↑IOP	↑IOP resolved 2 wk postop; required skeletal revision
27	6	EOMD†	Ø	Ø	Ø	
28	3	IOP, EOMD† (MR entrapment†)	EOMD,† CA	CA	Erythromycin ointment for 3 days; emergency repair for entrapment	CA resolved after 3 days, EOMD resolved 10 days postop

Abbreviations: CA, corneal abrasion; CR, commotio retinae; DR, diabetic retinopathy; EOMD, extraocular muscle dysfunction; H, hyphema; IR, inferior rectus; IOP, intraocular pressure; IRH, intraretinal hemorrhage; ME, macular edema; MH, microhyphema; MR, medial rectus; NLP, no light perception; OD, right eye; OHT, ocular hypertension; ON, optic neuropathy; OS, left eye; postop, postoperatively; PRH, preretinal hemorrhage; SRH, subretinal hemorrhage; VA, visual acuity; VH, vitreous hemorrhage.

*Bilateral cases have side delineated.

†OMS findings.

Reprinted from *Journal of Oral and Maxillofacial Surgery*. Peacock ZS, Boulos T, Miller JB, et al. Orbital Fractures and Ocular Injury: Is a Postoperative Ophthalmology Examination Necessary? *J Oral Maxillofac Surg*. 2014;72:1533–1540, Copyright 2014, with permission from American Association of Oral and Maxillofacial Surgeons.

fractures and had data from pre- and postoperative examinations by the oral and maxillofacial surgery and ophthalmology services available. The predictor variables included the service performing the ocular examination (oral and maxillofacial surgery or ophthalmology) and the number of fractures present. The outcome variables were the presence of pre- and postoperative ocular injuries. Logistic regression models were used to determine the relationship of the fracture number to ocular injury.

Results.—A total of 28 subjects had undergone repair of orbital fractures with preoperative and postoperative examinations performed by both services. Preoperative ocular injuries were found in 17 of the 28 subjects. Those detected by oral and maxillofacial surgeons were limited to changes in visual acuity, pupillary response, and extraocular muscle dysfunction in 11 subjects. Two subjects had new postoperative ocular findings that were considered minor and did not alter management. An increasing number of facial fractures was associated with an increased risk of ocular trauma. Those with 3 or more fractures had an odds ratio of 14.625 (95% confidence interval, 2.191 to 97.612, $P = .006$) for the presence of ocular injury.

Conclusions.—Operative repair of orbital fractures did not lead to new ocular injuries that would change the management. Thus, those without preoperative ocular injuries will not require a formal postoperative ophthalmology examination. However, the subjects with more fractures had an increased likelihood of ocular injuries (Table 4).

▶ This article looks at the need for a postoperative ophthalmic examination after repair of orbital fractures. This was a retrospective study done from 2005 to 2013 and included 28 patients. Surgical repair of the fracture was performed jointly by the oral-maxillofacial surgery department and ophthalmology. Patients all had an orbital floor fracture, and many had other facial fractures.

There were no significant new ocular injuries after surgery in any patient. One patient had a cornea abrasion, which resolved, and a second patient had decreased down gaze, which also resolved. The only concern I have with this study is the small number of patients included. This study suggests that a postoperative eye examination is not needed after orbital fracture repair.

I always check my patients' vision when they are awake after orbital fracture repair. With that in mind, any complaints of visual loss, severe pain, bleeding, and new diplopia should be evaluated postoperatively. It must be emphasized that a preoperative examination of the eye after trauma with an orbital fracture is still indicated to rule out injury to the eye itself and establish a baseline of the vision, motility, and other injuries.

R. B. Penne, MD

High-Frequency Radiowave Electrosurgery for Persistent Conjunctival Chemosis Following Cosmetic Blepharoplasty

Woo KI, Choi CY (Sungkyunkwan Univ School of Medicine, Seoul, South Korea)

Plast Reconstr Surg 133:1336-1342, 2014

Background.—Conjunctival chemosis often complicates cosmetic lower eyelid blepharoplasty. With the conventional approaches, including medical or surgical methods, irritative symptoms are produced and complete recovery is delayed. The authors introduced a new simple surgical approach for treating persistent conjunctival chemosis following cosmetic blepharoplasty.

Methods.—Eleven patients (12 eyes) with persistent chemosis lasting 6 weeks to 2 years were recruited for this study. Subconjunctival coagulation on the edematous conjunctiva was performed with a fine-needle electrode using a high-frequency radiowave electrosurgical unit in coagulation mode, and subconjunctival fluid drainage was performed by gentle pressure with a wet applicator. After the procedures, topical steroid and antibiotic eye drops were given four times per day for 1 month.

Results.—Chemosis in 11 eyes (91.7 percent) was resolved within 1 week and remained stable for a follow-up period of 6 months.

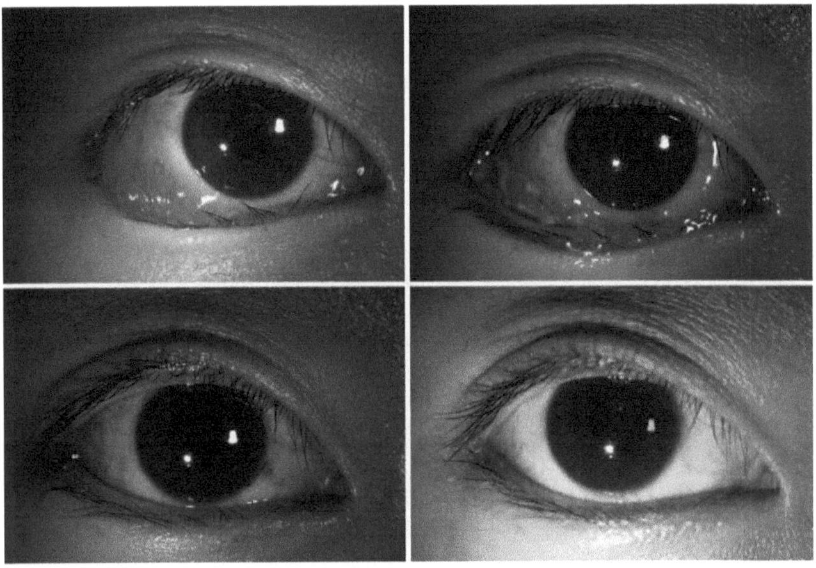

FIGURE 5.—Patient 4. High-frequency radiowave electrosurgery was performed for persistent conjunctival chemosis in a 23-year-old woman. (*Above, left*) Preoperative appearance shows marked conjunctival chemosis. (*Above, right*) One day postoperatively. (*Below, left*) One week postoperatively. (*Below, right*) One month postoperatively. (Reprinted from Woo KI, Choi CY. High-frequency radiowave electrosurgery for persistent conjunctival chemosis following cosmetic blepharoplasty. *Plast Reconstr Surg*. 2014;133:1336-1342, with permission from the American Society of Plastic Surgeons.)

Recurrence of chemosis and complications related to the procedure were not noted during the follow-up.

Conclusions.—A surgical approach with high-frequency radiowave electrosurgery produced a significant reduction of persistent chemosis and provided prompt symptom improvement. This procedure can be considered as a simple and safe method of treating persistent conjunctival chemosis following cosmetic blepharoplasty.

Clinical Question/Level of Evidence.—Therapeutic, IV (Fig 5).

▶ Chronic chemosis after blepharoplasty or after any eyelid and orbital procedures is rare. There are also rare patients who develop idiopathic chronic chemosis. Chronic chemosis can be frustrating for both the patient and doctor. This article offers a simple surgical technique to consider when conservative measures have failed.

The procedure uses a high-frequency radiowave electrosurgical unit with a fine-needle electrode handpiece. The procedure is done under topical anesthesia. The technique in the article is done under a microscope, but it would appear to be something that could be done with loupes. It worked in 11 of 13 patients with chronic chemosis, so I will definitely consider trying this in a patient with chronic chemosis. The technique from Fig 5 can be viewed with the following link: http://links.lww.com/PRS/A999.

R. B. Penne, MD

Surgical Debulking for Idiopathic Dacryoadenitis: A Diagnosis and a Cure

Mombaerts I, Cameron JD, Chanlalit W, et al (Univ Hosps Leuven, Belgium; Univ of Minnesota School of Medicine, Minneapolis; Srinakharinwirot Univ, Bangkok, Thailand; et al)

Ophthalmology 121:603-609, 2014

Purpose.—Idiopathic inflammatory tumor of the lacrimal gland, also called idiopathic dacryoadenitis, generally is treated with high-dose, long-term systemic corticosteroids, despite their limited success, high recurrence rate, and incidence of drug-induced side effects. This study describes the outcome of patients with idiopathic dacryoadenitis who were managed with surgical debulking.

Design.—Retrospective case series from 2 tertiary referral centers.

Participants.—Forty-six patients (46 lacrimal glands).

Methods.—Review of the clinical records, radiologic scans, and histopathologic specimens, with additional immunoglobulin G4 immunostaining.

Main Outcome Measures.—Clinical signs and symptoms at 2 months after the surgery and off medications.

Results.—Before referral, 41% (19 of 46) of the patients had received systemic high-dose corticosteroids, after which they all showed recurrence, of whom 26% (5 of 19) became dependent on corticosteroids. At referral, all patients underwent debulking surgery of the inflammatory lacrimal gland mass for diagnostic and therapeutic reasons. Additionally, intralesional or systemic low-dose corticosteroids were given during the operation or the first postoperative days in 54% (25 of 46) of the patients. At 2 months after the debulking surgery, a full clinical recovery was seen in 80% (37 of 46) of the patients. A recurrence occurred in 8% (3 of 37) of the patients 4 months and 2.2 and 4.6 years later. Surgical failure (20%; 9 of 46) was correlated with prior corticosteroid treatment ($P = 0.002$, Fisher exact test), but not with sclerosing inflammation present in 28% (13 of 46). The median follow-up time was 7.2 years (range, 0.7–18 years).

Conclusions.—Debulking biopsy procedures for idiopathic dacryoadenitis, in addition to being diagnostic, may be therapeutic.

▶ The idea of surgically debulking of the lacrimal gland for treatment of patients with idiopathic dacryoadenitis offers a nice alternative to the need for chronic steroid treatment with its potential side effects. If patients meet the criteria for diagnosis of idiopathic dacryoadenitis (Table 1 in the original article), they have an 80% chance of resolution of their symptoms by doing surgical debulking of the lacrimal gland. This was a retrospective study of 46 patients with idiopathic dacryoadenitis (Table 2 in the original article).

I believe this to be a reasonable approach to this disease. These patients all need a biopsy of their lacrimal gland and so will have surgery anyway. By doing a lacrimal gland debulking, not a complete excision, the chance of complications is reduced, and the surgery is only slightly more involved. The positive to this approach is that 80% of patients will be completely treated with this debulking and not require chronic steroids or other treatment. The other 20% can be treated with more traditional methods such as orbital radiation, methotrexate, or steroid injections. The other important point made in this study is that these patients should not receive a trial of steroids before surgery because it may alter the pathology.

This study will change my approach to idiopathic dacryoadenitis. I do some debulking when I do my lacrimal gland biopsy, but this gives me a reason to be more aggressive. The study suggests that the risk of dry eyes or worsening of dry eyes needs to be discussed, but in the 18 patients evaluated for this, no patients had worsening of their dry eyes after surgical debulking.

R. B. Penne, MD

Patient and Physician Perceptions of Medicare Reimbursement Policy for Blepharoplasty and Blepharoptosis Surgery

Bajric J, Levin JJ, Bartley GB, et al (Mayo Clinic, Rochester, MN)

Ophthalmology 121:1475-1479, 2014

Objective.—To describe patient preferences regarding payment for blepharoplasty and blepharoptosis repair and physician practices before and after the 2009 change in reimbursement for these 2 procedures by the Centers for Medicare and Medicaid Services (CMS).

Design.—Cross-sectional study.

Participants.—Fifty patients presenting for functional blepharoplasty and blepharoptosis repair at an academic oculoplastic practice and 198 members of the American Society of Ophthalmic Plastic and Reconstructive Surgery.

Methods.—A 5-question paper survey was administered to patients, and a 5-question web-based survey was distributed to 510 unique physician e-mail addresses obtained from the American Society of Ophthalmic Plastic and Reconstructive Surgery mailing list server in 2010.

Main Outcome Measures.—The surveys elicited patient knowledge and attitudes regarding the reimbursement policy of the CMS and physician knowledge and behaviors before and after the reimbursement policy change.

Results.—Ninety-one percent of patients would be opposed to having to pay out of pocket for blepharoplasty or having to wait at least 3 months after ptosis repair to have a blepharoplasty. When asked to choose between these options, 62% of the patients would rather have the 2 surgeries performed separately than pay out-of-pocket. Before the reimbursement policy change by the CMS, 77% of oculoplastic surgeons performed blepharoplasty and blepharoptosis repair in the same sitting, whereas 37% did so after the policy change ($P < 0.001$). Compared with before the

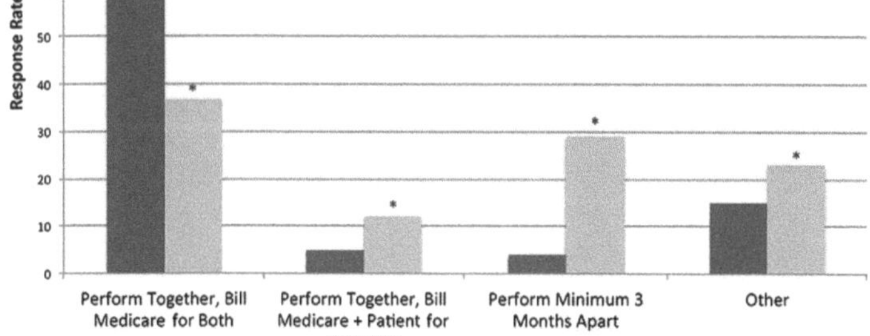

FIGURE 1.—Physician practices before and after the 2009 bundling of reimbursement for blepharoplasty and blepharoptosis repair by the Centers for Medicare and Medicaid Services. *$P < 0.05$. (Reprinted from Ophthalmology. Bajric J, Levin JJ, Bartley GB, et al. Patient and physician perceptions of medicare reimbursement policy for blepharoplasty and blepharoptosis surgery. *Ophthalmology.* 2014;121:1475-1479, Copyright 2014, with permission from the American Academy of Ophthalmology.)

TABLE 1.—Percent of Patients and Physicians Aware of Medicare Reimbursement Change

	Patients (n = 50)	Physicians (n = 198)
Aware	3 (6%)	179 (90%)
Unaware	45 (90%)	19 (10%)
Unsure	2 (4%)	–

– = Not applicable.

Reprinted from Ophthalmology. Bajric J, Levin JJ, Bartley GB, et al. Patient and physician perceptions of medicare reimbursement policy for blepharoplasty and blepharoptosis surgery. *Ophthalmology.* 2014;121:1475–1479, Copyright 2014, with permission from the American Academy of Ophthalmology.

policy change by the CMS, more surgeons performed the 2 procedures at least 3 months apart (4% before vs. 29% after, $P < 0.001$) and more often billed patients for a cosmetic blepharoplasty (5% before vs. 12% after, $P = 0.009$).

Conclusions.—Our study suggests that oculoplastic surgeons have made a change in the delivery of ptosis and blepharoplasty surgical services after the reimbursement policy change for these procedures by the CMS in 2009. This change, in which patients undergo separate surgical visits for ptosis repair and blepharoplasty, is not desirable to most patients (Fig 1, Table 1).

▶ This article surveys both patients' perceptions and oculoplastics surgeons' approach regarding payment for blepharoplasty and blepharoptosis when both are required. The brief background to this issue is these procedures were both reimbursed when done together before 2009, after which Medicare has no longer paid for both procedures when done at the same time. This has resulted in 3 options for the doctor and patient to consider. The 2 procedures can be done separately at least 3 months apart, patients can pay for the blepharoplasty on a cosmetic basis, or the surgeon can do the blepharoplasty and not be reimbursed.

Not surprising in the survey was that 90% of patients were unaware of this issue. This certainly means doctors need to spend time educating patients about this issue before the patient can make any decisions on how to proceed. Likewise, 91% of patients were opposed to both paying for the blepharoplasty procedure or waiting 3 months to have a second procedure. From the doctor side, the survey indicated that there was a much higher percent of doctors doing the 2 procedures separated by 3 months after 2009 (4% before vs 29% after), and more surgeons were billing patients for a cosmetic blepharoplasty.

The true value of this article is to bring this issue to everyone's attention. Although oculoplastic surgeons are well aware of this, the rest of ophthalmology may not be. The weakness of the article is that it was a survey and gives no actual numbers to the responses. I find when given the option of 2 procedures performed 3 months apart vs paying a fee, patients almost universally choose to pay the fee for the second procedure. This certainly may be biased based on practice location.

The end of the article does point out that the cost of 1 person doing a second procedure 3 months later is equal to the amount paid out for 5 people to have the second procedure at the same time as it was before 2009. Even with this information, it is unlikely Medicare will change this decision.

R. B. Penne, MD

Glucocorticoid Regimens for Prevention of Graves' Ophthalmopathy Progression Following Radioiodine Treatment: Systematic Review and Meta-Analysis

Shiber S, Stiebel-Kalish H, Shimon I, et al (Beilinson Hosp, Petah Tikva, Israel; Tel Aviv Univ, Israel)
Thyroid 24:1515-1523, 2014

Background.—Glucocorticoid (GC) therapy has been shown to prevent Graves' ophthalmopathy (GO) progression following radioactive iodine (RAI) treatment. However, the optimal regimen is controversial, with studies from recent years suggesting the use of lower doses and shorter GC treatment courses.

Methods.—We conducted a systematic review and meta-analysis of randomized controlled trials (RCTs) and retrospective controlled trials comparing GC regimens versus placebo, no treatment, or other GC regimens.

Results.—Eight trials evaluating 850 patients fulfilled inclusion criteria. In patients with preexisting GO, standard dose prednisone (0.4–0.5 mg/kg tapered over 3 months) was very effective for prevention of GO progression (OR 0.14 [CI 0.06–0.35], $p < 0.01$) in patients with mild to moderate GO. Two studies evaluated low-dose prednisone (0.2–0.3 mg/kg for 4–6 weeks) in patients with mild GO or risk factors, but were limited by not including patients with preexisting GO in the control groups. Therefore, the two low-dose groups were evaluated using indirect comparisons with control groups matched for age and clinical activity score, showing excellent efficacy versus no treatment or placebo (OR 0.20 [CI 0.07–0.60], $p = 0.004$) and no significant difference compared with standard dose (OR 1.7 [CI 0.52–5.52], $p = 0.47$). In patients without preexisting GO, steroid prophylaxis had no beneficial effect (OR 1.87 [CI 0.81–4.3]), though there were insufficient data regarding patients with risk factors for GO development. GC prophylaxis had no impact on hyperthyroidism resolution (OR 1.05 [CI 0.69–1.58]), and GC side effects were common but mild.

Conclusions.—Current evidence supports a three-tier approach for prevention of GO progression following RAI. Standard dose prednisone is the best validated regimen and should be used in patients with mild to moderate GO who have high risk of progression, while low dose prednisone can be used in patients with mild GO, and in patients without preexisting GO who have risk factors and are selected for GC prophylaxis. Patients

TABLE 1.—Included Studies

Study	Type	Pt (no.)	Treatment (Initial Dose)	Initiation	Duration	Follow-up	Mean Age (Years)
Bartalena 1998 (3)	RCT	145	PO prednisone (0.4 −0.5 mg/kg)	2–3 days after RAI	3 months	12 months	42
		150	No treatment				44
Bartalena 1989 (10)	RCT	26	PO prednisone (0.4 −0.5 mg/kg)	2–3 days after RAI	3 months	18 months	Both groups —49
		26	No treatment				
Vannucchi 2009 (9)	Retrospective	21	PO prednisone ($M = 36.5$ mg)*	1–2 days after RAI	8–10 weeks*	21 months	47
		9	IV methylprednisolone (500 mg twice/week)	7 days after RAI	1 month		53.2
		83	No treatment				45.2
Lai 2010 (11)	Retrospective	28	PO prednisone: low dose (0.22 ± 0.03 mg/kg)	1 day after RAI	6 weeks	6 months	51
		28	PO prednisone: high dose (0.36 ± 0.05 mg/kg)				47
		35	No treatment				NA
Jensen 2005 (12)	Retrospective	96	PO prednisolone (25 mg/day)	2 days before RAI	1 month	12 months	44.6
		111	No treatment				51.3
Vaisman 1997 (20)	RCT	25	PO prednisone (0.5 mg/kg)	The day of RAI	10–12 months	18 months	36*
		24	No treatment				
Gamstedt 1991 (18)	RCT	20	PO bethamethasone (6 mg)	3 weeks before RAI	7 weeks	12 months	55
		20	Placebo				62
Gamstedt 1986 (19)	RCT	20	PO bethamethasone (6 mg)	3 weeks before RAI	7 weeks	1 year	57
		23	No treatment				60

Allocation grading: A, adequate; B, unclear.
NA, not available; Y, yes; N, no.
Editor's Note: Please refer to original journal article for full references.
*Based on supplementary data provided by the authors.
Reprinted from Shiber S, Stiebel-Kalish H, Shimon I, et al. Glucocorticoid Regimens for Prevention of Graves' Ophthalmopathy Progression Following Radioiodine Treatment: Systematic Review and Meta-Analysis. *Thyroid*. 2014;24:1515-1523, with permission from Mary Ann Liebert, Inc. © 2014, American Thyroid Association.

without preexisting GO and without risk factors should not be treated with GC prophylaxis (Tables 1 and 2).

▶ There continues to be controversy around the use of radioactive iodine (RAI) to treat hyperthyroidism and Graves ophthalmopathy (GO). It has become generally accepted that glucocorticoids (GC) decrease the chance of progression of GO when patients undergo RAI treatment. The issue now is around the dosage and duration of treatment. This article makes an attempt to analyze the studies in the literature on GC treatment of patients undergoing RAI (Tables 1 and 2).

F (%)	Preexisting GO (%)	Smokers (%)	CAS (Mean)	Primary Outcome	Allocation Generation, Concealment	Binding	Sponsored y/n
81%	52%	60%	1.2 (*SD* = 1.2)	Hyperthyroidism resolution, GO progression	B,B	N	N
81%	48%	55%	1.1 (*SD* = 1.1)				
81%	81%	NA	NA	GO progression	A,B	N	N
77%	62%						
76%	36%	52%	1 (*SE* = 0.3)	GO progression			N
78%	55%	33%	2.1 (*SE* = 0.4)				
80%	28%	37%	0.6 (*SE* = 0.1)				
64%	79%	30%	1 (*SD* = 0.9)	GO progression			N
78%	71%	30%	1.3 (*SD* = 1)				
NA	NA						
85%	67%	42%	NA	Hyperthyroidism resolution			N
77%	0%	41%					
Total: 80%	100%	NA	NA "mild to moderate"	GO progression	A,A*	N	N
	100%						
85%	0%	NA	NA		B,B	Y	N
85%	0%						
70%	0%				B,B	N	N
78%	0%						

The problem is the large variability in the studies and trying to standardize the studies and results. Much of the article involves dealing with this variation.

The conclusions from this study are three-fold. First, patients with active GO undergoing RAI should be treated with GC. The risk of worsening of the GO went from 25% to 4% when patients were treated with GC. What is not clear is the optimal dose and duration of steroids to be used. Second, there is no benefit to treating patients without GO with GC. Patients with no GO but with risk factors such as smoking were also not shown to benefit from GC, but this is not in agreement with what many physicians do. Third, a study looking at lower doses and shorter duration of GC is needed.

I will continue to treat my patients who have GO and are to undergo RAI with GC. I tend to use a lower dose and shorter duration of GC treatment. I consider

TABLE 2.—Treatment Protocols

Corticosteroid Treatment Regimen	Study
Starting two to three days after RAI treatment, oral prednisone 0.4–0.5 mg/kg for one month, and then tapered off over two months	Bartalena 1998 (3) Bartalena 1989 (10)
Starting one to two days after RAI treatment, mean initial dose of prednisone 36.5 mg (8/21 patients 50 mg; 11/21 patients 25 mg; and 2/21 patients 35 mg) tapered off over 8–10 weeks	Vannucchi 2009 (9)
IV methylprednisolone: Starting seven days after RAI treatment, two weekly doses of 500 mg, then two weekly doses of 250 mg	
Prednisone—standard dose: Starting one day after RAI treatment, mean initial dose of 0.36 ± 0.05 mg/kg tapered off over six weeks	Lai 2010 (11)
Prednisone—low dose: Starting one day after RAI treatment, mean initial dose of 0.22 ± 0.03 mg/kg tapered off over six weeks	
Starting two days before RAI treatment, oral prednisolone 25 mg once daily for one month without tapering	Jensen 2005 (12)
Starting the day of RAI treatment, oral prednisone 0.5 mg/kg for four months, tapered off over 10–12 months	Vaisman 1997 (20)
Starting three weeks before RAI treatment, oral betamethasone 6 mg daily for five days, then reduced 0.5–1.5 mg weekly for a total of seven weeks	Gamstedt 1991 (18) Gamstedt 1986 (19)

Editor's Note: Please refer to original journal article for full references.

Reprinted from Shiber S, Stiebel-Kalish H, Shimon I, et al. Glucocorticoid Regimens for Prevention of Graves' Ophthalmopathy Progression Following Radioiodine Treatment: Systematic Review and Meta-Analysis. *Thyroid*. 2014;24:1515-1523, with permission from Mary Ann Liebert, Inc. © 2014, American Thyroid Association.

GC treatment in patients with no GO but who smoke and make the decision of whether to use GC on an individual basis.

R. B. Penne, MD

Serum selenium status in Graves' disease with and without orbitopathy: a case–control study

Khong JJ, Goldstein RF, Sanders KM, et al (The Univ of Melbourne, St Albans, Victoria, Australia)

Clin Endocrinol 80:905-910, 2014

Objective.—Selenium is effective in improving quality of life and reducing the progression of active Graves' orbitopathy. The effect of correcting relative selenium deficiency on improving Graves' orbitopathy is unknown, as baseline selenium levels have not previously been measured. The study aims to determine whether serum selenium levels are reduced in patients with Graves' disease with orbitopathy (GO) compared with without orbitopathy (GD).

Design.—A prospective, case-control study performed between 2009 and 2012 at endocrine and ophthalmology clinics in Australia.

Patients.—A total of 198 patients with Graves' disease participated in the study: 101 with Graves' orbitopathy and 97 without Graves' orbitopathy.

Measurements.—Serum selenium levels in both groups.

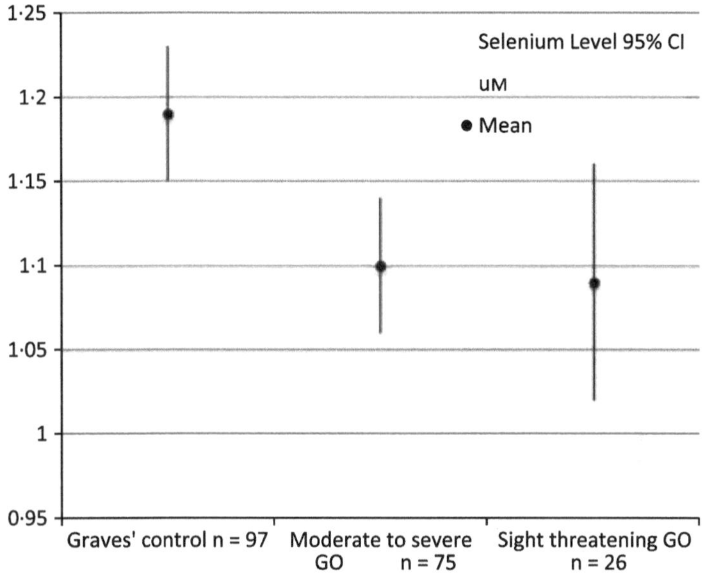

FIGURE 2.—Mean selenium levels and 95% confidence intervals for Graves' without orbitopathy, moderate-to-severe Graves' orbitopathy and sight-threatening Graves' orbitopathy, One-way ANOVA $P = 0{\cdot}003$. (Reprinted from Khong JJ, Goldstein RF, Sanders KM, et al. Serum selenium status in Graves' disease with and without orbitopathy: a case–control study. *Clin Endocrinol.* 2014;80:905-910, with acknowledgement of Wiley-Blackwell.)

Results.—Mean serum selenium levels were significantly lower in GO (1·10 ± 0·18 μM) than in GD (1·19 ± 0·20 μM) ($P = 0{\cdot}001$). Mean selenium levels appeared to decrease in parallel with increasing severity of GO; selenium level was 1·19 ± 0·20 μM in GD, 1·10 ± 0·19 μM in moderate-to-severe GO and 1·09 ± 0·17 μM in sight-threatening GO ($P = 0{\cdot}003$). Serum selenium levels remained significantly lower in GO after adjusting for age, smoking status, thyroidectomy, radioactive iodine treatment and residential location.

Conclusion.—Serum selenium levels are lower in patients with GO compared with GD in an Australian study population with marginal selenium status. Relative selenium deficiency may be an independent risk factor for orbitopathy in patients with Graves' disease (Fig 2).

▶ A European study published in the *New England Journal of Medicine*[1] in 2011 showed that selenium improved the quality of life and reduced progression of Graves' disease in study subjects. Those results have not been reproduced in the United States, and the fact that the study was done in an area where people tend to be selenium deficient has brought into question the value of selenium for the average person who is not selenium deficient. There has been no study that actually looked at selenium levels in patients with Graves' orbitopathy until this one.

This study showed that patients with Graves' orbitopathy had a lower serum selenium level compared with Graves' patients without orbitopathy. This may then suggest that selenium deficiency may be an independent risk factor for development of Graves' orbitopathy. This is intriguing, but there are many unanswered questions; more study is needed before this conclusion can be accepted. There is no universally accepted normal serum selenium value. The selenium levels found in different patient populations vary. Finally, there is a question whether the serum selenium level is really related to the tissue levels of selenium in all patients. For now, this is an interesting potential factor as we try to unravel the mysteries of Graves' orbitopathy.

R. B. Penne, MD

Reference

1. Marocci C, Kahaly GJ, Krassas GE, et al. Selenium and the course of mild Graves' orbitopathy. *N Engl J Med.* 2011;364:1920-1931.

Predicting the Need for Surgical Intervention in Pediatric Orbital Cellulitis

Smith JM, Bratton EM, DeWitt P, et al (Univ of Colorado, Aurora)
Am J Ophthalmol 158:387-394.e1, 2014

Purpose.—To investigate the predictive value of the complete ophthalmic examination at first presentation in foreseeing the need for surgery in patients with pediatric orbital cellulitis.

Design.—Retrospective observational case series.

Methods.—We reviewed 136 cases of radiographically confirmed orbital cellulitis between 2004 and 2012 at Children's Hospital Colorado. The presenting ophthalmic examinations, imaging results, medical and surgical interventions, and clinical complications were recorded. The main outcome measures were ophthalmic examinations on presentation, medical or surgical interventions, and complications.

Results.—The median age was 6.5 years. Of the patients, 56 (41%) underwent surgical intervention, and 80 patients (59%) were managed medically. Patients requiring surgery had higher rates of extraocular motility (EOM) restriction (78.6% vs 38.8% $P < 0.01$), proptosis (64.3% vs 21.2%, $P < 0.01$), elevated intraocular pressure (IOP) (35.7% vs 12.5%, $P < 0.01$), and age over 9 years (58.9% vs 20.0%, $P < 0.01$). Using any combination of the above risk factors at presentation, the probability of surgical intervention increases from 7% (95% confidence interval [CI] 1%-13%) with zero risk factors to 95% (95% CI 89%-100%) with 4 risk factors.

Conclusions.—In pediatric orbital cellulitis, the likelihood of surgical intervention can be estimated accurately based on the ophthalmic examination on initial presentation to the hospital. Risk factors for surgery include age older than 9 years, proptosis, EOM restriction, and elevated IOP. These factors may be used to identify patients at high risk for failure of medical management early in the clinical course (Fig 5, Tables 2-4).

▶ This is a retrospective observational case series that looks at factors that can be used to predict the need for surgical intervention in pediatric orbital cellulitis. The results found that 4 factors were predictive for the need to have surgery (Tables 2-4). These were age older than 9 years, proptosis, extraocular motility (EOM) restriction, and elevated intraocular pressure (IOP). Of the 136 patients, 41% required surgical intervention, and 59% were managed medically. The surgeries performed were mainly sinus drainage, orbital abscess drainage, or both. The exceptions were 3 patients who had emergent lateral canthotomy/cantholysis and 1 patient who required craniectomy for intracranial extension of an abscess.

I do not think anyone would be surprised that any one of these 4 factors suggests that the cellulitis is serious. There have been multiple studies looking at many of these 4 factors. The value in this article is that the need for surgery can be predicted on initial examination using these 4 factors. If the patient has all 4 factors on initial examination, he or she has a 96% chance of needing

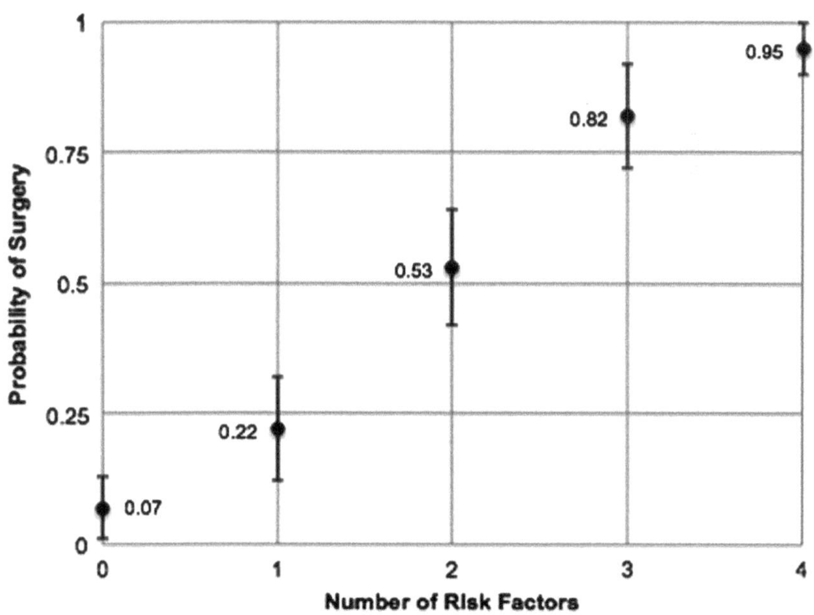

FIGURE 5.—Probability of surgical intervention in pediatric orbital cellulitis based on any combination of 4 risk factors at presentation. The risk factors are age older than 9 years, elevated intraocular pressure, extraocular motility restriction, and proptosis. (Reprinted from American Journal of Ophthalmology. Smith JM, Bratton EM, DeWitt P, et al. Predicting the need for surgical intervention in pediatric orbital cellulitis. *Am J Ophthalmol.* 2014;158:387-394.e1, Copyright 2014, with permission from Elsevier.)

TABLE 2.—Historical and Clinical Characteristics of Patients With Pediatric Orbital Cellulitis on Initial Presentation to the Hospital; Comparison of Findings in Medically and Surgically Managed Patients

Finding	All Patients (n = 136)	Medically Managed Patients (n = 80)	Surgically Managed Patients (n = 56)	*P* Value
Mean duration of eye symptoms prior to presentation	2.47 days	2.42 days	2.55 days	0.6128
Average age (years)	7.00 years	5.68 years	8.90 years	<0.0001
Age >9 years	49 (36%)	16 (20%)	33 (59%)	<0.0001
Male	87 (64%)	51 (64%)	36 (64%)	1.0
Antibiotic use in past 24 hours	71 (52%)	46 (58%)	25 (47%)	0.1926
Proptosis	53 (39%)	17 (21%)	36 (64%)	<0.0001
EOM restriction	75 (55%)	31 (39%)	44 (79%)	<0.0001
Elevated IOP	30 (22%)	10 (12%)	20 (36%)	0.0027
Decreased vision	13 (10%)	3 (4%)	10 (18%)	0.0140
Conjunctival chemosis	18 (13%)	6 (8%)	12 (21%)	0.0356
Abscess	83 (61%)	30 (38%)	53 (95%)	<0.0001

EOM = extraocular motility.

Reprinted from American Journal of Ophthalmology. Smith JM, Bratton EM, DeWitt P, et al. Predicting the need for surgical intervention in pediatric orbital cellulitis. *Am J Ophthalmol.* 2014;158:387-394.e1, Copyright 2014, with permission from Elsevier.

TABLE 3.—Univariable Analysis of Risk Factors for Surgical Intervention in Pediatric Orbital Cellulitis

	Odds Ratio	LCL	UCL	*P* Value
Age >9 years	5.74	2.66	12.41	<0.0001
Proptosis	6.67	3.08	14.44	<0.0001
EOM restriction	5.80	2.64	12.74	<0.0001
Chemosis	3.36	1.17	9.69	0.0234
Decreased vision	5.58	1.44	21.59	0.0120
Elevated IOP	3.89	1.63	9.25	0.0019
Abscess	29.44	8.36	103.75	<0.0001

EOM = extraocular motility; IOP = intraocular pressure; LCL = lower confidence interval; UCL = upper confidence interval.

Note: Each row in the table reports the odds ratio for surgical intervention for each risk factor. The table uses a univariable logistic regression model where the odds ratio of each risk factor is analyzed and reported independently of the other risk factors.

Reprinted from American Journal of Ophthalmology. Smith JM, Bratton EM, DeWitt P, et al. Predicting the need for surgical intervention in pediatric orbital cellulitis. *Am J Ophthalmol.* 2014;158:387-394.e1, Copyright 2014, with permission from Elsevier.

surgery. On the other extreme, if the patient had none of the 4 factors, the chance of needing surgery was 7%. The chance of needing surgery increases as the number of these 4 factors present on initial examination increases (Fig 5). Thus, if a patient has all 4 factors, there is little value in trying prolonged medical management, and surgery can be done sooner; hopefully, this offers a shorter hospital stay and faster recovery.

As with any study, application of these findings should be used as a guideline in clinical management, and clinical judgment must be applied for each

TABLE 4.—Multivariable Analysis of Risk Factors for Surgical Intervention in Pediatric Orbital Cellulitis

	Odds Ratio	LCL	UCL	*P* Value
Age >9 years	6.21	2.42	15.95	0.0001
Proptosis	5.97	2.24	15.92	0.0003
EOM restriction	2.27	0.86	6.00	0.0946
Elevated IOP	3.36	1.19	9.53	0.0212

EOM = extraocular motility; IOP = intraocular pressure; LCL = lower confidence interval; UCL = upper confidence interval.

Note: Each row in the table reports the odds ratio for surgical intervention for each risk factor. The table uses a multivariable logistic regression model where the odds ratio of each risk factor is reported after accounting for other listed risk factors.

Reprinted from American Journal of Ophthalmology. Smith JM, Bratton EM, DeWitt P, et al. Predicting the need for surgical intervention in pediatric orbital cellulitis. *Am J Ophthalmol*. 2014;158:387-394.e1, Copyright 2014, with permission from Elsevier.

individual patient. They are not an absolute. I do believe that these guidelines are something I will use in the future in managing children with orbital cellulitis.

R. B. Penne, MD

Management of Functional Epiphora in Patients With an Anatomically Patent Dacryocystorhinostomy

Shams PN, Chen PG, Wormald PJ, et al (Adelaide Univ, South Australia, Australia; Univ of Adelaide, South Australia, Australia; et al)

JAMA Ophthalmol 132:1127-1132, 2014

Importance.—Approximately 5% to 10% of patients continue to experience persistent epiphora following an anatomically successful dacryocystorhinostomy (DCR) for nasolacrimal duct obstruction or stenosis.

Objective.—To investigate the management and success rate of so-called "functional failure" of DCR for nasolacrimal duct obstruction by experienced lacrimal surgeons.

Design, Setting, and Participants.—Multicenter retrospective case series including 5 Australian and New Zealand centers. Participants included 61 patients (71% women [n = 46]; mean age, 66 years) with functional epiphora after 65 DCRs (69% transnasal) who were recruited over a mean of 7.6 years. Inclusion criteria included confirmed preoperative diagnosis of nasolacrimal duct obstruction or stenosis, age greater than 18 years, recurrent or persistent epiphora after DCR, an anatomically successful DCR, and follow-up longer than 6 months. Exclusion criteria included evidence of lacrimal hypersecretion, eyelid malposition, and punctal or canalicular abnormalities.

Main Outcomes and Measures.—The number, type, timing, and success of all clinical interventions performed for the management of functional epiphora after DCR.

Results.—Epiphora recurred a mean of 8.9 months after primary DCR; 89% of the cases (n = 58) had evidence of a patent ostium and 100% were patent on lacrimal irrigation. Intubation with a lacrimal stent was performed in 82% of the cases at the time of surgery, and all stents were removed a mean of 8 weeks postoperatively. Epiphora was reported immediately following DCR in 32% (n = 21) of the cases and within 6 weeks after removal of the stent in 31% (n = 20); late recurrence (>12 months after DCR) developed in 37% (n = 24) of the cases. In a total of 15% of the cases, participants declined any treatment following DCR. The remainder underwent a mean of 1.3 interventions (range, 1-3) during a mean of 23 to 41 months after primary DCR, following which 72% (n = 47) of the cases had a successful outcome; 12% (n = 8) failed to achieve improvement, and the patients declined further intervention. Thirty-nine interventions (60%) were intubation with a silicone stent with a 54% success rate. Almost half of those undergoing intubation elected to keep the stent permanently; 34% (n = 22) had an eyelid-tightening procedure with 50% success, and 15% (n = 10) required a Lester-Jones tube despite patent canaliculi, with a success rate of 90%.

Conclusions and Relevance.—Functional epiphora after DCR among patients with preoperative nasolacrimal duct obstruction or stenosis appears to be uncommon. Benefits can be achieved in most patients with intubation (transient or permanent) or eyelid tightening. More than one procedure is often required.

▶ Persistent tearing after a primary dacryocystorhinostomy (DCR) that is patent is a frustrating, and fortunately rare, problem. This article considers this problem and comes up with a nice treatment algorithm (Fig 2 in original article). It should be noted that the algorithm is not based on statistical findings in this retrospective study but rather on the authors' experience. However, I believe it is a rational approach to this problem.

The most common secondary procedure done was lacrimal intubation, which was done 39 times with a 54% success rate. Eyelid tightening was the second most common intervention, performed 22 times, and was 50% successful. Overall, 72% of patients has resolution of their tearing by having 1 to 3 additional procedures (Fig 1 in original article, Table 2 in original article).

This article offers a nice approach to patients who have a patent lacrimal system after DCR but continue to tear. In general, a second procedure will offer a 50% chance of resolution of tearing, and the patient may need up to 3 additional procedures.

R. B. Penne, MD

Elevated white blood cell count may predict risk of orbital implant exposure

Bee Y-S, Lin M-C, Sheu S-J, et al (Kaohsiung Veterans General Hosp, Taiwan; et al)

Can J Ophthalmol 49:45-49, 2014

Objective.—To determine the risk factors for primary implant exposure after enucleation and evisceration in infected eyes.

Design.—Retrospective, comparative case series.

Participants.—Patients who underwent enucleation or evisceration for infected eyes.

Methods.—Records of patients who underwent enucleation or evisceration for infected eyes with placement of solid sphere implants were reviewed. Preoperative white blood cell (WBC) count, microbiologic laboratory results, clinical features, medical treatment, and surgical methods were recorded to evaluate the risk for implant exposure.

Results.—Eighty-five infected eyes were collected. The mean age was 70.1 years. The positive culture rate was 69.4%. In 42 patients with endophthalmitis or panophthalmitis, the most common microorganisms were *Pseudomonas aeruginosa* in 6 cases (20.7%) and *Klebsiella pneumoniae* in 7 cases (24.1%). In 50 patients with keratitis or scleritis, the most common microorganisms were *P. aeruginosa* in 14 eyes (46.7%) and Fusarium in 4 eyes (13.3%). There was a 12.9% exposure rate for the 85 patients. Preoperative WBC count was significantly higher in patients with implant exposure compared with those without exposure ($p = 0.04$). Preoperative WBC count more than 9500 cells/L had significantly higher exposure ($p = 0.001$).

Conclusions.—Preoperative elevated WBC count was associated with higher risk for implant exposure. Primary implantation after enucleation or evisceration may be less safe in infected eyes with high preoperative WBC count.

▶ The placement of an orbital implant at the same time as the enucleation or evisceration for endophthalmitis saves the patient from a second surgical procedure. General surgical principles have questioned the placement of an implant into infected tissues. However, this has become an accepted approach with many surgeons. A number of these patients subsequently develop implant exposure/extrusion. This study looks at the potential variables that may help predict the risk of implant exposure.

The results in this article found preoperative white blood cell count (WBC) to be the only statistically significant variable that differentiated between the patients who developed exposure versus those that did not. A WBC count >9500 seemed to point to a greater risk of implant exposure.

The explanation for this difference is not clear to me or to the authors. It may suggest the infection is more severe with a higher WBC. It does make sense that a more severe infection may make implant exposure more likely. However, in endophthalmitis, the serum WBC is often normal and certainly not something we follow as we do for infections elsewhere in the body. For now, the WBC is something I will note and use as adjunct information when faced with a patient with endophthalmitis who requires an enucleation or evisceration.

R. B. Penne, MD

Bilateral Lacrimal Gland Disease: Clinical Features of 97 Cases

Tang SX, Lim RP, Al-Dahmash S, et al (SUNY Downstate Med Ctr, Brooklyn, NY; Wills Eye Inst, Philadelphia, PA; et al)

Ophthalmology 121:2040-2046, 2014

Objective.—Bilateral lacrimal gland (LG) disease is a unique presentation that can result from varied causes. We reviewed the diagnoses, clinical features, and outcomes of 97 patients with this entity.

Design.—Case series.

Participants.—Ninety-seven patients with bilateral LG disease.

Methods.—Retrospective review and statistical analysis using analysis of variance and the Fisher exact test.

Main Outcome Measures.—Patient demographics, clinical features, diagnostic testing, diagnosis, and treatment.

Results.—Patient age ranging from 8 to 84 years (mean, 46 years). The predominant gender was female (77%), and race included black (49%), white (38%), and Hispanic (12%) patients. Diagnoses fell into 4 categories: inflammatory (n = 51; 53%), structural (n = 20; 21%), lymphoproliferative (n = 19; 20%), and uncommon (n = 7; 7%) entities. The most common diagnoses included idiopathic orbital inflammation (IOI; n = 29; 30%), sarcoidosis (n = 19; 20%), prolapsed LG (n = 15; 15%), lymphoma (n = 11; 11%), lymphoid hyperplasia (n = 8; 8%), and dacryops (n = 5; 5%). Inflammatory conditions were more likely in younger patients ($P < 0.05$) and in those with pain ($P < 0.001$) and mechanical blepharoptosis ($P < 0.01$) at presentation, whereas lymphoma was more common in older patients ($P < 0.001$) without active signs of inflammation at presentation. Black patients were more likely to have sarcoidosis ($P < 0.01$). Laboratory results showed high angiotensin converting enzyme level being significantly more likely in patients with sarcoidosis ($P < 0.05$). However, sensitivity was limited to 45%, with 25% of patients diagnosed with IOI also demonstrating positive results. Corticosteroid therapy was the treatment of choice in 38 cases, corresponding to resolution of symptoms in 29% and improvement in an additional 32%. Overall, chronic underlying disease was found in 71% of patients, among whom 26% achieved a disease-free state, whereas 3% succumbed to their underlying disease.

Conclusions.—The cause of bilateral lacrimal gland disease most commonly was inflammatory, followed by structural and lymphoproliferative. Patient characteristics and clinical presentations were key features distinguishing between competing possibilities. Despite local control with

TABLE 5.—Bilateral Lacrimal Gland Diseases in 97 Patients: Outcomes

Diagnosis	Free of Disease	Alive with Disease	Dead of Disease
Total (n = 90)	**23 (26%)**	**64 (71%)**	3 (3%)
Inflammatory (n = 48)	**12 (25%)**	**36 (75%)**	0 (0%)
IOI (n = 27)	10 (37%)	17 (63%)	0 (0%)
Sarcoidosis (n = 18)	2 (11%)	16 (89%)	0 (0%)
Sjögren's syndrome (n = 3)	0 (0%)	3 (100%)	0 (0%)
Structural (n = 16)	**1 (6%)**	**15 (94%)**	**0 (0%)**
Lacrimal gland prolapse (n = 11)	1 (9%)	10 (91%)	0 (0%)
Dacryops (n = 5)	0 (0%)	5 (100%)	0 (0%)
Lymphoproliferative (n = 19)	**5 (26%)**	**12 (63%)**	**2 (11%)**
Lymphoma (n = 11)	3 (27%)	6 (55%)	2 (18%)*
Lymphoid hyperplasia (n = 8)	2 (25%)	6 (75%)	0 (0%)
Uncommon entities (n = 7)	**5 (71%)**†	**1 (14%)**†	**1 (14%)**
Rosai Dorfman disease (n = 3)	3 (100%)	0 (0%)	0 (0%)
Erdheim Chester disease (n = 2)	1 (50%)	1 (50%)	0 (0%)
Necrotizing granulomatous disease (n = 1)	1 (100%)	0 (0%)	0 (0%)
Extramedullary hematopoiesis (n = 1)	0 (0%)	0 (0%)	1 (100%)

IOI = idiopathic orbital inflammation.
Boldface represents treatment response of entire patient cohort.
*$P < 0.05$.
†$P < 0.01$.
Reprinted from Ophthalmology. Tang SX, Lim RP, Al-Dahmash S, et al. Bilateral Lacrimal Gland Disease: Clinical Features of 97 Cases. *Ophthalmology.* 2014;121:2040-2046, Copyright 2014, with permission from the American Academy of Ophthalmology.

corticosteroids or radiotherapy, underlying disease continued in 71% of patients and led to death in 3% (Table 5).

▶ Bilateral lacrimal gland disease is much less common than unilateral disease. This article offers some specific findings that help guide the clinical management of these patients. The rarity of this disease is evidenced by the fact that there were 23 contributors to the article to arrive at the 97 cases studied.

The differential diagnosis of bilateral lacrimal gland disease is in order of frequency: idiopathic orbital inflammation (IOI), sarcoidosis, lacrimal gland prolapse, and lymphoma (Table 5). The article also outlines a few useful characteristics. Inflammatory conditions were more likely to be seen in younger patients and have pain and mechanical ptosis. Lymphoma was found in older patients without signs of inflammation, and African Americans were more likely to be diagnosed with sarcoidosis. There is an obvious absence of epithelial tumors both benign and malignant in bilateral disease that would be part of a differential diagnosis in unilateral disease.

The workup of these patients involves clinical examination, laboratory examination, and imaging. This provides a basis for the differential diagnosis. However, the gold standard for making the diagnosis is biopsy. That does not mean this is necessary for every patient, but any patient who is older without inflammatory signs probably needs a biopsy. Also, any patient who does not respond appropriately to treatment should be biopsied. The chance that the disease may be lymphoid must always be considered.

R. B. Penne, MD

Dynamic Changes of Tear Fluid After Cosmetic Transcutaneous Lower Blepharoplasty Measured by Optical Coherence Tomography

Shao C, Fu Y, Lu L, et al (Shanghai Jiao Tong Univ School of Medicine, China)
Am J Ophthalmol 158:55-63.e1, 2014

Purpose.—To investigate the dynamic changes of tear fluid after cosmetic transcutaneous lower blepharoplasty.

Design.—Prospective, observational case series study.

Methods.—A total of 60 eyes of 30 patients with transcutaneous lower blepharoplasty were involved in the study. All subjects completed the Ocular Surface Disease Index questionnaire and underwent tear film break-up time measurements and the Schirmer test before surgery and 1 week, 1 month, and 3 months after surgery. Tear meniscus parameters measured by optical coherence tomography were recorded. Lower lid margin reflex distance was also measured. At each time point after surgery, these parameters were compared with the baseline parameters. The incidence of dry eye and chemosis after surgery was assessed.

Results.—The Ocular Surface Disease Index score increased significantly 1 week after surgery ($P < .01$). The Schirmer test values were significantly decreased 1 week postoperatively ($P < .01$), and they returned to baseline by 3 months. There was no significant change in tear film break-up time before and after surgery. The tear meniscus height, depth, and cross section area values were significantly increased at 1 week postoperatively, decreased at 1 month ($P < .01$), and returned to baseline at 3 months ($P > .05$). The cornea–lower eyelid angle significantly decreased at 1 week postoperatively ($P < .01$), increased at 1 month ($P < .01$), and returned to baseline by 3 months ($P > .05$). The lower lid margin reflex distance was increased 1 week after surgery ($P < .01$), and gradually recovered but had not returned to the baseline 3 months after surgery ($P < .01$). The increased tear meniscus height had a positive correlation with lower lid margin reflex distance. The incidence of dry eye and chemosis at 1 week postoperatively was 16.7% and 15%, respectively.

Conclusions.—Cosmetic transcutaneous lower blepharoplasty affects ocular surface and tear fluid, which leads to dryness, tearful eyes, and chemosis. However, this influence is temporary after surgery, and the symptoms resolve within 3 months. A positive correlation between tear meniscus height and lower lid margin reflex distance was observed. Assessment of the tear meniscus with optical coherence tomography provided a quick, noninvasive, and quantitative method to investigate the dynamic changes of the tear fluid after blepharoplasty (Figs 3 and 4).

▶ This is a prospective study looking at tears and tear function before and after lower lid transcutaneous blepharoplasty. The study evaluated a number of objective measurements of tear function and the subjective findings associated with dry eyes and exposure (Figs 3 and 4).

The subjective finding that the patient experiences and the objective changes that were measured showing tear fluid dysfunction were found to be similar and

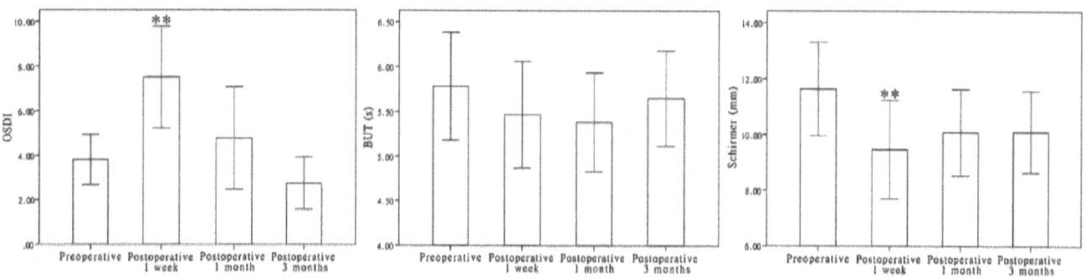

FIGURE 3.—Graph showing the mean difference in the value of Ocular Surface Disease Index (OSDI), tear film break-up time (BUT), and Schirmer I test before and after transcutaneous lower blepharoplasty. (**$P < .01$.) (Reprinted from American Journal of Ophthalmology. Shao C, Fu Y, Lu L, et al. Dynamic changes of tear fluid after cosmetic transcutaneous lower blepharoplasty measured by optical coherence tomography. *Am J Ophthalmol.* 2014;158:55-63.e1, Copyright 2014, with permission from Elsevier.)

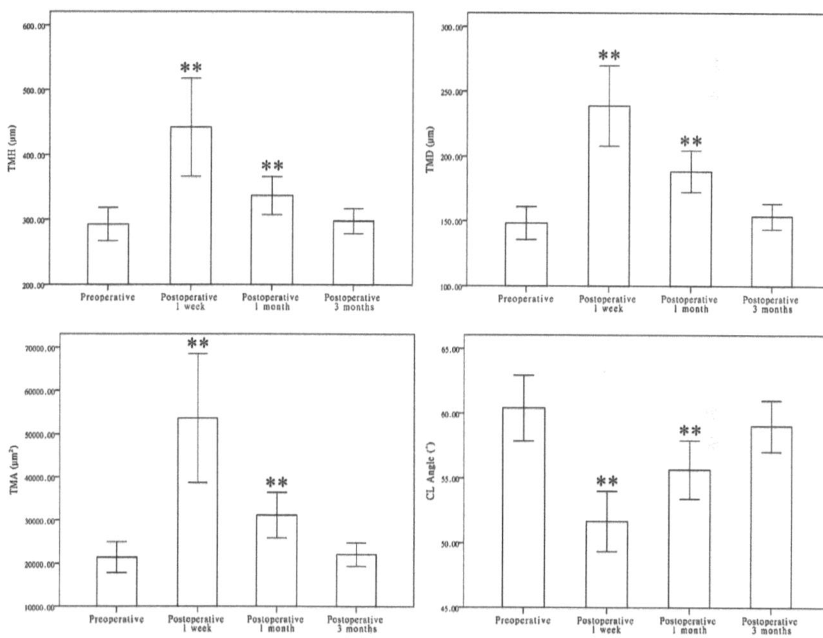

FIGURE 4.—Graph showing the mean difference in the value of tear meniscus height (TMH), tear meniscus depth (TMD), tear meniscus cross section area (TMA), and cornea–lower eyelid angle (CL Angle) before and after transcutaneous lower blepharoplasty. (**$P < .01$.) (Reprinted from American Journal of Ophthalmology. Shao C, Fu Y, Lu L, et al. Dynamic changes of tear fluid after cosmetic transcutaneous lower blepharoplasty measured by optical coherence tomography. *Am J Ophthalmol.* 2014;158:55-63.e1, Copyright 2014, with permission from Elsevier.)

related. The results showed signs and symptoms of dryness at 1 week and 1 month after surgery, but these signs and symptoms had resolved and returned to baseline at 3 months.

I do not find anything shown in this study surprising, but this does objectively show there is tear dysfunction after lower eyelid blepharoplasty. This dysfunction measured objectively seemed to follow the patients' subjective symptoms. The good news is that both the signs and symptoms of eye irritation after lower lid blepharoplasty resolve by 3 months, and patients tear function returns to their baseline.

The 1 point I take from this study is that we need to tell our patients undergoing lower lid external blepharoplasty that there is a good chance they will have postoperative eye irritation from dryness but that it will resolve by 3 months. How this relates to a lower lid transconjunctival blepharoplasty remains a question to be studied in the future.

R. B. Penne, MD

Surgical Timing and Postoperative Ocular Motility in Type B Orbital Blowout Fractures

Liao JC, Elmalem VI, Wells TS, et al (The Eye Inst, Milwaukee, WI; SUNY Downstate Med Ctr, Brooklyn, NY)

Ophthal Plast Reconstr Surg 31:29-33, 2015

Purpose.—To determine whether patients with Type B orbital blowout fractures (soft-tissue distortion disproportionate to bone-fragment displacement) repaired within 7 days of injury have statistically greater postoperative vertical binocular fusion than similar patients who undergo later surgery.

Methods.—Prospective and retrospective surgical case series. Inclusion criteria were orbital floor (with or without medial wall) blowout fracture repair, preoperative coronal orbital CT scans, and patient age of at least 12 years at time of postoperative binocular visual field.

Results.—Twenty-five patients met inclusion criteria. Ten patients (group 1) had surgery within 7 days of injury, and 15 patients (group 2) had surgery more than 7 days after injury. The total cohort had a median postoperative vertical binocular fusion of 90°. Group 1 had postoperative vertical binocular fusion averaging 100°. Nine of 10 patients (90%) were above and 1 of 10 (10%) were below the median for the entire cohort. Group 2 had postoperative vertical binocular fusion averaging 70°. Three of 15 patients (20%) were above and 12 of 15 patients (80%) were below the median for the entire cohort. The difference between the average postoperative vertical binocular fusion of the 2 groups was statistically significant by two-tailed unpaired t test with p value 0.0022.

Conclusions.—Patients with Type B orbital blowout fractures (soft-tissue distortion disproportionate to bone-fragment displacement) have statistically greater average postoperative vertical binocular fusion if repaired within 7 days of injury than similar patients who undergo later surgery (Figs 1 and 3).

▶ For many years, all orbital blowout fractures were lumped together when considering the timing for surgical repair. A 2-week window from the time of injury to time of repair was the standard of care for all orbital blowout fractures. In 1998, the white-eyed blowout fracture was recognized, and a small subset of fractures in young patients was recognized to have a much better chance of

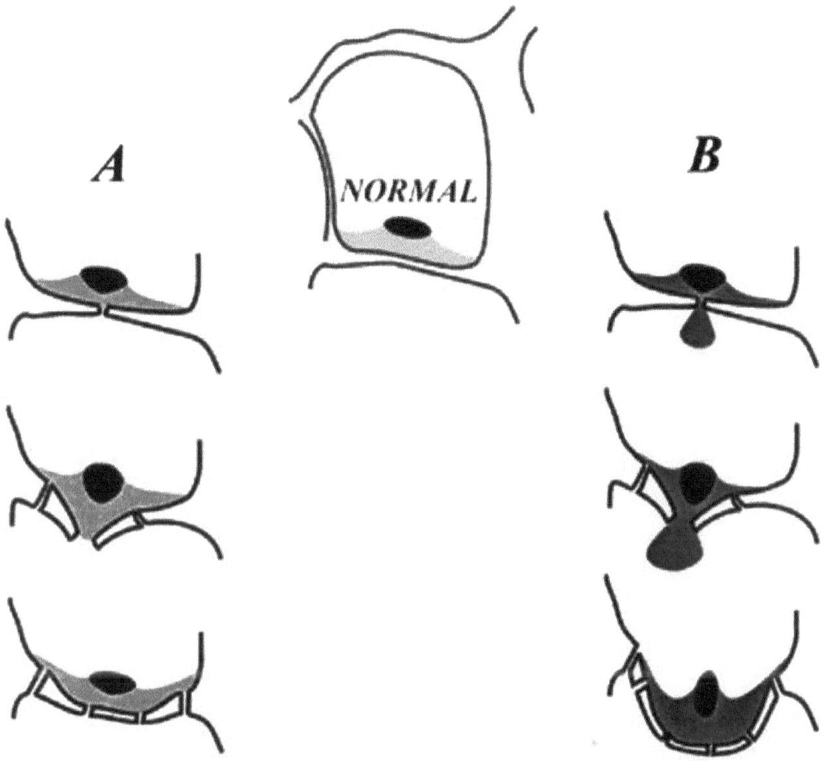

FIGURE 1.—Schematic classification of blowout fractures, based on lesser (A) or greater (B) soft-tissue distortion relative to bone fragment configuration. Reprinted with permission from Harris et al.[2] *Editor's Note*: Please refer to original journal article for full references. (Reprinted from Liao JC, Elmalem VI, Wells TS, et al. Surgical timing and postoperative ocular motility in type b orbital blowout fractures. *Ophthal Plast Reconstr Surg*. 2015;31:29-33, with permission from The American Society of Ophthalmic Plastic and Reconstructive Surgery, Inc.)

recovery of their ocular motility and alignment if they were repaired urgently. This report separates orbital blowout fractures in all patients, adults and children, based on orbital imaging. Orbital fractures with soft-tissue distortion disproportionate to bone fragment displacement (type B in the study, Figs 1 and 3) were found to have greater postoperative vertical binocular fusion if repaired within 7 days of injury when compared with similar patients who undergo later surgery.

As noted in the report, the great improvement in the resolution of orbital imaging has given orbital surgeons the chance to evaluate orbital fractures for potential muscle ischemia. This report suggests that these fractures should be repaired sooner for a better motility result. Further study is needed to determine the exact timing. For now, I believe that when recognizing a patient with a type B orbital blowout fracture, the repair should be scheduled as soon as it can be

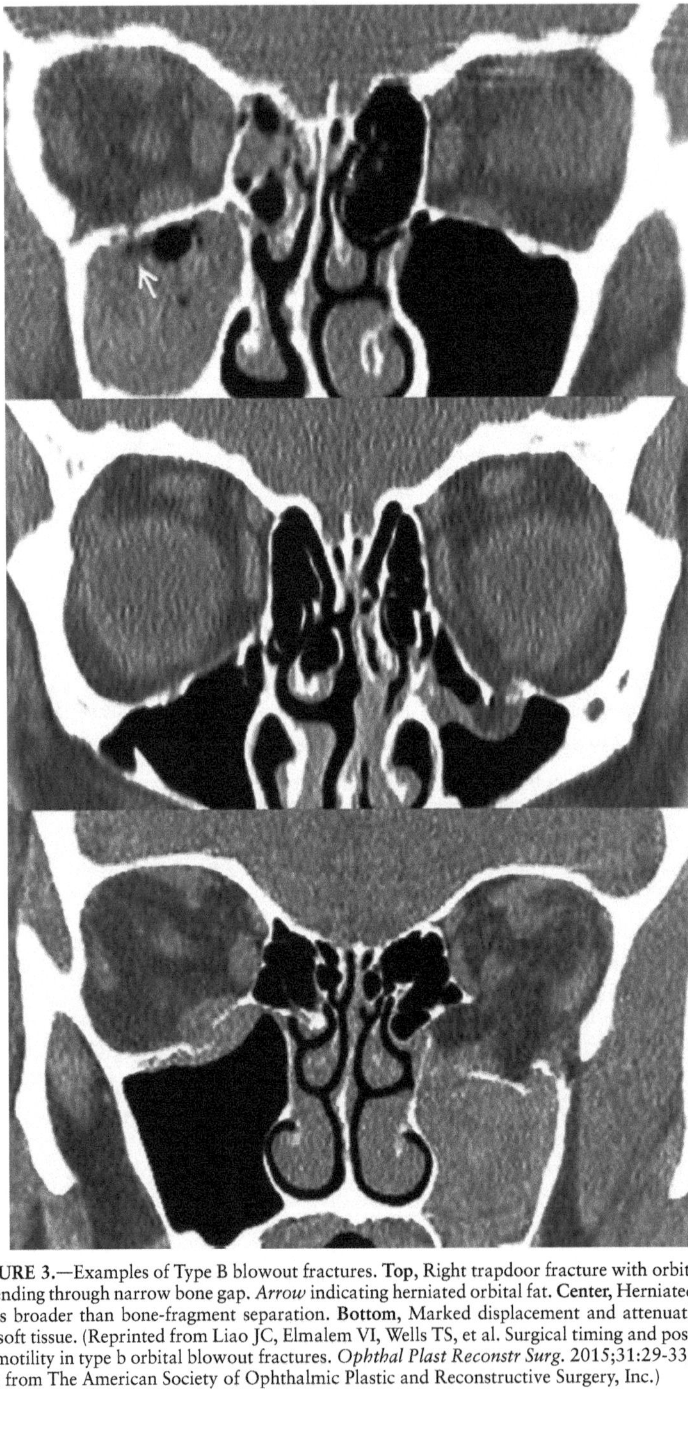

FIGURE 3.—Examples of Type B blowout fractures. **Top**, Right trapdoor fracture with orbital soft tissue extending through narrow bone gap. *Arrow* indicating herniated orbital fat. **Center**, Herniated left orbital fat is broader than bone-fragment separation. **Bottom**, Marked displacement and attenuation of left orbital soft tissue. (Reprinted from Liao JC, Elmalem VI, Wells TS, et al. Surgical timing and postoperative ocular motility in type b orbital blowout fractures. *Ophthal Plast Reconstr Surg*. 2015;31:29-33, with permission from The American Society of Ophthalmic Plastic and Reconstructive Surgery, Inc.)

done. It is not an emergent situation, such as a white-eyed blowout fracture, but doing surgery sooner may give a better outcome.

R. B. Penne, MD

The *tarsal belt* procedure for the correction of ectropion: description and outcome in 42 cases

Pascali M, Corsi A, Brinci L, et al (Univ of 'Tor Vergata', Rome, Italy)

Br J Ophthalmol 98:1691-1696, 2014

Background/Aims.—Ectropion correction is a challenge in plastic surgery. Correction of the lower lid area, including restoration of the shape and position of lid margin, is the surgical goal. In this study, we describe a new surgical technique, the *tarsal belt*, for the correction of ectropion and evaluation of the effective outcome and complications of this procedure.

Methods.—Between January 2008 and January 2012, a total of 42 patients aged between 48 and 75 years (average age 61.5 years) were treated with this technique. This procedure consists in a trans-tarsal mattress non-absorbable suture anchored to the periosteum of the lateral orbital rim, combined with a small wedge excision of a lateral portion of the tarsus close to the lateral canthal tendon. During the same period, 66 patients were treated with the standard lateral tarsal strip technique. Preoperative and postoperative Ectropion Grading Scale (EGS) was recorded to evaluate anatomical improvement. The average follow-up period was 24 months.

Results.—Rate of success was 100% for involutional and cicatricial ectropions, 90% for lid retraction and 87.5% for paralytic ectropions. Anatomical success according to EGS scale was obtained in 41 patients. Recurrence of ectropion occurred in only one patient 6 months after the first surgery and required a further operation with a larger posterior lamella resection and new *tarsal belt* suture.

Conclusions.—The *tarsal belt* seems to be effective to correct the horizontal and vertical instability of the lid. The suture supports the lower eyelid along the entire tarsal plate length and corrects the outward buckling of the tarsal plate.

▶ This article describes a new approach to the surgical correction of lower eyelid ectropion. I have not seen anything quite like this tarsal belt procedure (Figs 1 and 2 in the original article) described before, and it offers a unique way to address an ectropion.

The authors performed the tarsal belt procedure on 42 patients. The patients all had an entropion, but the etiology varied between involutional, paralytic, cicatricial, and lid retraction. When dividing up these 42 patients into these 4 categories, the numbers of each are small. Over the same period of time, 66 patients with ectropions had the ectropion addressed with a lateral tarsal strip procedure. There is no explanation as to what determined which patient had which procedure, but they were not randomized. All these factors as well as the small numbers preclude any comparison between the results of the tarsal belt and lateral tarsal strip in this study (Tables 1 and 2 in the original article).

The results were good, but the small numbers prevent any real conclusion. What I take away from this study is a new potential technique that I will consider for paralytic, cicatricial, or recurrent ectropions. I will not use it for my routine involutional ectropion patients. This procedure does seem to provide more support for the eyelid all the way across the tarsus rather than just pulling the eyelid tight laterally, which is what the lateral tarsal strip does. It is a more complicated procedure, which will take longer and involves more extensive eyelid dissection. Ultimately, how useful this procedure will be requires further study.

R. B. Penne, MD

Botulinum Toxin Type A Injection for Lateral Canthal Rhytids: Effect on Tear Film Stability and Tear Production

Ho M-C, Hsu W-C, Hsieh Y-T (Taipei Tzu Chi Hosp, Taiwan; et al)

JAMA Ophthalmol 132:332-337, 2014

Importance.—Botulinum toxin injection for lateral canthal rhytids has been reported to result in dry eye, but its effect on tear film stability and tear production has not been studied thoroughly.

Objective.—To investigate the effect of botulinum toxin type A on tear film stability and tear production after treatment of lateral canthal rhytids.

Design, Setting, and Participants.—We performed a clinical intervention study at a regional hospital in Taiwan of 58 women 30 to 60 years of age with lateral canthal rhytids from January 1 through December 31, 2011.

Interventions.—Botulinum toxin type A at 2 different preparations and doses (dose A: 3 injections of 2 U in 0.05 mL of normal saline per injection; dose B: 3 injections of 4 U in 0.05 mL of normal saline per injection) was injected at the lateral canthal areas. One eye of each study participant was randomly chosen for dose A, and the other eye received dose B.

Main Outcomes and Measures.—Baseline tear film break-up time (TBUT) and Schirmer tests without and with anesthesia were measured before and at 1 week, 1 month, 3 months, and 6 months after botulinum toxin injection. The TBUT and Schirmer test results were compared between different periods and doses.

Results.—The TBUT decreased significantly at 1 week after botulinum toxin type A injection ($P = .003$), and the effect persisted at 1 month and 3 months after treatment ($P = .01$ and .02, respectively). In younger participants, the TBUT recovered faster than in older patients. The results of the Schirmer tests without and with anesthesia decreased gradually, with significant reduction at 1 month after treatment ($P = .05$ and .02, respectively) and then recovered gradually. Both the TBUT and Schirmer test results decreased more in eyes that received dose B than in those that received dose A; however, none of the differences were statistically significant.

Conclusions and Relevance.—Tear film stability decreased as early as 1 week after botulinum toxin type A treatment for lateral canthal rhytids, and the effect persisted for more than 3 months. Tear production decreased to the trough at 1 month after treatment and then recovered gradually.

▶ This article looks at the affects of botulinum toxin type A when injected at the lateral canthus on tear function. The study evaluated these preinjection, at 1 week, 1 month, and 3 months after injection. The results were interesting. Both Schirmer scores and tear breakup time (TBUT) were decreased but in different ways. The Schirmer gradually decreased to a trough at 1 month and then improved. TBUT decreased sharply during the first week and then gradually improved over 6 months.

It would have been nice to have subjective testing of tear function done at the same time to see if ocular symptoms followed this pattern. It was not surprising that both TBUT and Schirmer scores were decreased with botulinum toxin injection. I was somewhat surprised that the effects lasted at least 3 months. Awareness of these findings would suggest that even simple botulinum toxin injection for lateral rhytids should be accompanied by a discussion that the patients' eyes may be drier and irritated for up to 3 months after injection.

R. B. Penne, MD

8 Pediatric Ophthalmology

Propranolol and Periocular Capillary Hemangiomas: Assessment of Refractive Effect

Glasman P, Chandna A, Nayak H, et al (Royal Liverpool Univ Hosp, UK; Alder Hey Children's Hosp, Liverpool, UK)

J Pediatr Ophthalmol Strabismus 51:165-170, 2014

Purpose.—To assess the effects of systemic propranolol on refractive error in infants with periocular capillary hemangiomas.

Methods.—A single-center study of consecutive patients with capillary hemangiomas treated with systemic propranolol. Refractive data were analyzed using Long's matrix formalism and the methods of Harris and Kaye.

Results.—Seventeen patients were included. At 6 months postoperatively, hemangioma size reduced from 3,214 to 1,806 mm^3 (standard deviation: 4,122 to 2,441). Mean refractive error in the affected eye significantly reduced: −1.25/0.38 × 36 (95% confidence intervals: −5.08/1.20 × 90 to 1.64/1.43 × 180, P =.048) with a smaller change (P =.06) in the unaffected eye of −1.01/+0.31 × 3.16 (95% confidence intervals: −4.02/+1.12 × 180 to +1.49/+0.51 × 90).

Conclusions.—Propranolol produced a clinically significant reduction in the infants' refractive error and anisometropia. The reduction in the total refractive error and anisometropia has not been evident in previous analyses, which have concentrated on the change in the "cylinder" as the principal outcome measure.

► Propranolol has become the more recently accepted treatment of periocular capillary hemangiomas in early childhood. Besides the cosmetic concerns of periocular capillary hemangiomas in young children, it can systematically interfere with the visual axis as well as cause changes in the refractive error of the involved eye, leading to amblyopia. It is not surprising that propanolol reduced the overall refractive error and, as a result, anisometropia of the involved eye. Of course, propanolol treatment requires close monitoring by a pediatrician for changes in blood pressure, pulse, and respiratory status.

L. B. Nelson, MD, MBA

Headache and Refractive Errors in Children

Roth Z, Pandolfo KR, Simon J, et al (Albany Med Ctr, NY)
J Pediatr Ophthalmol Strabismus 51:177-179, 2014

Purpose.—To investigate the association between uncorrected or miscorrected refractive errors in children and headache, and to determine whether correction of refractive errors contributes to headache resolution.

Methods.—Results of ophthalmic examination, including refractive error, were recorded at initial visit for headache. If resolution of headache on subsequent visits was not documented, a telephone call was placed to their caregivers to inquire whether headache had resolved.

Results.—Of the 158 patients, 75.3% had normal or unchanged eye examinations, including refractions. Follow-up data were available for 110 patients. Among those, 32 received new or changed spectacle correction and 78 did not require a change in refraction. Headaches improved in 76.4% of all patients, whether with (71.9%) or without (78.2%) a change in refractive correction. The difference between these two groups was not statistically significant ($P = .38$).

Conclusions.—Headaches in children usually do not appear to be caused by ophthalmic disease, including refractive error. The prognosis for improvement is favorable, regardless of whether refractive correction is required.

▶ Referrals to a pediatric ophthalmologist for children with headaches are a common occurrence. Often the primary care physician is concerned whether the headache is related to an ophthalmologic condition, such as a treatable refractive error. It is unusual for refractive errors to cause headaches, as was confirmed by the authors. Of course, any child with headaches should have an appointment and thorough medical evaluation. If there appears to be any ocular condition, then an appropriate ophthalmologic referral is warranted.

L. B. Nelson, MD, MBA

Frequency of Choroidal Abnormalities in Pediatric Patients With Neurofibromatosis Type 1

Goktas S, Sakarya Y, Ozcimen M, et al (Konya Training and Res Hosp, Turkey; et al)
J Pediatr Ophthalmol Strabismus 51:204-208, 2014

Purpose.—To investigate the frequency of choroidal abnormalities in pediatric patients with neurofibromatosis type 1 detected by infrared reflectance imaging.

Methods.—The fundus of 38 eyes of 19 patients with neurofibromatosis type 1 was examined using infrared reflectance imaging with optical coherence tomography. Forty eyes of 20 age-matched controls were examined similarly. Each patient was evaluated for the presence and the number of choroidal abnormalities. The correlation between the total number of choroidal abnormalities and the patient's age was studied.

Results.—A total of 19 patients (11 females, 8 males) were included. The mean age of the neurofibromatosis group was 8.63 ± 3.15 years (range: 4 to 16 years) and that of the control group was 9.05 ± 3.27 years (range: 4 to 15 years). Choroidal nodules appearing as bright patchy nodules were detected in 15 (78.9%) of 19 patients with neurofibromatosis type 1 and 1 (5%) of 20 control subjects. In terms of the frequency of choroidal abnormalities, the difference was significant between the patients with neurofibromatosis type 1 and the controls ($P < .001$). There was a positive correlation between the number of choroidal abnormalitiesin both eyes and the patient's age ($r = 0.701$, $P = .001$).

Conclusions.—Choroidal abnormalities are frequent in neurofibromatosis type 1. Choroidal abnormalities detected by infrared reflectance imaging with optical coherence tomography can be used to diagnose neurofibromatosis type 1.

▶ Ophthalmologists are frequently consulted to assist in the diagnosis of neurofibromatosis type 1 (NF-1). The diagnosis of NF-1 is especially challenging in young children because many clinical findings are not present during childhood but develop with age. The ocular examination includes assessing the visual acuity, performing a slit-lamp examination to determine the presence of iris nodules, and evaluating the appearance of the optic nerve. An optical coherence tomography infrared reflectance is used for imaging deeper ocular structures, such as the choroid. Multiple patchy and bright choroidal abnormalities have been found using this technique. This noninvasive procedure has the potential to become the eighth criteria used by physicians in the clinical diagnosis of NF-1.

L. B. Nelson, MD, MBA

Risk Factors for Amblyopia in the Vision in Preschoolers Study

Pascual M, for the Vision In Preschoolers (VIP) Study Group (Drexel Univ, Philadelphia, PA; et al)

Ophthalmology 121:622-629.e1, 2014

Objective.—To evaluate risk factors for unilateral amblyopia and for bilateral amblyopia in the Vision in Preschoolers (VIP) study.

Design.—Multicenter, cross-sectional study.

Participants.—Three- to 5-year-old Head Start preschoolers from 5 clinical centers, overrepresenting children with vision disorders.

Methods.—All children underwent comprehensive eye examinations, including threshold visual acuity (VA), cover testing, and cycloplegic retinoscopy, performed by VIP-certified optometrists and ophthalmologists who were experienced in providing care to children. Monocular threshold VA was tested using a single-surround HOTV letter protocol without correction, and retested with full cycloplegic correction when retest criteria were met. Unilateral amblyopia was defined as an interocular difference in best-corrected VA of 2 lines or more. Bilateral amblyopia was defined as best-corrected VA in each eye worse than 20/50 for 3-year-olds and worse than 20/40 for 4- to 5-year-olds.

Main Outcome Measures.—Risk of amblyopia was summarized by the odds ratios and their 95% confidence intervals estimated from logistic regression models.

Results.—In this enriched sample of Head Start children (n = 3869), 296 children (7.7%) had unilateral amblyopia, and 144 children (3.7%) had bilateral amblyopia. Presence of strabismus ($P < 0.0001$) and greater magnitude of significant refractive errors (myopia, hyperopia, astigmatism, and anisometropia; $P < 0.00001$ for each) were associated independently with an increased risk of unilateral amblyopia. Presence of strabismus, hyperopia of 2.0 diopters (D) or more, astigmatism of 1.0 D or more, or anisometropia of 0.5 D or more were present in 91% of children with unilateral amblyopia. Greater magnitude of astigmatism ($P < 0.0001$) and bilateral hyperopia ($P < 0.0001$) were associated independently with increased risk of bilateral amblyopia. Bilateral hyperopia of 3.0 D or more or astigmatism of 1.0 D or more were present in 76% of children with bilateral amblyopia.

Conclusions.—Strabismus and significant refractive errors were risk factors for unilateral amblyopia. Bilateral astigmatism and bilateral hyperopia were risk factors for bilateral amblyopia. Despite differences in selection of the study population, these results validated the findings from the Multi-Ethnic Pediatric Eye Disease Study and Baltimore Pediatric Eye Disease Study.

▶ It is not surprising that strabismus and significant refractive errors were risk factors for unilateral amblyopia. Although strabismus is usually obvious to parents, resulting in early referral, unrelated refractive errors are asymptomatic, requiring a more uniform screening program to detect. Unilateral refractive errors are usually first diagnosed after a formal visual screening test performed initially followed by a referral to a pediatric ophthalmologist. Some pediatrician groups use a photoscreener to determine refractive errors, which require further referral.

L. B. Nelson, MD, MBA

Outcomes of Strabismus Surgery with or without Trainee Participation as Surgeon

Mehta VJ, Utz VM, Traboulsi EI, et al (Vanderbilt Univ, Nashville, TN; Cole Eye Inst, Cleveland, OH; Abrahamson Eye Inst, Cincinnati, OH; et al)
Ophthalmology 121:2066-2069, 2014

Purpose.—To compare success rates of strabismus surgery that involves trainees versus those performed solely by staff surgeons.

Design.—Retrospective, comparative case series.

Subjects.—Patients undergoing eye muscle surgery for primarily horizontal deviations.

Methods.—Retrospective comparative case series of 543 patients (921 eyes) undergoing eye muscle surgery, with or without trainee participation, for horizontal deviations.

Main Outcome Measures.—Success in surgery defined as residual horizontal deviations of 10 prism diopters or less.

Results.—Trainees were involved in surgeries on 396 patients (672 eyes), whereas only staff surgeons operated on 147 patients (249 eyes). After minimum follow-up of 8 weeks, there was no overall significant difference between the success rates of procedures that involved trainees as surgeons and those that did not ($P = 0.59$).

Conclusions.—The involvement of trainees as operators in surgeries on horizontal eye muscles does not result in a worse outcome than surgeries exclusively performed by staff. With a shift toward competency-based education and more scrutiny of patient outcomes, these data further support the quality of surgical care provided by trainees.

▶ It was not surprising to me that the involvement of second-year ophthalmology residents or pediatric fellows as the primary operators in strabismus surgery did not result in a worse outcomes than surgeries performed exclusively by staff. With proper supervision of trainees by pediatric ophthalmology fellowship-trained staff, surgical outcomes should not be negatively affected. Appropriate teaching or proper surgical techniques should facilitate successful outcomes in which trainees are the primary operators of strabismus surgery. It is important for the staff to determine appropriate cases to be performed by trainees depending on their skill level and expertise in the operating room.

L. B. Nelson, MD, MBA

Dual application versus single application of povidone-iodine in reducing surgical site contamination during strabismus surgery

Benson CE, Rogers KL, Suh DW, et al (The Univ of Nebraska Med Ctr, Omaha, Nebraska)

J AAPOS 18:347-350, 2014

Purpose.—To investigate the contamination rates in patients undergoing strabismus surgery who received a single versus a dual application of povidone-iodine.

Methods.—Patients undergoing strabismus surgery were divided into two groups of approximately equal size. Prior to surgery, the surgical sites for both groups were prepared by applying 4 drops of povidone-iodine 5% directly into the conjunctival fornices, after which the eyelashes were cleaned with cotton tips soaked with povidone-iodine 5%. Sterile gauze pads soaked with povidone-iodine 5% were used to clean the periocular skin. After lid speculum placement, the patients in the dual application group received an additional 2 drops of povidone-iodine in the conjunctival fornices. Intraoperatively, the conjunctiva, sclera, needles/sutures, and lid speculum were cultured. Gram stain and cultures were obtained and quantified. Contamination was defined as any bacterial growth on blood agar plates at 2 days.

Results.—A total of 104 patients (aged 7 months to 79 years) were included. The single application group had a 25% contamination rate of surgical site and sutures; the dual application group, a 10% contamination rate. This difference was statistically significant ($P = 0.03$). The rate of eyelid speculum contamination was unaffected by additional applications (12.5% contamination rate in both groups [$P = 0.5$]). The additional application of povidone-iodine affected the contamination rate of the conjunctival incision site the most, with a decrease from 20.5% to 5% ($P = 0.02$).

Conclusions.—In our study cohort a second application of povidone-iodine significantly decreased the rate of contamination of the surgical site and sutures. It did not affect contamination of the lid speculum.

▶ A majority of pediatric ophthalmologists are using preoperative application of povidone–iodine just before strabismus surgery to reduce the risk of postoperative infection. Although the authors did show that a second application of povidone–iodine reduced the contamination from 25% to 10%, whether this second application ultimately reduces postoperative infection is unknown. Additional studies involving a larger number of strabismus surgeries performed at multiple centers are needed to determine the effectiveness of a second application of povidone–iodine to reduce the risk of infection after strabismus surgery.

L. B. Nelson, MD, MBA

Treatment of age-related distance esotropia with unilateral lateral rectus resection

Yadav S, Young J, Voas-Clarke C, et al (Royal Liverpool Univ Hosp, UK)
J AAPOS 18:446-448, 2014

Purpose.—To report the results of a series of patients who underwent lateral rectus resection of a single muscle using nonadjustable sutures to correct acquired concomitant esotropia (age-related distance esotropia).

Methods.—The medical records of patients with symptomatic age-related distance esotropia who were treated by unilateral lateral rectus resection were retrospectively reviewed. Pre- and postoperative near and distance prism diopter measurements were compared.

Results.—The average age of the patients was 79.8 years (range, 68-90 years). The mean lateral rectus resection was 4.9 ± 1.3 mm. All patients had complete resolution of diplopia after surgery. Median distance esotropia measurements in primary gaze were reduced from 16.0^{Δ} preoperatively to 0^{Δ} postoperatively ($P < 0.005$) at final follow-up. Any preoperative near esotropia was also completely resolved.

Conclusions.—In this patient cohort, age-related distance esotropia was effectively managed solely with unilateral lateral rectus resection.

▶ Age-related distance esotropia is not an uncommon clinical scenario in adult strabismus. Even though these patients present with normal ductions and versions and are comitant in all distance measurements, imaging studies should be performed before surgical correction to rule out any intracranial abnormality. Although unilateral lateral rectus resection was successful, I have performed an appropriate unilateral medical rectus recession with equal success in these patients. The advantage of a medical rectus recession is that recessions are easier and require less anesthesia time than resections. Many of these patients with this type of esotropia are elderly with medical problems, which necessitates local anesthesia. In this setting, a recession is again a better option than a resection.

L. B. Nelson, MD, MBA

Functional Burden of Strabismus: Decreased Binocular Summation and Binocular Inhibition

Pineles SL, Velez FG, Isenberg SJ, et al (Univ of California, Los Angeles; et al)

JAMA Ophthalmol 131:1413-1419, 2013

Importance.—Binocular summation (BiS) is defined as the superiority of visual function for binocular over monocular viewing. Binocular summation decreases with age and large interocular differences in visual acuity. To our knowledge, BiS has not heretofore been well studied as a functional measure of binocularity in strabismus.

Objective.—To evaluate the effect of strabismus on BiS using a battery of psychophysical tasks that are clinically relevant and easy to use and to determine whether strabismus is associated with binocular inhibition in extreme cases.

Design.—Case-control study.

Setting.—University-based eye institute.

Participants.—Strabismic patients recruited during 2010 to 2012 from a preoperative clinic and control participants with no history of eye disease other than refractive error.

Intervention.—A battery of psychophysical and electrophysiological tests including Early Treatment Diabetic Retinopathy Study visual acuity, Sloan low-contrast acuity (LCA) (2.5% and 1.25%), Pelli-Robson contrast sensitivity, and sweep visual evoked potential contrast sensitivity.

Main Outcome and Measure.—Binocular summation was calculated as the ratio between binocular and better-eye individual scores.

Results.—Sixty strabismic and 80 control participants were prospectively examined (age range, 8-60 years). Mean BiS was significantly lower in the strabismic patients than controls for LCA (2.5% and 1.25%, P=.005 and <.001, respectively). For 1.25% LCA, strabismic patients had a mean BiS score less than 1, indicating binocular inhibition (ie, the binocular score was less than that of the better eye's monocular score). There was no significant difference in BiS for contrast thresholds on Early Treatment Diabetic Retinopathy Study visual acuity, Pelli-Robson contrast sensitivity, or sweep visual evoked potential contrast sensitivity. Regression analysis revealed a significant worsening of BiS with strabismus for 2.5% (P=.009) and 1.25% (P=.002) LCA, after accounting for age.

Conclusions and Relevance.—Strabismic patients demonstrate subnormal BiS and even binocular inhibition for LCA, suggesting that strabismus impairs visual function more than previously appreciated. This may explain why strabismic patients who are not diplopic close 1 eye in visually demanding situations. This finding clarifies the visual deficits impacting quality of life in strabismic patients and may represent a novel measure by which to evaluate and monitor function in strabismus.

▶ It is not unusual for adult strabismus patients to complain of difficulty focusing, even when they do not have diplopia. These patients commonly close 1 eye when they need to focus clearly. When asked as to why they close their 1 eye, they will respond that it makes them "see better." The authors have demonstrated that these adult strabismus patients have normal binocular summation suggesting that strabismus impairs visual function, which may explain why they close 1 eye in visually demanding situations. Therefore, many adult strabismus patients, even without diplopia, not only experience psychosocial aspects to the daily life but an impairment in their visual function.

L. B. Nelson, MD, MBA

Masked Bilateral Superior Oblique Palsy in Children

Dotan G, Roarty JD, Baker JD (Tel Aviv Univ, Israel; Wayne State Univ, Detroit, MI)

J Pediatr Ophthalmol Strabismus 51:333-336, 2014

Purpose.—Following surgery on an eye for unilateral superior oblique palsy, it is a well-recognized postoperative occurrence for the unoperated eye to develop superior oblique palsy, commonly referred to as masked bilateral superior oblique palsy. The purpose of this study was to describe this postoperative finding in children following unilateral inferior oblique weakening surgery.

Methods.—A retrospective review of records of children who underwent unilateral inferior oblique weakening surgery at Children's Hospital of Michigan, Detroit, Michigan, from 1987 to 2005, including information on the development of masked bilateral superior oblique palsy with contralateral inferior oblique overaction requiring a second surgical intervention.

Results.—Of 50 children (25 boys and 25 girls, mean age: 5.6 years) who underwent unilateral inferior oblique weakening surgery (47 recessions and 3 myectomies), 9 (18%) manifested masked bilateral superior oblique palsy postoperatively, requiring subsequent surgical weakening of the inferior oblique muscle in the unoperated eye. Preoperative primary position hypertropia in children who were eventually diagnosed as having masked bilateral superior oblique palsy (5.56 ± 4.22 prism diopters [PD]) was significantly smaller compared to children with unilateral superior oblique palsy (10.4 ± 6.5 PD, $P = .012$), and preoperative primary position hypertropia of less than 5 PD was associated with an odds ratio of 8.2 (95% confidence interval: 1.7 to 38.5, $P = .008$) for requiring reoperation.

Conclusions.—Masked bilateral superior oblique palsy is a possible outcome after surgery for the correction of pediatric unilateral superior oblique palsy. Parents should be informed of this possible outcome, especially when primary position hypertropia is less than 5 PD.

▶ The term *masked bilateral superior oblique palsy* is often applied to the occurrence of a hypertropia in the unoperated eye after unilateral inferior oblique-weakening surgery. This phenomenon certainly occurs in clinical practice. The authors concluded that it seems to occur more frequently when the preoperative primary portion hypertropia is quite small—less than 5 prism diopters. When performing unilateral weakening of the inferior oblique muscle in a setting of a small unilateral hypertropia, a similar clinical finding may occur in the opposite eye requiring surgery often several months after the initial surgery. This finding may occur even when a slight overreaction of the contralateral inferior oblique muscle is not present preoperatively.

L. B. Nelson, MD, MBA

Physician Use of White Coats in Pediatric Ophthalmology

DeBenedictis CN, Liu GT, Nelson LB, et al (Thomas Jefferson Univ, Philadelphia, PA; Pediatric Ophthalmic Consultants, NY)

J Pediatr Ophthalmol Strabismus 51:13-16, 2014

Purpose.—Recent literature reports that patients and parents of pediatric patients prefer their physician to wear a white coat and to address them informally. This study aims to characterize current practice patterns of pediatric ophthalmologists regarding their use of white coats and salutations during outpatient pediatric encounters.

Methods.—An eight-question survey was e-mailed to members of the American Academy of Pediatric Ophthalmology and Strabismus in 2012. The questions focused on clinical setting, use of white coats in out-patient encounters, and preferred language used to address the patient's parents. Surveys not completed in full were excluded from data analysis.

Results.—Of approximately 1,266 members who received the survey, 606 completed the survey. Five hundred ninety-nine surveys were included in the data analysis. Sixty-three percent of attending physicians and 80% of fellows reported they did not routinely wear white coats while examining outpatient children. Forty-six percent of attending physicians and 48% of fellows addressed the patient's parents as "mom" or "dad". There was no significant association between wearing a white coat and type of practice setting, practice characteristics, or location in a children's hospital for attending physicians or fellows.

Conclusions.—Contrary to preferences expressed by patients and their parents, a majority of pediatric ophthalmologists do not routinely wear white coats during pediatric outpatient examinations. Practice patterns appear to be in line with previously reported parental greeting preferences.

▶ I was surprised by a recent study in which Reddy et al[1] found that 57% of parents prefer their children's physician to wear a white coat during an outpatient pediatric ophthalmology examination. I was always of the opinion that most pediatric ophthalmologists did not wear white coats while examining children. It was my feeling that children were more fearful and stressed when the physician wore a white coat. With this dilemma in mind, several faculty from the Departments of Pediatric Ophthalmology and Ocular Genetics of Wills Eye Hospital developed an 8-question, multiple-choice, close-ended questionnaire that was emailed to all members of the American Association of Pediatric Ophthalmology and Strabismus list-serv, once in January 2012 and again in February 2012. The response confirmed my opinion that most pediatric ophthalmologists do not routinely wear white coats during pediatric outpatient examinations.

L. B. Nelson, MD, MBA

Reference

1. Reddy AK, Coats DK, Yen KG. An evidence-based approach to physician etiquette in pediatric ophthalmology. *J Pediatric Ophthalmology Strabismus*. 2011;48: 336-340.

Surgical Outcomes Following Rectus Muscle Plication: A Potentially Reversible, Vessel-Sparing Alternative to Resection

Chaudhuri Z, Demer JL (Univ of California, Los Angeles)
JAMA Ophthalmol 132:579-585, 2014

Importance.—Extraocular muscle strengthening is a common treatment for strabismus. Plication is an alternative procedure for strengthening muscles with less tissue trauma than resection.

Objective.—To compare the surgical dose effect of plication with that of resection.

Design, Setting, and Participants.—Retrospective comparison of surgical outcomes in an academic pediatric ophthalmology and strabismus practice from July 25, 2005, through March 28, 2013, with a mean follow-up of 137 days for plication and 1243 days for resection. A single surgeon performed all procedures. Twenty-two consecutive patients underwent bilateral horizontal rectus plication or plication combined with antagonist recession (13 with esotropia and 9 with exotropia; mean [SD] age, 38 [21] years). Thirty-one consecutive patients underwent bilateral resection or resection combined with antagonist recession (12 with esotropia and 19 with exotropia; mean [SD] age, 28 [24] years). Six patients underwent vertical rectus plication.

Exposures.—Rectus resection or plication performed by folding the anterior tendon posteriorly under the muscle margins oversewn to the poles of the scleral insertion, avoiding the anterior ciliary arteries.

Main Outcomes and Measures.—Postoperative binocular alignment at the first postoperative and last available examinations.

Results.—Lateral rectus plication (mean [SD], 6.5 [2.2] mm) and resection (6.6 [1.6] mm) were performed for similar magnitudes of esotropia (27.9 [13.4] prism diopters [PD] for plication, 29.0 [15.2] PD for resection; $P = .44$). Mean (SD) initial correction by lateral rectus plication was 5.17 (0.29) PD/mm, slightly less than the 95% CI (5.51-7.75 PD/mm) for resection (6.63 [0.50] PD/mm). Medial rectus plication (mean [SD], 4.9 [0.9] mm) vs resection (5.1 [1.1] mm) was performed for similar magnitudes of exotropia (32.8 [14.2] PD for plication, 31.2 [15.6] PD for resection; $P = .33$). Mean (SD) initial correction by medial rectus plication (7.10 [1.65] PD/mm) was within the 95% CI (4.65-9.87 PD/mm) for resection (7.26 [1.23] PD/mm). Initial and late effects were similar. Ciliary circulation observed at surgery remained patent after plication. Plication was cosmetically acceptable and did not produce conspicuous tissue elevations.

Conclusions and Relevance.—Horizontal rectus muscle plication is a rapidly performed, technically simple surgical procedure to strengthen the rectus muscles, with an equivalent (per millimeter) in surgical effect to that of medial rectus resection for treatment of esotropia and exotropia. Plication diminishes surgical trauma and does not intentionally sacrifice ciliary circulation, with the potential for reversal by suture release in the first postoperative days.

▶ Plication of a rectus muscle is a possible alternative to resection with the potential of preserving ciliary circulation and the possibility of reversal if necessary. For years, I have performed placation and scleral suture placement of the superior oblique tendon as a technique for superior oblique tuck with success. Comparing plication with resection with accompanying recession should be performed. Also comparing these 2 techniques unilaterally will help confirm the validity of the plication technique. Using scleral suture placement at the insertion instead of just folding the muscle on itself may reduce the possibility of conjunctival congestion in the long-term postoperative period.

L. B. Nelson, MD, MBA

A Survey of Children's Reported Experience in Outpatient Pediatric Ophthalmology Clinics

Tan NET, Lim WS, Jain S (Royal Free London NHS Foundation Trust, UK)
J Pediatr Ophthalmol Strabismus 51:270-273, 2014

Purpose.—Patient-reported experience measures influence contemporary health care. To monitor the experience of children in health care, some inherent difficulties must be overcome. The authors sampled the opinion of children in outpatient pediatric ophthalmology clinics.

Methods.—Questionnaires were designed and distributed to children ages 2 to 16 years in pediatric ophthalmology clinics over three sites.

Results.—Ninety-three forms were completed by children ages 2 to 16 years. The average duration of clinic visits was 69 minutes. Children commented that helpful staff improved their experience. Waiting times and boredom were negative issues raised consistently. Children particularly enjoyed visual acuity testing, which they also described as the most challenging aspect of the clinic. On average, patients found eye drops only mildly painful.

Conclusions.—Various areas for service improvement were identified from this study, including the value of keeping children occupied and minimizing waiting times. It was not clear to children which healthcare professionals they were seeing and this was an area of confusion. Adolescent patients felt the clinic was too childish. Sampling children's opinions through questionnaires had some limitations in terms of some inconsistencies of response, incomplete questionnaires, and multiple answers, but overall provided useful information specific to the clinics.

▶ Several aspects of the visit to a pediatric ophthalmologist can determine the quality of the experience from the child's perspective. The more positive the experience, the more likely a child will cooperate during a pediatric ophthalmology examination. The authors have outlined factors reported by children in a survey that can influence their experience in a pediatric ophthalmology setting. One of the concerns of the children was the length of the waiting time. Even when the office setting provides toys, movies, and other materials to occupy a child's attention, it is important to shorten the waiting as much as possible. This may involve scheduling other infrastructural changes to accomplish the shortest waiting time. It is not surprising that a number of children found that visual acuity testing was the most difficult part of the examination. During visual acuity testing, children must make decisions, in a sense "perform," in front of their parents or guardians, and it can at times be intimidating. Putting drops in children's eyes is often not a pleasant experience for the child, and therefore, it is important to explain the process and the expectations ahead of time. Finally, it is necessary for all staff in the clinical setting to be friendly, helpful, and understanding to both the child's and the caretaker's needs.

L. B. Nelson, MD, MBA

Comparison of Contact Lens and Intraocular Lens Correction of Monocular Aphakia During Infancy: A Randomized Clinical Trial of HOTV Optotype Acuity at Age 4.5 Years and Clinical Findings at Age 5 Years

The Infant Aphakia Treatment Study Group (Emory Univ School of Medicine, Atlanta, GA; Emory Univ School of Public Health, Atlanta, GA; Univ of Alabama at Birmingham; et al)

JAMA Ophthalmol 132:676-682, 2014

Importance.—The efficacy and safety of primary intraocular lens (IOL) implantation during early infancy is unknown.

Objective.—To compare the visual outcomes of patients optically corrected with contact lenses vs IOLs following unilateral cataract surgery during early infancy.

Design, Setting, and Participants.—The Infant Aphakia Treatment Study is a randomized clinical trial with 5 years of follow-up that involved 114 infants with unilateral congenital cataracts at 12 sites. A traveling examiner assessed visual acuity at age 4.5 years.

Interventions.—Cataract surgery with or without primary IOL implantation. Contact lenses were used to correct aphakia in patients who did not receive IOLs. Treatment was determined through random assignment.

Main Outcomes and Measures.—HOTV optotype visual acuity at 4.5 years of age.

Results.—The median logMAR visual acuity was not significantly different between the treated eyes in the 2 treatment groups (both, 0.90 [20/159]; $P = .54$). About 50% of treated eyes in both groups had visual acuity less than or equal to 20/200. Significantly more patients in the IOL group had at least 1 adverse event after cataract surgery (contact lens, 56%; IOL, 81%; $P = .02$). The most common adverse events in the IOL group were lens reproliferation into the visual axis, pupillary membranes, and corectopia. Glaucoma/glaucoma suspect occurred in 35% of treated eyes in the contact lens group vs 28% of eyes in the IOL group ($P = .55$). Since the initial cataract surgery, significantly more patients in the IOL group have had at least 1 additional intraocular surgery (contact lens, 21%; IOL, 72%; $P < .001$).

Conclusions and Relevance.—There was no significant difference between the median visual acuity of operated eyes in children who underwent primary IOL implantation and those left aphakic. However, there were significantly more adverse events and additional intraoperative procedures in the IOL group. When operating on an infant younger than 7 months of age with a unilateral cataract, we recommend leaving the eye aphakic and focusing the eye with a contact lens. Primary IOL implantation should be reserved for those infants where, in the opinion of the surgeon, the cost and handling of a contact lens would be so burdensome as to result in significant periods of uncorrected aphakia.

Trial Registration.—clinicaltrials.gov Identifier: NCT00212134

▶ I am not surprised that there was no significant difference between the median visual acuity of operated eyes in children who underwent primary intraocular lens (IOL) implantation and those aphakic patients using contact lenses. Although the placement of an IOL lens has been successful for older children, teens, and adults, it does not seem that the visual results for infantile cataracts are more successful than using a contact lens. One particular advantage of primary IOL placement in infantile cataract patients was the possibility that there would be a more accurate correction of the refractive error. However, this potential scenario has not succeeded. Although the investigators in the study did reasonably well achieving their target postoperative refractive error, of concern is the variable and unpredictable change in refractive error during later childhood. This study does provide the ophthalmologist with the ability to inform parents properly of the various treatment options and the issues involved in pediatric aphakic correction.

L. B. Nelson, MD, MBA

Fusion Maldevelopment (Latent/Manifest Latent) Nystagmus Syndrome: Effects of Four-Muscle Tenotomy and Reattachment

Dell'Osso LF, Orge FH, Jacobs JB, et al (CASE Med School, Cleveland, OH)

J Pediatr Ophthalmol Strabismus 51:180-188, 2014

Purpose.—To examine the waveform and clinical effects of the four-muscle tenotomy and reattachment procedure in fusionmal development nystagmus syndrome (FMNS) and to compare them to those documented in infantile nystagmus syndrome (INS) and acquired nystagmus.

Methods.—Both infrared reflection and high-speed digital video systems were used to record the eye movements in a patient with FMNS (before and after tenotomy and reattachment). Data were analyzed using the eXpanded Nystagmus Acuity Function (NAFX) that is part of the OMtools software. Model simulations and predictions were performed using the authors' behavioral ocular motor system model in MATLAB Simulink (The MathWorks, Inc., Natick, MA).

Results.—The model predicted, and the patient's data confirmed, that the tenotomy and reattachment procedure produces improvements in FMN waveforms across a broader field of gaze and decreases the Alexander's law variation. The patient's tenotomy and reattachment plots of NAFX after surgery versus gaze angle were higher and had lower slope than before surgery. Clinically, despite moderate improvements in both peak measured acuity and stereoacuity, dramatic improvements in the patient's abilities and lifestyle resulted.

Conclusions.—The four-muscle tenotomy and reattachment nystagmus surgery produced beneficial therapeutic effects on FMN waveforms that are similar to those demonstrated in INS and acquired nystagmus. These results support the authors' prior recommendation that tenotomy and reattachment nystagmus should be added to required strabismus procedures in patients who also have FMNS (ie, perform tenotomy and reattachment on all unoperated muscles in the plane of the nystagmus). Furthermore, when strabismus surgery is not required, four-muscle tenotomy and reattachment may be used to improve FMN waveforms and visual function.

▶ Before 2000, there was no surgical treatment for patients with nystagmus who did not have associated strabismus or an eccentric gaze angle and null position. Positive therapeutic effects of the 4-muscle tenotomy and reattachment procedure, including a generalized broadening of the null position and an improvement in central vision, have been demonstrated by a variety of investigators. The results have been documented by extensive eye movement recordings. It is currently an accepted treatment option for such patients, and although it is being performed throughout the United States and worldwide, it is performed primarily in only a few academic centers. Further clinical studies will be necessary to show the positive effects of the 4-muscle tenotomy and reattachment in patients with or without the fusion maldevelopment nystagmus syndrome and associated anomalous head posture or strabismus.

L. B. Nelson, MD, MBA

Resident and Fellow Participation in Strabismus Surgery: Effect of Level of Training and Number of Assistants on Operative Time and Cost

Winter TW, Olson RJ, Larson SA, et al (Univ of Iowa)

Ophthalmology 121:797-801, 2014

Objective.—To investigate the effect of the level of training and number of assistants on operative time for uncomplicated, 2-muscle, horizontal strabismus surgery at an academic institution.

Design.—Comparative case series.

Participants.—A total of 993 children and adults between the ages of 6 months and 75 years.

Methods.—Retrospective chart review of strabismus surgeries performed between July 1, 2008, and December 31, 2012, by any of 3 attending surgeons assisted by a resident in the postgraduate year 3 (PGY3), fellow in the postgraduate year 5 (PGY5), or both.

Main Outcome Measures.—Operative time (minutes) and associated operative cost (dollars).

Results.—There were 373 cases with 1 assistant and 44 cases with 2 assistants. Of all cases with 1 assistant, there were 200 cases with a PGY3 assistant an average operative time of 62.5 minutes (standard deviation [SD], 15.1) and 173 cases with a PGY5 assistant an average operative time of 59.0 minutes (SD, 14.7); the difference of 3.5 minutes was statistically significant ($P = 0.02$). The average operative time for all cases with 2 assistants (both PGY3 and PGY5) was 10.6 minutes longer than all cases with 1 assistant ($P = 0.0002$). No statistically significant variation in operative times was demonstrated when comparing cases with a PGY3 ($P = 0.29$) and PGY5 ($P = 0.44$) assistant in their respective first and last halves of the academic year, but operative times within individual quarters of the academic year were significant for PGY3 ($P = 0.03$) but not for PGY5 ($P = 0.24$) assistant cases. Operative times were significantly different for individual PGY3 ($P = 0.03$) but not PGY5 ($P = 0.22$) assistant cases. Cost per PGY3 assistant per year for additional operative time is $3141.95.

Conclusions.—Operative time in strabismus surgery increased with PGY3 participation and further increased with both assistants over either assistant alone. Operative times earlier in the year did not vary from those later in the year for PGY3 or PGY5 assistants. The difference in quarterly and individual PGY3 but not PGY5 assistant operative times suggests that efficiency in strabismus surgery varies by assistants with less experience or interest.

▶ Unfortunately, many ophthalmology residency programs do not have a wet laboratory in strabismus to standardize teaching of surgical techniques and instrumentation in strabismus surgery. The development of a wet laboratory and a standardized surgical curriculum has been shown to decrease resident complications during cataract surgery, which supports the need for a similar one for strabismus surgery. The finding that there was no decrease in operative times between the early versus late postgraduate year (PGY)3 assistants is difficult to evaluate considering the lack of information as to the actual assistant participation in such strabismus cases. Again, the finding that PGY5 assistants were not faster later in their training suffers the same issue as the PGY3 situation in that there is no information provided regarding the amount of actual surgery participation. Perhaps as the PGY5 assistants gain further surgical experience, the attending surgeon allows these trainees more surgical participation in each strabismus surgery case.

L. B. Nelson, MD, MBA

9 Neuro-ophthalmology

Effect of Disease Stage on Progression of Hydroxychloroquine Retinopathy

Marmor MF, Hu J (Stanford Univ School of Medicine, Palo Alto, CA)

JAMA Ophthalmol 132:1105-1112, 2014

Importance.—Hydroxychloroquine sulfate retinopathy can progress after the drug is stopped. It is not clear how this relates to the stage of retinopathy or whether early screening with modern imaging technology can prevent progression and visual loss.

Objective.—To determine the relationship between progression of retinopathy and the severity of disease using objective data from optical coherence tomography and assess the value of early screening for the toxic effects of hydroxychloroquine.

Design, Setting, and Participants.—Clinical findings in patients with hydroxychloroquine retinopathy were monitored with repeated anatomical and functional examinations for 13 to 40 months after the drug was stopped in a referral practice in a university medical center. Eleven patients participated, with the severity of toxic effects categorized as *early* (patchy parafoveal damage shown on field or objective testing), *moderate* (a 50%-100% parafoveal ring of optical coherence tomography thinning but intact retinal pigment epithelium), and severe (visible bull's-eye damage).

Main Outcomes and Measures.—Visual acuity, white 10-2 visual field pattern density plots, fundus autofluorescence, spectral-density optical coherence tomography cross sections, thickness (from cube diagrams), and ellipsoid zone length.

Results.—Visual acuity and visual fields showed no consistent change. Fundus autofluorescence showed little or no change except in severe cases in which the bull's-eye damage expanded progressively. Optical coherence tomography cross sections showed little visible change in early and moderate cases but progressive foveal thinning (approximately 7 μm/y) and loss of ellipsoid zone (in the range of 100 μm/y) in severe cases, which was confirmed by quantitative measurements. The measurements also showed some foveal thinning (approximately 4 μm/y) and deepening of parafoveal loss in moderate cases, but the breadth of the ellipsoid zone remained constant in both early and moderate cases. A few cases showed a suggestion of ellipsoid zone improvement.

Conclusions and Relevance.—Patients with hydroxychloroquine retinopathy involving the retinal pigment epithelium demonstrated progressive damage on optical coherence tomography for at least 3 years after the drug was discontinued, including loss of foveal thickness and cone structure.

Cases recognized before retinal pigment epithelium damage retained foveal architecture with little retinal thinning. Early recognition of hydroxychloroquine toxic effects before any fundus changes are visible, using visual fields and optical coherence tomography (along with fundus autofluorescence and multifocal electroretinography as indicated), will greatly minimize late progression and the risk of visual loss.

▶ This study found that patients diagnosed early with hydroxychloroquine retinopathy—before involvement of the retinal pigment epithelium (RPE)—remained relatively stable on optical coherence tomography (OCT) for the next few years. Those with involvement of the RPE showed progressive damage on OCT for at least 3 years after the drug was discontinued, including loss of foveal thickness and cone structure. Vision may have worsened a little in 2 patients but visual fields remained stable.

Intuitively, finding hydroxychloroquine toxicity earlier leads to less visual loss. This study verifies that by OCT measurements of foveal thickness and loss of ellipsoid zone, those who discontinue the medication with early toxicity remain stable, whereas those with severe involvement continue to have progressive deterioration for the next 3 years. Although the study is small and follow-up was only 2 years to slightly more than 3 years, it emphasizes the need for appropriate monitoring of patients for early diagnosis and discontinuation of the medication.

M. L. Moster, MD

Opportunistic Infections of the Retina in Patients With Aquaporin-4 Antibody Disease

George JS, Leite MI, Kitley JL, et al (Univ of Oxford, UK)

JAMA Neurol 71:1429-1432, 2014

Importance.—Patients with neuromyelitis optica who have aquaporin-4 antibodies are being identified and receiving immunosuppressant treatment earlier and more aggressively as a result of increasing awareness of the importance of preventing relapses responsible for the high morbidity and mortality associated with the disease. To our knowledge, opportunistic retinal infection in patients with aquaporin-4 antibodies who are receiving immunosuppressants has not been reported to date.

Observations.—We describe 2 patients with aquaporin-4 antibodies who were receiving conventional doses of first-line immunosuppressive therapy. Both patients presented with vision loss that was initially thought to be optic neuritis attacks. The subsequent diagnoses were ocular toxoplasmosis and cytomegalovirus retinitis.

Conclusions and Relevance.—Retinal opportunistic infections can occur in patients with aquaporin-4 antibodies who are receiving relatively low levels of immunosuppression, may mimic optic neuritis, and are a potentially reversible cause of vision loss when treated promptly.

▶ The default diagnosis in a patient with visual loss who has aquaporin-4 antibodies and either classic neuromyelitis optica (NMO) or a variant would be an episode of optic neuritis. However, this article describes 1 case of cytomegalovirus retinitis and 1 of ocular toxoplasmosis and highlights the importance of a thorough ophthalmic examination in anyone with visual loss. This is reminiscent of the patient with multiple sclerosis (MS) who is on natalizumab and has what mimics an exacerbation but really has progressive multifocal leukoencephalopathy (PML). Of course, the treatments in both these situations are dramatically different. On the one hand, an exacerbation of NMO or MS may require treatment with steroids and boosting up the immunosuppression. On the other hand, an infection with PML or infectious retinitis must be treated with anti-infectious agents and not increasing the immunosuppression.

We must emphasize to our neurology colleagues that anyone with visual loss needs a thorough funduscopic examination—we have had cases called central retinal artery occlusion that were retinal detachment or called optic neuritis that were really central serous retinopathy.

M. L. Moster, MD

Microcystic Macular Edema: Retrograde Maculopathy Caused by Optic Neuropathy

Abegg M, Dysli M, Wolf S, et al (Univ of Bern, Switzerland)

Ophthalmology 121:142-149, 2014

Purpose.—To investigate retrograde axonal degeneration for its potential to cause microcystic macular edema (MME), a maculopathy that has been previously described in patients with demyelinating disease. To identify risk factors for MME and to expand the anatomic knowledge on MME.

Design.—Retrospective case series.

Participants.—We included 117 consecutive patients and 180 eyes with confirmed optic neuropathy of variable etiology. Patients with glaucoma were excluded.

Methods.—We determined age, sex, visual acuity, etiology of optic neuropathy, and the temporal and spatial characteristics of MME. Eyes with MME were compared with eyes with optic neuropathy alone and to healthy fellow eyes. With retinal layer segmentation we quantitatively measured the intraretinal anatomy.

Main Outcome Measures.—Demographic data, distribution of MME in the retina, and thickness of retinal layers were analyzed.

Results.—We found MME in 16 eyes (8.8%) from 9 patients, none of whom had multiple sclerosis or neuromyelitis optica. The MME was restricted to the inner nuclear layer (INL) and had a characteristic perifoveal circular distribution. Compared with healthy controls, MME was associated with significant thinning of the ganglion cell layer and nerve fiber layer, as well as a thickening of the INL and the deeper retinal layers. Youth is a significant risk factor for MME.

Conclusions.—Microcystic macular edema is not specific for demyelinating disease. It is a sign of optic neuropathy irrespective of its etiology. The distinctive intraretinal anatomy suggests that MME is caused by retrograde degeneration of the inner retinal layers, resulting in impaired fluid resorption in the macula.

► In this retrospective study, the authors searched their databases for patients with a history of optic neuropathy who underwent macular optical coherence tomography testing. They found that 16 of 180 eyes had microcystic macular edema (MME) limited to the inner nuclear layer. A striking finding was the perifoveal location of the MME in all eyes. The cause of the optic neuropathy included compressive (9), vascular (3), hereditary (2), and idiopathic (2), and the proportions did not differ from the non-MME eyes. The shortest time to develop MME was 4 months, and the longest time was several years. The authors make a compelling argument that this represents a retrograde degenerative process.

This article demonstrates that MME is not likely part of the pathophysiologic process of inflammatory optic neuropathy as previously proposed (first for multiple sclerosis [MS] and then for neuromyelitis optica [NMO]), but a nonspecific secondary change occurring in optic neuropathy. It was seen in compressive, vascular, and hereditary causes of optic neuropathy, but further clinical details on these patients was not provided. If it were part of the primary inflammatory process in optic neuritis from MS or NMO, one would not expect to see it in these other optic neuropathies.

The authors excluded glaucoma cases "to better match patients with MS in whom MME had been first described." I do not understand how ischemic, compressive, and hereditary optic neuropathy are better matches for patients with MS, but that does not detract from the findings in this study. Indeed, MME has now been described in a group of glaucoma patients as well.[1]

M. L. Moster, MD

Reference

1. Wolff B, Basdekidou C, Vasseur V, Mauget-Faysse M, Sahel JA, Vignal C. Retinal inner nuclear layer microcystic changes in optic nerve atrophy: a novel spectral-domain OCT finding. *Retina.* 2013;33:2133-2138.

Marked Recovery of Vision in Children With Optic Pathway Gliomas Treated With Bevacizumab

Avery RA, Hwang EI, Jakacki RI, et al (Children's Natl Med Ctr, Washington, DC; Children's Hosp of Pittsburgh, PA)

JAMA Ophthalmol 132:111-114, 2014

Importance.—Children with optic pathway gliomas (OPGs) frequently experience vision loss from their tumors. Standard front-line treatment using carboplatin-based chemotherapy typically produces only a modest benefit (eg, stabilization or 0.2 logMAR improvement) in visual acuity (VA). Bevacizumab is a monoclonal antibody that targets vascular endothelial growth factor and acts primarily as an anti-angiogenic agent. Recent reports suggest a qualitative improvement in vision after bevacizumab-based treatment in children with OPGs.

Observations.—We report 4 cases of pediatric OPGs (2 neurofibromatosis type 1—related and 2 sporadic cases) that received treatment with bevacizumab due to progressive VA or visual field (VF) loss despite prior treatment with chemotherapy or proton-beam radiation. All 4 subjects demonstrated a marked improvement in their VA, VF, or both while receiving bevacizumab-based therapy. Three patients had complete resolution of their VA or VF loss in at least 1 eye—2 of whom had previously received bevacizumab therapy.

Conclusions and Relevance.—Given that most patients with OPG-related visual impairment will show modest or no visual improvement with standard treatment, the incorporation of bevacizumab in these cases may greatly improve visual outcomes and should be considered in appropriate clinical situations.

▶ Four patients with progressive visual loss from optic nerve glioma had improvement of visual acuity, visual field, or both on bevacizumab therapy. Although an anecdotal report of only 4 patients, this article demonstrates hope for visual recovery in children with optic glioma who have had visual and radiographic progression after treatment with chemotherapy and radiation. Particularly encouraging is that the improvement was also seen in 3 children who had prior bevacizumab treatment as part of their treatment regimen.

It is likely reasonable to try bevacizumab in a child with progressive visual loss from glioma. Where bevacizumab ultimately fits in the global treatment of these patients awaits further clinical trials, particularly in light of a previous series of patients who developed optic neuropathy while on treatment with bevacizumab for glioblastoma elsewhere in the brain.

M. L. Moster, MD

Safety and Effects of the Vector for the Leber Hereditary Optic Neuropathy Gene Therapy Clinical Trial

Koilkonda RD, Yu H, Chou T-H, et al (Univ of Miami, FL; et al)
JAMA Ophthalmol 132:409-420, 2014

Importance.—We developed a novel strategy for treatment of Leber hereditary optic neuropathy (LHON) caused by a mutation in the nicotinamide adenine dinucleotide dehydrogenase subunit IV (*ND4*) mitochondrial gene.

Objective.—To demonstrate the safety and effects of the gene therapy vector to be used in a proposed gene therapy clinical trial.

Design and Setting.—In a series of laboratory experiments, we modified the mitochondrial *ND4* subunit of complex I in the nuclear genetic code for import into mitochondria. The protein was targeted into the organelle by agency of a targeting sequence (allotopic expression). The gene was packaged into adeno-associated viral vectors and then vitreally injected into rodent, nonhuman primate, and ex vivo human eyes that underwent testing for expression and integration by immunohistochemical analysis and blue native polyacrylamide gel electrophoresis. During serial follow-up, the animal eyes underwent fundus photography, optical coherence tomography, and multifocal or pattern electroretinography. We tested for rescue of visual loss in rodent eyes also injected with a mutant G11778A *ND4* homologue responsible for most cases of LHON.

Exposure.—Ocular infection with recombinant adeno-associated viral vectors containing a wild-type allotopic human *ND4* gene.

Main Outcomes and Measures.—Expression of human *ND4* and rescue of optic neuropathy induced by mutant human *ND4*.

Results.—We found human *ND4* expressed in almost all mouse retinal ganglion cells by 1 week after injection and *ND4* integrated into the mouse complex I. In rodent eyes also injected with a mutant allotopic *ND4*, wild-type allotopic *ND4* prevented defective adenosine triphosphate synthesis, suppressed visual loss, reduced apoptosis of retinal ganglion cells, and prevented demise of axons in the optic nerve. Injection of *ND4* in the ex vivo human eye resulted in expression in most retinal ganglion cells. Primates undergoing vitreal injection with the *ND4* test article and followed up for 3 months had no serious adverse reactions.

Conclusions and Relevance.—Expression of our allotopic *ND4* vector in the ex vivo human eye, safety of the test article, rescue of the LHON mouse model, and the severe irreversible loss of visual function in LHON support clinical testing with mutated G11778A mitochondrial DNA in our patients.

▶ Most patients with Leber hereditary optic neuropathy (LHON) carry the G11778A mutation, which affects the ND4 gene. The authors packaged "normal" and "mutant" human ND4 genes into an adeno-associated viral vector (AAVV). Either normal ND4 AAVV or control AAVV was injected intravitreally in mouse eyes. Three days later, the mutant ND4 AAVV, which has been shown to cause an optic neuropathy in mice similar to LHON, was injected. Rhesus monkeys underwent injection of control AAVV. Two enucleated human eyes received injections of normal ND4 AAVV.

This article describes all the steps that have been taken in animal studies and ex vivo human eyes demonstrating the efficacy of this genetic therapy.

Mouse and human eyes showed human ND4 expression in nearly all retinal ganglion cells within a week. Mouse eyes preinjected with normal ND4 AAVV maintained significantly better pattern electroretinogram amplitudes, retinal nerve fiber layer, and adenosine triphosphate synthesis than eyes preinjected with control AAVV. No complications occurred from control AAVV in primate eyes except a mild vitritis at 1 month. No important adverse effects were seen in the animals treated with normal ND4 AAVV.

The work described provides justification for proceeding with a phase 1 clinical trial in humans with LHON, which has already begun. Positive results would have more widespread beneficial implications for other diseases with mitochondrial inheritance.

M. L. Moster, MD

Optic Neuropathy Induced by Experimentally Reduced Cerebrospinal Fluid Pressure in Monkeys

Yang D, Fu J, Hou R, et al (Capital Med Univ, Beijing, China; et al)
Invest Ophthalmol Vis Sci 55:3067-3073, 2014

Purpose.—To examine the influence of experimentally reduced cerebrospinal fluid pressure (CSFP) on retinal nerve fiber layer (RNFL) thickness and neuroretinal rim area of the optic nerve head.

Methods.—This experimental study included nine monkeys that underwent implantation of a lumbar-peritoneal cerebrospinal fluid (CSF) shunt. In the study group ($n = 4$ monkeys), the shunt was opened to achieve a CSF of approximately 40 mm H_2O, while the shunt remained closed in the control group ($n = 5$ monkeys). At baseline and in monthly intervals thereafter, optical coherence tomographic and photographic images of the optic nerve head and RNFL were taken of all monkeys.

Results.—Two out of four monkeys in the study group showed bilaterally a progressive reduction in RNFL thickness between 12% and 30%, reduction in neuroretinal rim area and volume, and increase in cup-to-disc area ratios. A third monkey developed a splinter-like disc hemorrhage in one eye. The fourth monkey in the study group did not develop morphologic changes during follow-up, nor did any monkey in the control group.

Conclusions.—Experimental and chronic reduction in CSF in monkeys was associated with the development of an optic neuropathy in some monkeys.

▶ In this study, investigators implanted a programmable lumboperitoneal shunt (LPS) into 9 rhesus monkeys. The valve was not opened in 5 control monkeys, and the valve was set to achieve a cerebrospinal fluid pressure (CSFP) of 4 cm H_2O in 4 monkeys. The CSFP, measured intraoperatively, declined in the study animals from 7.4 mm Hg (10 cm H_2O) at baseline to less than 2 mm Hg (2.7 cm H_2O) for the study. The CSFP did not change significantly in the control animals. Retinal nerve fiber layer (RNFL) thickness, optic nerve head area, neuroretinal rim area, and cup-to-disc ratio were measured monthly for 1 year. At 1-year follow up, 2 of the 4 monkeys had progressive thinning of the mean RNFL of 20 to 30 microns. The area of the neuroretinal rim significantly decreased and the cup-to-disc ratio significantly increased. The other 2 study animals and the control animals had no appreciable changes in the study parameters, but 1 low-pressure monkey had a disc hemorrhage. The intraocular pressure did not change over the study period in either group, and no morphologic changes of the lamina cribrosa were observed.

This article is of interest in light of a small developing literature finding that in glaucoma the important issue may be translaminar pressure difference rather than absolute IOP. In patients with NTG, the CSFP is lower than high-pressure glaucoma and normal controls. However, the patients reported in the literature only had a single ICP measurement, in contrast to the ongoing monitoring in these monkeys. It would be nice to know whether the IOP was also low in the monkeys that did not develop RNFL thinning or cupping. At baseline, IOP was similar in control and experimental monkeys, but this information for follow-up is not mentioned.

Animal studies like this one will help clarify the true importance of translaminar pressure differences in both glaucoma and papilledema patients.

M. L. Moster, MD

Therapeutic Outcomes of High-Dose Intravenous Steroids in the Treatment of Dysthyroid Optic Neuropathy

Currò N, Covelli D, Vannucchi G, et al (Ospedale Maggiore Policlinico, Milan, Italy)

Thyroid 24:897-905, 2014

Background.—While pulsed intravenous methylprednisolone (iv-MP) has been shown to be effective and well tolerated in moderate to severe Graves' orbitopathy (GO), limited data are available on dysthyroid optic neuropathy (DON). The objective of this retrospective study was to investigate the efficacy of iv-MP in the treatment of DON and to seek parameters predictive of response.

Methods.—Twenty-four DON patients (40 eyes) treated with iv-MP from 2007 to 2012 were included in the study. Concurrent neurological or ophthalmologic diseases or signs of corneal exposure were considered as exclusion criteria. Iv-MP was administered daily for three consecutive days and repeated the following week. At six months, eyes not requiring surgery to preserve visual function were considered as responsive to treatment. Visual acuity, color sensitivity, visual field, and optic discs were analyzed at two and four weeks, and at 3, 6, and 12 months after treatment. Activity of GO was graded using a clinical activity score (CAS). Visual and clinical characteristics of the eyes responsive to iv-MP were studied by comparison to those of nonresponsive eyes.

Results.—At six months, 17 of 40 (42.5%) eyes had complete visual recovery and were spared from surgical decompression. At two weeks, visual acuity, color sensitivity, and visual field improved significantly in almost all eyes, but GO inactivated (CAS <4) only in the eyes that permanently responded to iv-MP ($p < 0.01$). The CAS at two weeks was a good predictor of response (cutoff ≥4 66.7% sensitivity, 76.9% specificity). Optic disc swelling at diagnosis was highly predictive for unresponsiveness to iv-MP (34% sensitivity, 100% specificity). At baseline, high CAS (cutoff >5

40.2% sensitivity, 94.1% specificity) and severely altered visual field mean defect (cutoff ≤6.31 dB 73.9% sensitivity, 58.8% specificity) were associated with unresponsiveness to steroids. No major side effects were observed.

Conclusions.—High-dose iv-MP was effective in permanently restoring visual function in about 40% of the eyes treated. When successful, it generally induced inactivation of the orbital disease within two weeks and normalization of visual function within one month. The presence of optic disc swelling at diagnosis and persistent active disease at two weeks were good predictors of unresponsiveness to steroids.

▶ There is little written about the use of pulsed doses of methylprednisolone in compressive optic neuropathy, and although this is a retrospective, nonrandomized, and noncontrolled study, it adds some useful clinical information that is quite practical.

Twenty-four patients with dysthyroid optic neuropathy (DON) received intravenous (IV) steroids (either 500 mg or 1000 mg pulsed methylprednisolone) daily for 3 days and repeated 1 week later, followed by an oral or IV taper. The primary outcome was "not requiring decompressive surgery by 6 months later." Forty-two percent (17 of 40 eyes) were able to avoid surgery with complete recovery and no further relapse, but the time of final follow-up is not mentioned. Three patients had 1 responsive eye and the other requiring surgery (12.5%).

Two features predicted a poor response to the pulsed steroid therapy. Those with optic disc edema at presentation all failed and required surgery. Additionally, by using the Clinical Activity Score (CAS), 70% those with still active disease at 2 weeks required surgery, compared with only 20% with CAS inactive disease. The CAS is the sum of 10 items: 2 symptoms (orbital pain at rest or with eye movement), 5 signs of orbital inflammation and/or congestion (soft tissue swelling, lid redness, conjunctival redness, chemosis, and swelling of the caruncle), and 3 signs of deterioration (worsening of proptosis, ductions, and visual acuity). Active disease was defined as ≥4 or 10. Interestingly, smoking history did not influence the response to steroids.

Despite its limitations, this article has some practical information we can use in the office today. First, one may have an excellent response of DON to pulsed steroids. Second, if disc edema is present, response is likely to be poor. Finally if the disease activity is still present at 2 weeks posttreatment, long-term response is less likely.

M. L. Moster, MD

Factors associated with optic nerve sheath diameter during exposure to hypobaric hypoxia

Strapazzon G, Brugger H, Dal Cappello T, et al (EURAC Inst of Mountain Emergency Medicine, Bolzano, Italy; et al)
Neurology 82:1914-1918, 2014

Objective.—To monitor the changes in optic nerve sheath diameter (ONSD) induced by acute exposure to hypobaric hypoxia and to investigate factors associated with these changes, including development of acute mountain sickness.

Methods.—In this cohort study, neurologic signs and symptoms, cardiovascular parameters, and ultrasonography of ONSD were prospectively assessed in 19 healthy lowlanders at baseline and after ascent to 3,830 m (3 hours, 9 hours, 24 hours, 48 hours, 72 hours, and 8 days) by blinded investigators. Potential confounding factors (e.g., altitude variations, physical effort) were minimized. A multivariate analysis of factors associated with ONSD was performed by means of generalized estimating equations.

Results.—ONSD increased with exposure to altitude in all participants ($p < 0.001$). The increase between 9 and 24 hours was larger in patients who developed acute mountain sickness ($p = 0.001$). There was no influence of sex, oxygen saturation, or acclimatization on ONSD.

Conclusion.—Both physiologic and pathologic responses to hypobaric hypoxia were independently associated with changes in ONSD. Studies on a larger cohort, at a range of altitudes, and with baseline neuroimaging techniques are necessary to further understand the clinical significance of increased ONSD during exposure to hypobaric hypoxia.

▶ This small study demonstrated an increase in optic nerve sheath diameter (ONSD) within 3 hours of reaching 3830 m altitude by helicopter with further increase at 24 hours and a parabolic pattern of return to normal, decreasing slightly at 72 hours and then stable until 8 days. The 3 patients who developed acute mountain sickness (AMS) had a greater increase in ONSD between 9 and 24 hours than those without AMS. If these findings hold up in larger studies, orbital ultrasound may be used clinically to predict AMS presymptomatically with possible earlier intervention.

This article is another example in which examination of the eye provides insights into neurologic disease.

M. L. Moster, MD

Prospective randomized trial of venous angioplasty in MS (PREMiSe)

Siddiqui AH, Zivadinov R, Benedict RH, et al (State Univ of New York)

Neurology 83:441-449, 2014

Objective.—We report the results of the investigation of safety and efficacy of venous angioplasty in patients with multiple sclerosis (MS) with findings of extracranial venous anomalies, considered hallmarks of chronic cerebrospinal venous insufficiency (CCSVI), in a 2-phase study (ClinicalTrials.gov NCT01450072).

Methods.—Phase 1 was an open-label safety study (10 patients); phase 2 was sham-controlled, randomized, and double-blind (10 sham procedure, 9 treated). All study patients fulfilled venous hemodynamic screening criteria indicative of CCSVI. Assessment was at 1, 3, and 6 months postprocedure with MRI, clinical, and hemodynamic outcomes. Primary endpoints were safety at 24 hours and 1 month, venous outflow restoration >75% at 1 month, and effect of angioplasty on new lesion activity and relapse rate over 6 months. Secondary endpoints included changes in disability, brain volume, cognitive tests, and quality of life.

Results.—No perioperative complications were noted; however, one patient with history of syncope was diagnosed with episodic bradycardia requiring placement of a pacemaker before discharge. Doppler evidence-based venous hemodynamic insufficiency severity score (VHISS) was reduced >75% compared to baseline in phase 1 (at 1 month) but not phase 2. In phase 2, higher MRI activity (cumulative number of new contrast-enhancing lesions [19 vs 3, $p = 0.062$] and new T2 lesions [17 vs 3, $p = 0.066$]) and relapse activity (4 vs 1, $p = 0.389$) were identified as nonsignificant trends in the treated vs sham arm over 6 months. Using analysis of covariance, significant cumulative new T2 lesions were related to larger VHISS decrease ($p = 0.028$) and angioplasty ($p = 0.01$) over the follow-up. No differences in other endpoints were detected.

Conclusion.—Venous angioplasty is not an effective treatment for MS over the short term and may exacerbate underlying disease activity.

Classification of Evidence.—This is a Class I study demonstrating that clinical and imaging outcomes are no better or worse in patients with MS identified with venous outflow restriction who receive venous angioplasty compared to sham controls who do not receive angioplasty. This study also includes a Class IV phase 1 study of safety in 10 patients receiving the angioplasty procedure.

▶ In 2009, Zamboni published an unmasked study showing that 90% of patients with multiple sclerosis have venous outflow abnormalities in the internal jugular and/or azygous vein and that angioplasty improved clinical and magnetic resonance imaging (MRI) outcomes.[1] The condition is known as chronic cerebrospinal venous insufficiency (CCSVI). Since then, many other papers have been published, mostly not supportive of the original study. In 2012, the US Food and Drug Administration issued a warning about the lack of proof of benefit and the dangers of the procedure including stroke and death. Nonetheless, interventional radiologists and others have performed venous angioplasty on thousands of patients worldwide.

The Prospective Randomized Trial of Venous Angioplasty in MS (PREMiSe) trial is the first randomized double-blind trial to compare venous angioplasty with a sham angioplasty for patients with findings of CCSVI. The findings showed no clinical benefit at 6 months for the treatment. In fact, there was a trend toward increased MRI disease activity in those receiving the treatment. Additionally, self-reported improvements were seen in the sham group and the treated group, suggesting a placebo effect of treatment. Although a small study of only 19 patients, it is the first to provide class I evidence against venous angioplasty for MS, and unless proven beneficial in future class I studies, the procedure should likely be abandoned.

M. L. Moster, MD

Reference

1. Zamboni P, Galeotti R, Menegatti E, et al. A prospective open-label study of endovascular treatment of chronic cerebrospinal venous insufficiency. *J Vasc Surg.* 2009;50:1348-1358.e1–3.

Clinical features of MS associated with Leber hereditary optic neuropathy mtDNA mutations

Pfeffer G, Burke A, Yu-Wai-Man P, et al (Inst of Genetic Medicine, Newcastle, UK; Univ College London, UK; et al)
Neurology 81:2073-2081, 2013

Objective.—To determine whether the association between multiple sclerosis (MS) and Leber hereditary optic neuropathy (LHON) (known as "Harding disease") is a chance finding, or the 2 disorders are mechanistically linked.

Methods.—We performed a United Kingdom–wide prospective cohort study of prevalent cases of MS with LHON mitochondrial DNA (mtDNA) mutations. The new cases were compared with published cases, enabling a comprehensive clinical description. We also performed a meta-analysis of studies screening patients with MS for LHON mtDNA mutations to find evidence of a genetic association.

Results.—Twelve new patients were identified from 11 pedigrees, and 44 cases were identified in the literature. The combined cohort had the following characteristics: multiple episodes of visual loss, predominance for women, and lengthy time interval before the fellow eye is affected (average 1.66 years), which is very atypical of LHON; conversely, most patients presented without eye pain and had a poor visual prognosis, which is unusual for optic neuritis associated with MS. The number of UK cases of LHON-MS fell well within the range predicted by the chance occurrence of MS and the mtDNA mutations known to cause LHON. There was no association between LHON mtDNA mutations and MS in a meta-analysis of the published data.

Conclusions.—Although the co-occurrence of MS and LHON mtDNA mutations is likely to be due to chance, the resulting disorder has a distinct phenotype, implicating a mechanistic interaction. Patients with LHON-MS have a more aggressive course, and prognostication and treatment should be guarded.

▶ This study describes the clinical presentation of the overlap of patients with multiple sclerosis (MS) and an Leber hereditary optic neuropathy (LHON) mutation. Based on the rarity of the association, it provides support to the notion that LHON does not cause an MS-like illness but rather that the relatively common illness of MS occurs in some patients who also have LHON.

Intriguing are the phenotypic features that are different from either MS or LHON and in some ways an average of both. For instance, the ratio of women to men of 2.1 to 1 is much greater than in LHON but less than in MS. The visual loss had features of both LHON and MS and not typical for either. Four of 12 patients had pain, 5 patients had more than 2 episodes, and 4 patients had some degree of recovery. Half the patients ended with visual acuity less than 20/400. One patient had bilateral simultaneous visual loss. When sequential visual loss occurred, the interval was more than 1 year in 7 patients and up to 17 years in 1 patient, much greater than the typical days to months in LHON patients.

The authors concluded that the LHON-MS phenotype, which is distinct from either disorder, may have several possible causes. One possibility is that having the mtDNA mutation modifies the MS phenotype. The other is that the genetic and environmental factors that predispose to MS precipitates acute LHON in carriers, mostly women, who would have otherwise remained asymptomatic.

This study has limitations of being based on a survey of neurologists voluntarily responding with reports of both LHON and MS in the same patient. Therefore, it may underestimate the number of cases.

M. L. Moster, MD

Effects of Bacille Calmette-Guerin after the first demyelinating event in the CNS

Ristori G, Romano S, Cannoni S, et al (S. Andrea Hosp-site, Rome, Italy; et al)
Neurology 82:41-48, 2014

Objective.—To evaluate Bacille Calmette-Guérin (BCG) effects after clinically isolated syndromes (CIS).

Methods.—In a double-blind, placebo-controlled trial, participants were randomly assigned to receive BCG or placebo and monitored monthly with brain MRI (6 scans). Both groups then entered a preplanned phase with IM interferon-β-1a for 12 months. From month 18 onward, the patients took the disease-modifying therapies (DMTs) that their neurologist considered indicated in an open-label extension phase lasting up to 60 months.

Results.—Of 82 randomized subjects, 73 completed the study (33 vaccinated and 40 placebo). During the initial 6 months, the number of cumulative lesions was significantly lower in vaccinated people. The relative risks were 0.541 (95% confidence interval [CI] 0.308-0.956 $p = 0.03$) for gadolinium-enhancing lesions (the primary endpoint), 0.364 (95% CI 0.207-0.639 $p = 0.001$) for new and enlarging T2-hyperintense lesions, and 0.149 (95% CI 0.046-0.416 $p = 0.001$) for new T1-hypointense lesions. The number of total T1-hypointense lesions was lower in the BCG group at months 6, 12, and 18: mean changes from baseline were -0.09 ± 0.72 vs 0.75 ± 1.81 ($p = 0.01$), 0.0 ± 0.83 vs 0.88 ± 2.21 ($p = 0.08$), and -0.21 ± 1.03 vs 1.00 ± 2.49 ($p = 0.02$). After 60 months, the cumulative probability of clinically definite multiple sclerosis was lower in the BCG + DMT arm (hazard ratio = 0.52, 95% CI 0.27-0.99

$p < 0.05$), and more vaccinated people remained DMT-free (odds ratio = 0.20, 95% CI 0.04-0.93 $p = 0.04$).

Conclusions.—Early BCG may benefit CIS and affect its longterm course.

Classification of Evidence.—BCG, as compared to placebo, was associated with significantly reduced development of gadolinium-enhancing lesions in people with CIS for a 6-month period before starting immunomodulating therapy (Class I evidence).

▶ This study of 1 dose of Bacille Calmette-Guérin (BCG) in addition to subsequent disease-modifying therapy in patients with clinically isolated syndrome found a decrease in active MRI lesions and in subsequent clinical exacerbations. All MRI parameters (Gadolinium enhancing T1, T2, and T1 hypointense) were better in patients receiving BCG. The number of exacerbations and the rate of conversion to clinically definite MS over 5 years were decreased as well.

Although this study provides class I evidence, having been a randomized double-blind placebo-controlled trial, there are limitations as pointed out by the authors and an accompanying editorial. First, the sample size was small. Second, only the first portion of the clinical trial was controlled with the care after 18 months in the hands of the treating neurologists.

Both the authors and editorial writers speculate on what mechanisms may be at play in the immune response to BCG that might provide the clinical benefits seen. If these results are borne out in future studies, BCG will provide a reasonably priced, reasonably safe, and quite easily tolerated adjunctive treatment for patients with clinically isolated syndrome and possibly for patients with clinically definite multiple sclerosis as well.

M. L. Moster, MD

Effect of Acetazolamide on Visual Function in Patients With Idiopathic Intracranial Hypertension and Mild Visual Loss: The Idiopathic Intracranial Hypertension Treatment Trial

The NORDIC Idiopathic Intracranial Hypertension Study Group Writing Committee (Univ of Iowa; Univ of Rochester School of Medicine & Dentistry, NY; et al)

JAMA 311:1641-1651, 2014

Importance.—Acetazolamide is commonly used to treat idiopathic intracranial hypertension (IIH), but there is insufficient information to establish an evidence base for its use.

Objective.—To determine whether acetazolamide is beneficial in improving vision when added to a low-sodium weight reduction diet in patients with IIH and mild visual loss.

Design, Setting, and Participants.—Multicenter, randomized, double-masked, placebo-controlled study of acetazolamide in 165 participants with IIH and mild visual loss who received a low-sodium weight-reduction diet. Participants were enrolled at 38 academic and private practice sites in North America from March 2010 to November 2012 and followed up for 6 months (last visit in June 2013). All participants met the modified Dandy criteria for IIH and had a perimetric mean deviation (PMD) between −2 dB and −7 dB. The mean age was 29 years and all but 4 participants were women.

Interventions.—Low-sodium weight-reduction diet plus the maximally tolerated dosage of acetazolamide (up to 4 g/d) or matching placebo for 6 months.

Main Outcomes and Measures.—The planned primary outcome variable was the change in PMD from baseline to month 6 in the most affected eye, as measured by Humphrey Field Analyzer. Perimetric mean deviation is a measure of global visual field loss (mean deviation from age-corrected normal values), with a range of 2 to −32 dB; larger negative values indicate greater vision loss. Secondary outcome variables included changes in papilledema grade, quality of life (Visual Function Questionnaire 25 [VFQ-25] and 36-Item Short Form Health Survey), headache disability, and weight at month 6.

Results.—The mean improvement in PMD was greater with acetazolamide (1.43 dB, from −3.53 dB at baseline to −2.10 dB at month 6; n = 86) than with placebo (0.71 dB, from −3.53 dB to −2.82 dB; n = 79); the difference was 0.71 dB (95% CI, 0 to 1.43 dB; $P = .050$). Mean improvements in papilledema grade (acetazolamide: −1.31, from 2.76 to 1.45; placebo: −0.61, from 2.76 to 2.15; treatment effect, −0.70; 95% CI, −0.99 to −0.41; $P < .001$) and vision-related quality of life as measured by the National Eye Institute VFQ-25 (acetazolamide: 8.33, from 82.97 to 91.30; placebo: 1.98, from 82.97 to 84.95; treatment effect, 6.35; 95% CI, 2.22 to 10.47; $P = .003$) and its 10-item neuro-ophthalmic supplement (acetazolamide: 9.82, from 75.45 to 85.27; placebo: 1.59, from 75.45 to 77.04; treatment effect, 8.23; 95% CI, 3.89 to 12.56; $P < .001$) were also observed with acetazolamide. Participants assigned to acetazolamide also experienced a reduction in weight (acetazolamide: −7.50 kg, from 107.72 kg to 100.22 kg; placebo: −3.45 kg, from 107.72 kg to 104.27 kg; treatment effect, −4.05 kg, 95% CI, −6.27 to −1.83 kg; $P < .001$).

Conclusions and Relevance.—In patients with IIH and mild visual loss, the use of acetazolamide with a low-sodium weight-reduction diet compared with diet alone resulted in modest improvement in visual field function. The clinical importance of this improvement remains to be determined.

Trial Registration.—clinicaltrials.gov Identifier: NCT01003639.

▶ The NORDIC IIHTT is an important clinical trial of acetazolamide in idiopathic intracranial hypertension (IIH). Acetazolamide has been the standard of care for treatment of mild visual loss in patients with IIH for years. However, we now have evidence from this multicenter, double-masked, randomized, controlled clinical trial that acetazolamide provides modest improvement in visual function as measured by perimetric mean deviation. There was also improvement in grade of papilledema and quality-of-life measures.

There are numerous limitations of this study, some nicely outlined in the accompanying editorial by Jonathan Horton, MD. First, those enrolled most often had only mild visual loss, limiting the ability to show benefit. This was necessary because those with more severe visual loss who are more likely to benefit would not be eligible for a placebo arm of the study. Indeed, those with more severe papilledema had more benefit than those with milder papilledema. Additionally, a weight loss program was included, and those on acetazolamide lost more weight than those on placebo.

M. L. Moster, MD

High prevalence of IgG4-related lymphoplasmacytic infiltrative disorder in 25 patients with orbital inflammation: a retrospective case series

Deschamps R, Deschamps L, Depaz R, et al (Fondation Ophtalmologique Adolphe de Rothschild, Paris, France)
Br J Ophthalmol 97:999-1004, 2013

Aims.—To evaluate retrospectively the prevalence of positive IgG4-immunostaining in orbital tissue of patients with idiopathic orbital inflammation and to compare the clinical, radiographic and pathologic features among patients with and without IgG4-positive cells.

Patients and Methods.—25 patients with biopsy-proven idiopathic orbital inflammation examined from January 2006 through December 2011 were included. Immunohistochemistry with IgG and IgG4 immunostaining from biopsy specimens of all patients was performed. Tissue with more than 10 IgG4-positive plasma cells per high-power field and with a ratio of IgG4+/IgG+ plasma cells of more than 40% was scored as positive. Histopathologic features, demographic and clinical data, radiologic findings, treatment and follow-up information for each patient were analysed.

Results.—Immunohistochemical staining showed 10 cases (40%) were IgG4 positive. The symptoms and signs included eyelid or periocular swelling/mass in all, pain (3/10), extraocular muscle restriction (3/10), proptosis (5/10) and/or decreased vision (4/10). Demographic and clinical findings of these patients did not differ from those with IgG4-negative cells. The presence of positive IgG4-immunostaining in orbital tissue was significantly associated with characteristic pathological features (more background fibrosis, lymphoid hyperplasia, plasma cells and phlebitis).

Conclusions.—Finally, 40% of patients with biopsy-proven orbital inflammation were classified as IgG4-RD, with typical histological features, but without specific clinical or radiological findings.

▶ This article points out that Immunoglobulin (Ig) G4-related disease (IgG4RD) in the orbit may present identically to idiopathic orbital inflammatory syndrome (IOIS). IgG4RD often has inflammation at many sites and often requires treatment beyond steroids, with good preliminary results with rituximab. Therefore, it is important to consider this entity in our IOIS patients.

A problem with interpreting this article is the lack of a standard definition for IgG4 positivity. This article used the criteria of more than 10 IGG4+ cells per high-power field and a ratio of IgG4+/IgG+ cells of 40%. Although others have used this cutoff in the literature, it is somewhat arbitrary. In fact, had they used the more stringent cutoff of >100 IgG4+ cells per high-power field, there would have only been 1 case considered positive. Additionally, in this retrospective series, serum IgG4 levels were not available, which, if available, would help support the diagnosis.

There is no mention of whether the patients were on steroids before biopsy, which could affect the results.

We often use pain as a criterion distinguishing IOIS from lymphoma or other infiltrative lesions. Therefore, it is surprising to see such a low percentage with pain in both the IgG4+ (30%) and IgG4 – (33%) groups in this series. It is also surprising to see a similar number of bilateral cases, regardless of IgG4 status. One would have expected more bilateral cases with IgG4 positivity.

Because IgG4RD has ramifications for the possibility of systemic inflammation outside the orbit and the presentation seems identical to IOIS in many cases, this article will decrease my threshold for ordering serum IgG4 levels in future patients with orbital disease.

M. L. Moster, MD

Giant Cell Arteritis: Diagnostic Accuracy of MR Imaging of Superficial Cranial Arteries in Initial Diagnosis—Results from a Multicenter Trial

Klink T, Geiger J, Both M, et al (Inselspital-Bern Univ Hosp, Switzerland; Univ Med Ctr Freiburg, Germany; Univ Hosp Schleswig-Holstein, Kiel, Germany; et al)

Radiology 273:844-852, 2014

Purpose.—To assess the diagnostic accuracy of contrast material–enhanced magnetic resonance (MR) imaging of superficial cranial arteries in the initial diagnosis of giant cell arteritis (GCA).

Materials and Methods.—Following institutional review board approval and informed consent, 185 patients suspected of having GCA were included in a prospective three–university medical center trial. GCA was diagnosed or excluded clinically in all patients (reference standard [final clinical diagnosis]). In 53.0% of patients (98 of 185), temporal artery biopsy (TAB) was performed (diagnostic standard [TAB]). Two observers independently evaluated contrast-enhanced T1-weighted MR images of superficial cranial arteries by using a four-point scale. Diagnostic accuracy, involvement pattern, and systemic corticosteroid (sCS) therapy effects were assessed in comparison with the reference standard (total study cohort) and separately in comparison with the diagnostic standard TAB (TAB subcohort). Statistical analysis included diagnostic accuracy parameters, interobserver agreement, and receiver operating characteristic analysis.

Results.—Sensitivity of MR imaging was 78.4% and specificity was 90.4% for the total study cohort, and sensitivity was 88.7% and specificity was 75.0% for the TAB subcohort (first observer). Diagnostic accuracy was comparable for both observers, with good interobserver agreement (TAB subcohort, $\kappa = 0.718$; total study cohort, $\kappa = 0.676$). MR imaging scores were significantly higher in patients with GCA-positive results than in patients with GCA-negative results (TAB subcohort and total study cohort, $P < .001$). Diagnostic accuracy of MR imaging was high in patients without and with sCS therapy for 5 days or fewer (area under the curve, ≥0.9) and was decreased in patients receiving sCS therapy for 6–14 days. In 56.5% of patients with TAB-positive results (35 of 62), MR imaging displayed symmetrical and simultaneous inflammation of arterial segments.

Conclusion.—MR imaging of superficial cranial arteries is accurate in the initial diagnosis of GCA. Sensitivity probably decreases after more than 5 days of sCS therapy; thus, imaging should not be delayed.

Clinical Trial Registration No.—DRKS00000594.

▶ Although temporal artery biopsy (TAB) is uniformly recommended by neuroophthalmologists, a search for less invasive tests has been underway for some time.

In this study, patients suspected of having giant cell arteritis (GCA) underwent neuroimaging, and masked reviewers evaluated the magnetic resonance imaging (MRI) scans for temporal and occipital artery mural thickening and enhancement. About half went on to have a temporal artery biopsy (TAB). Averaging the results between the 2 masked reviewers, positive scans showed a sensitivity of approximately 80% and a specificity of approximately 87% for the entire cohort. The sensitivity and specificity were very different based on whether the diagnosis was made with or without a TAB. Looking at the group that underwent TAB, the sensitivity of MRI was about 90%, and specificity was 75%. Among the subgroup that did not have a TAB, MRI sensitivity was about 64% and specificity was about 91%. It is interesting that the sensitivity of MRI was much lower in those diagnosed without a TAB in this study. Perhaps these patients who have not been biopsied and were diagnosed by clinical criteria did not actually have GCA.

MRI of the temporal and occipital arteries is a relatively noninvasive technique that makes sense for patients undergoing MRI anyway. As of now, it will not replace a TAB, and if an MRI is not planned, I would be reluctant to recommend it because it should not deter the performance of a TAB. I think it will have a role as an ancillary test, such as intravenous fluorescein angiography or orbital color Doppler. It may also be helpful in deciding on which side to perform the TAB.

M. L. Moster, MD

Co-occurrence of Acute Retinal Artery Occlusion and Acute Ischemic Stroke: Diffusion-Weighted Magnetic Resonance Imaging Study

Lee J, Kim SW, Lee SC, et al (Yonsei Univ College of Medicine, Seoul, South Korea)

Am J Ophthalmol 157:1231-1238, 2014

Purpose.—To evaluate the co-occurrence of acute ischemic stroke and acute retinal artery occlusion (RAO).

Design.—Retrospective observational case series.

Methods.—We included 33 consecutive patients with acute RAO who underwent diffusion-weighted magnetic resonance imaging within 7 days of the onset of visual symptoms. The causes of RAO were classified according to the Trial of Org 10172 in Acute Stroke Treatment (TOAST) criteria, which are based on clinical features and the results of etiological evaluations for atherosclerosis, cardioembolism and other prothrombotic conditions. We evaluated the prevalence of accompanying acute ischemic stroke in subjects with acute RAO and examined the relationships with etiological parameters.

Results.—Acute ischemic stroke was detected in 8 (24.2%) subjects with RAO. Among these subjects, 3 (37.5%) patients did not exhibit any neurologic symptoms or signs. Most of the infarction patterns were small, multiple and scattered. All of the subjects with RAO who were positive for lesions on diffusion-weighted imaging had identifiable causes, whereas only 36% of the subjects who were negative for lesions had identifiable etiologies ($P = .003$). Carotid stenosis or cardioembolic sources were found more commonly in cases of central retinal artery occlusion (CRAO; 7/18, 38.9%) than in cases of branch retinal artery occlusion (BRAO; 1/15 6.7%, $P = .046$).

Conclusions.—Acute cerebral infarctions frequently accompany RAO. We recommend diffusion-weighted imaging for patients with RAO because the presence of lesions on diffusion-weighted imaging is accompanied by a significantly increased probability of identifying the cause.

▶ This study demonstrates that asymptomatic cerebral ischemia seen on magnetic resonance imaging (MRI) with diffusion-weighted imaging (DWI) may accompany retinal artery ischemia—both central retinal artery occlusion (RAO) and branch RAO. The presence of cerebral ischemia was more often associated with a definitive etiology being found for the ischemia, such as embolic cardiac disease. This and prior findings in other studies showing that asymptomatic brain infarcts are associated with an increased risk of subsequent clinical infarct prompted the authors to recommend MRI with DWI on all RAO patients. This concurs with the American Heart Association/American Stroke Association guidelines, which do not distinguish retinal artery ischemia from hemispheric ischemia.

The recommendations that patients with RAO be evaluated at an emergency department or outpatient stroke unit rather than a slow elective outpatient workup make sense and are appropriately amplified in the accompanying editorial by Biousse.[1] However, if the article is not read carefully, one can be misled into thinking that 24.2% of patients with isolated branch or central RAO have acute ischemic stroke. Indeed, 5 of the 8 patients in this study with DWI changes had hemispheric brain symptoms as well, most often unilateral weakness. Despite this possible overestimation of asymptomatic cerebral ischemia, it is important for the ophthalmologic and neurologic communities to take transient or permanent monocular visual loss more seriously and treat it as an emergency, similar to cerebral transient ischemic attack or infarct.

M. L. Moster, MD

Reference

1. Biousse V. Acute retinal arterial ischemia: an emergency often ignored. *Am J Ophthalmol.* 2014;157:1119-1121.

Blood Biomarkers for Brain Injury in Concussed Professional Ice Hockey Players

Shahim P, Tegner Y, Wilson DH, et al (Sahlgrenska Univ Hosp, Mölndal, Sweden; Luleå Univ of Technology, Sweden; Quanterix Corp, Lexington, MA; et al)
JAMA Neurol 71:684-692, 2014

Importance.—Lack of objective biomarkers for brain damage hampers acute diagnosis and clinical decision making about return to play after sports-related concussion.

Objectives.—To determine whether sports-related concussion is associated with elevated levels of blood biochemical markers of injury to the central nervous system and to assess whether plasma levels of these biomarkers predict return to play in professional ice hockey players with sports-related concussion.

Design, Setting, and Participants.—Multicenter prospective cohort study involving all 12 teams of the top professional ice hockey league in Sweden, the Swedish Hockey League. Two hundred eighty-eight professional ice hockey players from 12 teams contesting during the 2012-2013 season consented to participate. All players underwent clinical preseason baseline testing regarding concussion assessment measures. Forty-seven players from 2 of the 12 ice hockey teams underwent blood sampling prior to the start of the season. Thirty-five players had a concussion from September 13, 2012, to January 31, 2013; of these players, 28 underwent repeated blood sampling at 1, 12, 36, and 144 hours and when the players returned to play.

Main Outcomes and Measures.—Total tau, S-100 calcium-binding protein B, and neuron-specific enolase concentrations in plasma and serum were measured.

Results.—Concussed players had increased levels of the axonal injury biomarker total tau (median, 10.0 pg/mL; range, 2.0-102 pg/mL) compared with preseason values (median, 4.5 pg/mL; range, 0.06-22.7 pg/mL) ($P < .001$). The levels of the astroglial injury biomarker S-100 calcium-binding protein B were also increased in players with sports-related concussion (median, 0.075 μg/L; range, 0.037-0.24 μg/L) compared with preseason values (median, 0.045 μg/L; range, 0.005-0.45 μg/L) ($P < .001$). The highest biomarker concentrations of total tau and S-100 calcium-binding protein B were measured immediately after a concussion, and they decreased during rehabilitation. No significant changes were detected in the levels of neuron-specific enolase from preseason values (median, 6.5 μg/L; range, 3.45-18.0 μg/L) to postconcussion values (median, 6.1 μg/L; range, 3.6-12.8 μg/L) ($P = .10$).

Conclusions and Relevance.—Sports-related concussion in professional ice hockey players is associated with acute axonal and astroglial injury. This can be monitored using blood biomarkers, which may be developed into clinical tools to guide sport physicians in the medical counseling of athletes in return-to-play decisions.

▶ It is important to have an objective test that identifies concussion and can provide prognostic information. In this article, the authors found that plasma total tau levels were elevated in professional hockey players with concussion. This elevation persisted for several days and correlated well with the duration of postconcussion syndrome (PCS) symptoms. Plasma S-100B levels were also increased in players with concussion from baseline, but they were no different from S-100B levels after a game in which no concussions occurred.

A biomarker that does not rely on the athlete's performance is crucial because some athletes purposely perform poorly on baseline cognitive examinations to avoid being diagnosed with concussion during the season.

The finding of elevated tau and the correlation of the level with time to recovery may improve the ability to appropriately counsel athletes with concussions. Objective biomarkers will also be helpful in caring for patients with concussions who may have nonphysiologic symptoms.

M. L. Moster, MD

Clinical import of Horner syndrome in internal carotid and vertebral artery dissection

Lyrer PA, Cervical Artery Dissection and Ischemic Stroke Patients (CADISP) Study Group (Basel Univ Hosp, Switzerland; et al)
Neurology 82:1653-1659, 2014

Objective.—To study the prognostic importance of Horner syndrome (HS) in patients with internal carotid artery dissection (ICAD) or vertebral artery dissection (VAD).

Methods.—In this observational study, characteristics and outcome of patients with ICAD or VAD from the CADISP (Cervical Artery Dissection and Ischemic Stroke Patients) database were analyzed. The presence of HS was systematically assessed using a standardized questionnaire. Patients with HS (HS+) were compared with HS- patients. Crude odds ratios (ORs) with 95% confidence intervals and ORs adjusted for age, sex, center, arterial occlusion, bilateral dissection, stroke severity, and type of antithrombotic treatment were calculated.

Results.—We analyzed 765 patients (n = 496 with ICAD, n = 269 with VAD, n = 303 prospective, n = 462 retrospective). HS was present in 191 (38.5%) of the patients with ICAD and 36 (13.4%) of the patients with VAD ($p < 0.001$). HS+ ICAD patients presented less often with stroke or TIA ($p < 0.001$), less often had bilateral ($p = 0.019$) or occlusive ($p = 0.001$) dissections, and had fewer severe strokes ($p = 0.041$) than HS– ICAD patients. HS+ ICAD patients had a better functional 3-month outcome than those without HS (ORcrude = 4.0 [2.4-6.7]), and also after adjustment for outcome-relevant covariates (OR adjusted = 2.0 [1.1-4.0]). HS+ ICAD patients were less likely to have new strokes than HS– ICAD patients ($p = 0.039$). HS+ VAD patients more often had vessel occlusion ($p = 0.014$) than HS– patients but did not differ in any of the other aforementioned variables.

Conclusion.—In patients with ICAD, HS is an easily assessable marker that might indicate a more benign clinical course. HS had no prognostic meaning in patients with VAD.

▶ This study of patients with cervical artery dissections looked at the difference in the number of patients with stroke based on whether they had Horner syndrome (HS) at presentation. About 85% of the internal carotid artery dissection (ICAD) patients without HS and 37% of those with HS had a stroke or transient ischemic attack at baseline.

In clinical practice, we often see isolated HS as the presentation of ICAD. In the past, almost all of these patients were treated with anticoagulation, but there has been a move toward antiplatelet agents in the stroke community even in acute cases, and patients have done relatively well with either treatment. This study looked at the prognosis in the presence or absence of HS (not necessarily isolated), and the main finding was that there were fewer and less severe strokes if HS was present. They postulate that an HS presentation may represent a more benign tear in the outer wall of the ICA, compared with those that are closer to the inner wall that spare the sympathetic fibers. The findings are consistent with previous reports of a less frequent stroke risk with HA than other presentations. Nonetheless, stroke risk is still high, and it is hard to predict who is at risk; we still have to figure out the optimal treatment.

Not surprisingly, in vertebral artery dissection, the presence of HS made little difference because in those cases, the HS is a manifestation of the brainstem infarct, rather than related to any fibers in the vertebral artery.

M. L. Moster, MD

Isolated Third, Fourth, and Sixth Cranial Nerve Palsies from Presumed Microvascular versus Other Causes: A Prospective Study

Tamhankar MA, Biousse V, Ying G-S, et al (Univ of Pennsylvania, Philadelphia; Emory Univ, Atlanta, GA; Brigham and Women's Hosp, Boston, MA)

Ophthalmology 120:2264-2269, 2013

Purpose.—To estimate the proportion of patients presenting with isolated third, fourth, or sixth cranial nerve palsy of presumed microvascular origin versus other causes.

Design.—Prospective, multicenter, observational case series.

Participants.—A total of 109 patients aged 50 years or older with acute isolated ocular motor nerve palsy.

Testing.—Magnetic resonance imaging (MRI) of the brain.

Main Outcome Measures.—Causes of acute isolated ocular motor nerve palsy (presumed microvascular or other) as determined with early MRI and clinical assessment.

Results.—Among 109 patients enrolled in the study, 22 had cranial nerve III palsy, 25 had cranial nerve IV palsy, and 62 had cranial nerve VI palsy. A cause other than presumed microvascular ischemia was identified in 18 patients (16.5%; 95% confidence interval, 10.7–24.6). The presence of 1 or more vasculopathic risk factors (diabetes, hypertension, hypercholesterolemia, coronary artery disease, myocardial infarction, stroke, and smoking) was significantly associated with a presumed microvascular cause ($P = 0.003$, Fisher exact test). Vasculopathic risk factors were also present in 61% of patients (11/18) with other causes. In the group of patients who had vasculopathic risk factors only, with no other significant medical condition, 10% of patients (8/80) were found to have other causes, including midbrain infarction, neoplasms, inflammation, pituitary apoplexy, and giant cell arteritis (GCA). By excluding patients with third cranial nerve palsies and those with GCA, the incidence of other causes for isolated fourth and sixth cranial nerve palsies was 4.7% (3/64).

Conclusions.—In our series of patients with acute isolated ocular motor nerve palsies, a substantial proportion of patients had other causes, including neoplasm, GCA, and brain stem infarction. Brain MRI and laboratory workup have a role in the initial evaluation of older patients with isolated acute ocular motor nerve palsies regardless of whether vascular risk factors are present.

► This is a thought-provoking article that calls into question the common practice of following elderly patients with presumed vasculopathic cranial nerve palsies without neuroimaging.

Although on initial calculation, 16.5% had an etiology that was not microvascular, the authors appropriately claim that for most of them—those with cranial nerve III palsy—there is no controversy and all neuroophthalmologists will agree on imaging.

In analyzing the message of this article, we should concentrate on those areas where there is controversy (fourth and sixth nerve palsies), in which 3 of 64 were found to have structural lesions, and see what difference it would have made had they not been immediately imaged. The first was a patient with vasculopathic risk factors and a midbrain infarct in whom the treatment of risk factors is identical with or without a small, likely lacunar, infarct. The second was a woman with petroclival meningioma subsequently treated with surgery. In her case, when the diplopia did not resolve in a few months, she could have been imaged and subsequently treated with surgery. The third case was a man with lymphoma. He too could have been diagnosed when he worsened or did not recover within the following few months. One could make the case that in this 1 patient out of 64 who had imaging, earlier treatment might have made a difference.

One valid point the authors make is that demyelinating disease may present with a cranial neuropathy. Because we are seeing patients with MS over age 50, those of us who are comfortable following elderly patients without imaging may want to begin scanning patients who are less than 60 years old.

The authors point out the importance of MRI in reassuring those who want to know there is no lesion. Although this is true, there is another group of patients who want reassurance that they do not need an MRI. Explaining to my patients that there is a small risk of a lesion and that I am willing to follow them and not order an MRI reassures this segment of our patient population.

So for me, I will likely scan a few more patients and perhaps follow only those who are a little older, but I am not yet ready to order MRI for all patients.

M. L. Moster, MD

Effect of chlorzoxazone in patients with downbeat nystagmus: a pilot trial

Feil K, Claaßen J, Bardins S, et al (Univ Hosp Munich, Germany)

Neurology 81:1152-1158, 2013

Objective.—Downbeat nystagmus (DBN) is the most frequent form of acquired persisting fixation nystagmus with different symptoms such as unsteadiness of gait, postural instability, and blurred vision with reduced visual acuity (VA) and oscillopsia. However, different symptomatic therapeutic principles are required, such as 3,4-diaminopyridine and 4-aminopyridine, that effectively suppress DBN. Chlorzoxazone (CHZ) is a nonselective activator of small conductance calcium-activated potassium (SK) channels that modifies the activity of cerebellar Purkinje cells. We evaluated the effects of this agent on DBN in an observational proof-of-concept pilot study.

Methods.—Ten patients received CHZ 500 mg 3 times a day for 1 or 2 weeks. Slow-phase velocity of DBN, VA, postural sway, and the drug's side effects were evaluated. Recordings were conducted at baseline, 90 minutes after first administration, and after 1 or 2 weeks.

Results.—Mean slow-phase velocity significantly decreased from a baseline of 2.74°/s ± 2.00 to 2.29°/s ± 2.12 (mean ± SD) 90 minutes after first administration and to 2.04°/s ± 2.24 ($p < 0.001$; post hoc both $p = 0.024$) after long-term treatment. VA significantly increased and postural sway in posturography showed a tendency to decrease on medication. Fifty percent of patients did not report any side effects. The most common reported side effect was abdominal discomfort and dizziness.

Conclusions.—The treatment with the SK-channel activator CHZ is a potentially new therapeutic agent for the symptomatic treatment of DBN.

Classification of Evidence.—This study provides Class IV evidence that CHZ 500 mg 3 times a day may improve eye movements and visual fixation in patients with DBN.

▶ Chlorzoxazone, 500 mg 3 times daily, improved function in 10 patients with downbeat nystagmus in this study. The authors measured slow phase velocity, visual acuity, and postural sway at baseline and after 1 to 2 weeks of treatment. They found a mean improvement of 44% in slow phase velocity, a marginal change in visual acuity, and no change in postural sway.

A new nystagmus treatment is always welcome, especially one reasonably priced and widely available (chlorzoxazone is commonly known in the United States as Parafon Forte, a muscle relaxant). What is hard to glean from this report but of utmost importance is whether the responders felt any symptomatic improvement. The "bellyache" side effect of chlorzoxazone is not worth it (50% of patients) if it doesn't provide much relief.

Chlorzoxazone is now added to a few other off-label medications that may help with downbeat nystagmus, including 4-aminopyridine, 3,4 diaminopyridine, and clonazepam.

M. L. Moster, MD

Education in medical billing benefits both neurology trainees and academic departments

Waugh JL (Boston Children's Hosp, MA)

Neurology 83:1856-1861, 2014

The objective of residency training is to produce physicians who can function independently within their chosen subspecialty and practice environment. Skills in the business of medicine, such as clinical billing, are widely applicable in academic and private practices but are not commonly addressed during formal medical education. Residency and fellowship training include limited exposure to medical billing, but our academic department's performance of these skills was inadequate: in 56% of trainee-generated outpatient notes, documentation was insufficient to sustain the chosen billing level. We developed a curriculum to improve the accuracy of documentation and coding and introduced practice changes to address our largest sources of error. In parallel, we developed tools that increased the speed and efficiency of documentation. Over 15 months, we progressively eliminated note devaluation, increased the mean level

billed by trainees to nearly match that of attending physicians, and increased outpatient revenue by $34,313/trainee/year. Our experience suggests that inclusion of billing education topics into the formal medical curriculum benefits both academic medical centers and trainees.

▶ Although this study was in a neurology department, the implications would be similar in ophthalmology or other residencies as well. In response to billing audits that found errors in 56% of patient encounters in resident's clinic, the Division of Pediatric Neurology at Boston Children's Hospital embarked on a program to train the residents in proper documentation. This included 4 hours of lectures and individualized structured feedback for each resident. Initial errors included in declining order: inadequate review of systems, insufficient documentation to justify billing as a new patient, medical decision making, physical examination, undercoding, overcoding, and medical history. After the training, accuracy improved from 44% sustaining the audit to 93%. Financially, this resulted in an increase in revenue of $34,313 per trainee per year.

In addition to the obvious financial benefit to academic departments and medical centers, this type of training during residency will certainly help the transition from training to practice.

As the accompanying editorial by Kaminski and Busis emphasized, we best educate residents in the "3 legs that support the health care delivery platform: the art, science and business of medicine."

M. L. Moster, MD

10 Imaging

Spontaneous Lateral Sphenoid Cephaloceles: Anatomic Factors Contributing to Pathogenesis and Proposed Classification

Settecase F, Harnsberger HR, Michel MA, et al (Univ of California, San Francisco; Univ of Utah, Salt Lake City; Med College of Wisconsin, Milwaukee; et al)

AJNR Am J Neuroradiol 35:784-789, 2014

Spontaneous lateral sphenoid cephaloceles arise from bony defects in the lateral sphenoid, in the absence of predisposing factors such as trauma, surgery, mass, or congenital skull base malformation. We reviewed CT and MR imaging findings and clinical data of 26 patients with spontaneous lateral sphenoid cephaloceles to better understand anatomic contributions to pathogenesis, varying clinical and imaging manifestations, and descriptive terminology. Two types of spontaneous lateral sphenoid cephaloceles were identified. In 15 of 26 patients, a type 1 spontaneous lateral sphenoid cephalocele was noted, herniating into a pneumatized lateral recess of the sphenoid sinus, and typically presenting with CSF leak and/or headache. In 11 of 26 patients, a type 2 spontaneous lateral sphenoid cephalocele was noted, isolated to the greater sphenoid wing without extension into the sphenoid sinus, presenting with seizures, headaches, meningitis, cranial neuropathy, or detected incidentally. All patients had sphenoid arachnoid pits, and 61% of patients had an empty or partially empty sella, suggesting that altered CSF dynamics may play a role in their genesis.

▶ Spontaneous lateral sphenoid cephaloceles are associated with bony defects in the lateral sphenoid, in the absence of predisposing factors, including prior trauma or surgery, mass, or congenital malformation. These are believed to be acquired lesions resulting from a combination of physiologic factors (including altered cerebrospinal fluid dynamics) and anatomic factors (including presence of bone defects) and have been shown to be associated with certain imaging features—pneumatization of the lateral recess of the sphenoid sinus, arachnoid pits, and empty or partially empty sella. These observations are supported by the current study. Additionally, in this retrospective study, the authors have attempted to explain the relationship of varying clinical presentation to anatomic location of the cephaloceles and have proposed a classification for the same. In addition to being retrospective in nature, the study lacks descriptive clinical details, especially regarding workup of seizure or headache symptoms and features of idiopathic intracranial hypertension.

K. Talekar, MD

Volumetric Assessment of Optic Nerve Sheath and Hypophysis in Idiopathic Intracranial Hypertension

Hoffmann J, Schmidt C, Kunte H, et al (Charité-Universitätsmedizin Berlin, Germany; et al)

AJNR Am J Neuroradiol 35:513-518, 2014

Background and Purpose.—Idiopathic intracranial hypertension is a headache syndrome characterized by increased CSF pressure. Compression of the hypophysis and distension of the optic nerve sheath are reliable imaging signs. The purpose of the study was to validate, in patients with idiopathic intracranial hypertension, MR imaging–based volumetric measurements of the optic nerve sheath and hypophysis as an objective observation method for more accurate diagnosis and posttreatment follow-up.

Materials and Methods.—Twenty-three patients with idiopathic intracranial hypertension as well as age-, sex-, and body mass index–matched controls underwent volumetric measurements of the optic nerve, optic nerve sheath, and hypophysis on high-resolution T2-weighted MR images by using a 7-cm surface coil, followed by correlation with CSF opening pressures and clinical symptom scores of visual disturbances and headache.

Results.—Mean values of optic nerve sheath ($341.86 \pm 163.69\ mm^3$ versus $127.56 \pm 53.17\ mm^3$, $P < .001$) and hypophysis volumes ($554.59 \pm 142.82\ mm^3$ versus $686.60 \pm 137.84\ mm^3$, $P < .05$) differed significantly between healthy and diseased subjects. No significant differences between mean optic nerve volumes were observed. Receiver operating characteristic analysis showed optic nerve sheath volumes of $>201.30\ mm^3$ (sensitivity, 86.96%; specificity, 91.30%) and hypophysis volumes of $<611.21\ mm^3$ (sensitivity, 78.26%; specificity, 69.57%) to be indicative of idiopathic intracranial hypertension diagnosis. In patients with idiopathic intracranial hypertension, no correlations were found between optic nerve sheath and hypophysis volumes and CSF opening pressures or clinical scores of visual disturbances and headache.

Conclusions.—Semiautomated volumetric measurement of optic nerve sheath and hypophysis has the potential to more accurately diagnose and follow patients with idiopathic intracranial hypertension.

▶ Idiopathic intracranial hypertension is a headache syndrome associated with elevated intracranial pressure in the absence of an intracranial space-occupying lesion. It is usually a diagnosis of exclusion and is based on clinical symptoms such as headache and visual disturbances with elevated cerebrospinal fluid pressures and papilledema. Radiologic examinations have been traditionally performed to help exclude intracranial pathologies that cause headache, such as mass, hydrocephalus, and cerebral edema. More recently, neuroimaging findings, including compression of the pituitary (empty/partially empty sella), flattening of the posterior globe, and dilated optic nerve sheath have been described as imaging criteria for diagnosis of idiopathic intracranial hypertension. Additionally, transverse sinus stenoses and rarely spontaneous sphenoid cephalocele have been shown to be associated with idiopathic intracranial hypertension. However, these findings can be subtle and may be absent, especially in the early stages of the disease process; additionally, these findings have a subjective component. In this article, the authors explore the potential of magnetic resonance imaging-based volumetric measurements as an objective method to diagnose idiopathic intracranial hypertension by comparing pituitary, optic nerve sheath, and optic nerve volumes, measured on high-resolution magnetic resonance images, in patients with idiopathic intracranial hypertension and age-, sex-, and body mass index-matched controls; they report significant differences between the volumes of the optic nerve sheath and pituitary between patients and controls.

K. Talekar, MD

11 Ocular Oncology

Banning the Handshake From the Health Care Setting

Sklansky M, Nadkarni N, Ramirez-Avila L (David Geffen School of Medicine at UCLA, Los Angeles, CA; et al)

JAMA 311:2477-2478, 2014

Background.—Although the handshake is an important cultural, social, political, and even financial entity, in health care the handshake carries the distinction of having great potential for transmitting communicable diseases. Preventing such transmission may transcend the importance of the handshake, but the course toward eliminating it from society will be rocky and difficult.

Disease Transmission Via Handshake.—The handshake began as a gesture of peace but has evolved into an international symbol of greeting or departure, reconciliation, respect, friendship, peace, congratulations, sportsmanship, or formal agreement. Health care practitioners often begin and end their encounters with patients using a handshake, which can have an important impact on the way the physician is seen by others. However, the hands of health care workers can serve as vectors for the transmission of organisms and disease. Hands become contaminated from patients, then the contaminants are passed along during patient encounters and environmental contact. Bacteria and viruses can survive for varying periods of time on the hands of health care workers. Although hand hygiene is emphasized as a fundamental way to prevent hospital-acquired infections and measures are in place in most health care facilities to allow health care providers to practice good hand hygiene routinely, compliance with these measures is only about 40%. Patients and visitors have even lower rates of compliance. In addition, the alcohol-based hand sanitizers are not universally effective, with some pathogens, such as *Clostridium difficile*, not affected by these rubs.

Proposed Alternatives.—Based on the experience of banning the widely accepted practice of smoking back in the 1960s, it will require widespread media and educational efforts coupled with the development and promotion of effective alternatives to achieve a handshake ban and replacement. Appropriate signage may be needed, such as "Handshake-free zone to protect your health and the health of those you meet." Among the possible replacements for shaking hands that will not spread infection or disease are the hand wave, placing the right palm over the heart, bowing, the Namaste gesture, the wai gesture, and the salaam (peace) gesture. All have cultural significance and may convey the respect and acknowledgement that a handshake traditionally offers.

Conclusions.—To ban handshakes from the health care environment will require specific education of the public about how pathogens and diseases are transmitted. This must then be combined with a suitable replacement gesture that will also require widespread acceptance and educational support. Underlying all these efforts is a thorough understanding that not shaking hands will protect the health of patients and care givers.

▶ The handshake is a widely accepted greeting in our culture and is expected from physicians in patient interactions. Recently, however, there has been increasing concern about the risk of infection transmission via the handshake. In this article, the authors cite several recent studies finding inadequacies in the current practice regarding handshakes and recommend an alternative system.

Studies find that handshakes transmit pathogens.[1,2] *Clostridium difficile* spores (a common cause of diarrhea) have been found to transmit via the handshake.[2] Moreover, alcohol rub, the most common method of hand hygiene, has been found to lack efficacy against certain pathogens, including *C difficile*.[3] Only an average of 40% of health care personnel is compliant with hand hygiene guidelines.[4] This finding considerably increases the risk for handshake-related infection transmission. Thus, the authors recommend that we institute an alternative greeting in place of the handshake. Alternatives include a hand wave, head nod, or placing the hand over the heart as a greeting. The authors acknowledge that the handshake is deeply embedded in our culture, and avoiding it could offend patients, but this can change with proper patient education.

Other recent articles have dealt with similar concerns regarding physicians' clothing and belongings, such as neckties, long-sleeve shirts, stethoscopes, and even pens.[5] Bacteria such as *Staphylococcus aureus* have been isolated from physicians' stethoscopes[6] and neckties.[7] These concerns have prompted recommendations for reform regarding the hygiene of personal objects from many institutions. In June 2009, the American Medical Association (AMA) House of Delegates passed a resolution to encourage the "adoption of hospital guidelines for dress codes that minimize transmission of nosocomial infections."[8] The AMA resolution is measured and does not recommend a ban on any specific mode of dress. In the United Kingdom, however, government policies are more stringent and recommend a "bare beneath the elbows" dress code that bans neckties, white coats, and jewelry and requires short sleeve shirts such as hospital scrubs.[5]

Although some authors argue that physician hygiene in the United States should be reformed, others feel that these measures are excessive. They argue that the risk of infection is small, and these changes will disrupt the doctor–patient relationship.[9] A handshake preceding a social interaction enhances trust and promotes a more favorable impression,[10] and this would likely be lost if handshakes were avoided. They also argue that all personal attire has bacteria on it, and we must accept small risks that are impossible to avoid.

Further studies are necessary to determine whether health care practitioners should make these changes.

Y. C. Ziemba, BTL
C. L. Shields, MD

References

1. Hamburger M. Transfer of beta hemolytic streptococci by shaking hands. *Am J Med.* 1947;2:23-25.
2. Ghareeb PA, Bourlai T, Dutton W, McClellan WT. Reducing pathogen transmission in a hospital setting: handshake versus fist bump: a pilot study. *J Hosp Infect.* 2013;85:321-323.
3. Jabbar U, Leischner J, Kasper D, et al. Effectiveness of alcohol-based hand rubs for removal of Clostridium difficile spores from hands. *Infect Control Hosp Epidemiol.* 2010;31:565-570.
4. Erasmus V, Daha TJ, Brug H, et al. Systematic review of studies on compliance with hand hygiene guidelines in hospital care. *Infect Control Hosp Epidemiol.* 2010;31:283-294.
5. Dancer SJ. Pants, policies and paranoia. *J Hosp Infect.* 2010;74:10-15.
6. Jones JS, Hoerle D, Riekse R. Stethoscopes: a potential vector of infection? *Ann Emerg Med.* 1995;26:296-299.
7. McGovern B, Doyle E, Fenelon LE, FitzGerald SF. The necktie as a potential vector of infection: are doctors happy to do without? *J Hosp Infect.* 2010;75:136-137.
8. American Medical Association (AMA). *American Medical Association House of Delegates.* Chicago, IL: AMA; 2009. Resolution 720: hospital dress codes for the reduction of nosocomial transmission of disease.
9. Eisenbeis JF, Sappington JM. The necktie in medicine: professional or a double windsor fomite? *Mo Med.* 2010;107:368-369.
10. Stewart G, Dustin S, Barrick M, Darnold T. Exploring the handshake in employment interviews. *J Appl Psychol.* 2008;93:1139-1146.

Iris stromal cyst management with absolute alcohol-induced sclerosis in 16 patients

Shields CL, Arepalli S, Lally EB, et al (Thomas Jefferson Univ, Philadelphia, PA)

JAMA Ophthalmol 132:703-708, 2014

Importance.—The management of symptomatic iris stromal cyst is challenging using methods of aspiration with or without adjunctive cryotherapy, intracameral cautery, or photocoagulation. Failed cases often require surgical resection, with risks for epithelial downgrowth, glaucoma, blindness, and loss of the eye.

Objective.—To study the safety and efficacy of the management of iris stromal cysts with aspiration and alcohol irrigation to induce cyst sclerosis.

Design, Setting, and Participants.—Interventional case series at a tertiary referral center among 16 patients.

Exposures.—Microscopically monitored transcorneal aspiration of cysts was performed with a 30-gauge needle on a 3-way T-extension into a 3-mL syringe, followed by immediate infusion of absolute alcohol from a separate 1-mL syringe through the other arm of the T-extension. Subsequent alcohol aspiration and repetition of the cycle was performed until the collapsed cyst wall appeared gray.

Main Outcomes and Measures.—Cyst involution, visual acuity, and treatment complications.

Results.—The iris stromal cysts were primary congenital (n = 6), primary acquired (n = 4), or secondary (n = 6). The cysts had a median basal diameter of 12 mm and a thickness of 4 mm, occupying 50% or more of the anterior or posterior chamber in each case. Treatment was administered following failure of simple aspiration (n = 16) and additional methods (n = 8). During a median follow-up period of 5 years, treatment was successful in 14 of 15 patients (1 patient was lost to follow-up). Cyst sclerosis with stabilization (n = 1) or involution (n = 13) was achieved following 1 (n = 10), 2 (n = 2), or 3 (n = 2) procedures. The single failure occurred in a 3-year-old child with cyst recurrence and severe photophobia requiring resection. Visual acuity remained stable or had improved in 14 patients and was reduced in 1 patient because of cataract. Complications included transient corneal edema (n = 4) and transient anterior chamber inflammation (n = 1), which resolved following topical corticosteroid therapy. No evidence was seen of treatment-related glaucoma, epithelial downgrowth, tissue necrosis, cataract, posterior segment toxic effects, or need for enucleation.

Conclusions and Relevance.—Microscopically monitored aspiration and absolute alcohol-induced sclerosis of iris stromal cysts is safe and effective, with cyst involution obtained in 93% (14 of 15) of patients.

▶ Iris tumors are typically classified by architecture as either cystic or solid. Cystic iris tumors are further defined by the tissue involved, whether it is iris pigment epithelium (IPE) or iris stromal tissue. The IPE cysts tend to remain relatively asymptomatic and stable over time, whereas iris stromal cysts tend to be symptomatic with vision loss and often enlarge within the anterior chamber, leading to complications. Complications include visual impairment and cyst rupture with secondary glaucoma, anterior uveitis, and epithelial downgrowth. Enlarging or ruptured cysts may necessitate surgical resection or enucleation.[1,2] Surgical management can resolve some problems but can also cause problems such as astigmatism, amblyopia, cataract, and retinal detachment. In most cases, medical management of iris stromal cysts is preferable.

Systemic cysts, such as those in the liver, kidney, and lung, can be managed effectively with sclerosing agents. More recently, the use of sclerosing agents in the management of intraocular cysts has been investigated. In 2003, Behrouzi and Khodadoust[3] published a study of 99 eyes with iris stromal cysts following treatment with intracystic ethanol irrigation. They found cyst involution in 94% after 1 treatment, 97% after 2 treatments, and 99% after 3 treatments.[3]

In this study, Shields et al investigated 16 cases of iris stromal cysts that were treated with absolute alcohol-induced sclerosis, with a modified technique from Behrouzi and Khodadoust.[3] Using a 30-gauge needle, the cyst was entered at the limbal cornea where the cyst was adherent to the endothelium. The cyst contents were aspirated and then alcohol infused and aspirated once the cyst wall appeared gray (1–2 minutes). After several alcohol infusions in a single session, final cyst aspiration was performed, and the anterior chamber was infused with balanced salt solution for cyst tamponade. In this study, 12 patients required 1 treatment, 2 patients required 2 treatments, and 2 patients required 3 treatments to achieve permanent cyst involution. Fourteen of 16 patients (93%) had involution of cysts at median 5-year follow-up. Only 1 patient showed recurrence and requested surgical management, and 1 patient was lost to follow-up. Complications included 4 eyes with corneal edema that showed partial or complete resolution with topical corticosteroids. After treatment, visual acuity improved in 8, remained stable in 6, and decreased in 1 patient secondary to cataract progression.

Iris stromal cysts are benign and can occur in infants, leading to serious eye complications. Cyst enlargement and rupture can threaten vision and the integrity of the eye. Management with alcohol-sclerosing agents offers a minimally invasive approach that, if performed carefully, offers a high probability of long-term involution with minimal complications.

P. Mellen, BS
C. L. Shields, MD

References

1. Shields CL, Shields PW, Manalac J, Jumroendararasame C, Shields JA. Review of cystic and solid tumors of the iris. *Oman J Ophthalmol.* 2013;6:159-164.
2. Shields JA, Shields CL. *Intraocular Tumors: An Atlas and Textbook.* 2nd ed. Philadelphia, PA: Lippencott Williams & Wilkins; 2008:46-57.
3. Behrouzi Z, Khodadoust A. Epithelial iris cysts treatment with intracystic ethanol irrigation. *Ophthalmology.* 2003;110:1601-1605.

Proposed Lexicon for Anatomic Landmarks in Normal Posterior Segment Spectral-Domain Optical Coherence Tomography: The IN•OCT Consensus

Staurenghi G, for the International Nomenclature for Optical Coherence Tomography (IN•OCT) Panel (Luigi Sacco Hosp Univ of Milan, Italy; et al)

Ophthalmology 121:1572-1578, 2014

Purpose.—To develop a consensus nomenclature for the classification of retinal and choroidal layers and bands visible on spectral-domain optical coherence tomography (SD-OCT) images of a normal eye.

Design.—An international panel with expertise in retinal imaging (International Nomenclature for Optical Coherence Tomography [IN•OCT] Panel) was assembled to define a consensus for OCT imaging terminology.

Participants.—A panel of retina specialists.

Methods.—A set of 3 B-scan images from a normal eye was circulated to the panel before the meeting for independent assignment of nomenclature to anatomic landmarks in the vitreous, retina, and choroid. The outputs were scrutinized, tabulated, and used as the starting point for discussions at a roundtable panel meeting. The history of anatomic landmark designations over time was reviewed for the various cellular layers of the ocular structures that are visible by SD-OCT. A process of open discussion and negotiation was undertaken until a unanimous consensus name was adopted for each feature.

Main Outcome Measures.—Definitions of normal eye features showed by SD-OCT.

Results.—Definitions for various layers changed frequently in the literature and were often inconsistent with retinal anatomy and histology. The panel introduced the term "zone" for OCT features that seem to localize to a particular anatomic region that lacks definitely proven evidence for a specific reflective structure. Such zones include the myoid, ellipsoid, and the interdigitation zones.

Conclusions.—A nomenclature system for normal anatomic landmarks seen on SD-OCT outputs has been proposed and adopted by the IN•OCT Panel. The panel recommends this standardized nomenclature for use in future publications. The proposed harmonizing of terminology serves as a basis for future OCT research studies.

▶ Optical coherence tomography (OCT) is an imaging method that uses interferometry and light scattering to produce cross-sectional images of tissues in vivo. Its efficacy depends on differences in reflectivity among different layers of tissue. Spectral domain-OCT (SD-OCT) was first introduced as a method of visualization of the retinal layers in 1991 and has become a necessary component in the armamentarium for retinal and glaucoma assessment. OCT has increased in its value across clinics as the technology has become more advanced, leading to speed, sensitivity, and resolution improvements. In 1991, the first OCT imaging of the eye with the time domain method identified only the retinal pigment epithelium (RPE).[1] Subsequently, in 1997, finer anatomic outer nuclear and photoreceptor layers of the retina were identified on OCT using reflectivity as the differentiating characteristic.[2] Then, in 2001, "ultra-high resolution OCT" was able to capture 3 distinct bands in the outer retina, believed to be outer segments, RPE, and choriocapillaris.[3] More recently, faster and higher resolution OCT have allowed resolution in identification of 4 lines in the outer retina and alternating bands in the inner retina, clarifying errors in anatomic attribution made previously.

The development of advanced OCT imaging has coincided with its increased use in clinical and surgical ophthalmology. Unfortunately, there have been anatomic discrepancies regarding terminology of hyperreflective and hyporeflective bands and layers. Disorganized and nonuniversal nomenclature interferes with scientific communication.

To improve OCT nomenclature, a task force was convened with OCT experts to define anatomic structures on labeled OCT scans to provide a consensual standard lexicon. Using 2 standard OCT scans, the experts identified 18 anatomic zones, each representing a different reflective region on OCT. Following an independent naming exercise, the experts met at the "Roundtable International Nomenclature for Optical Coherence Tomography Panel Meeting" to agree on consensus terminology. Three new zones were defined, including the myoid, ellipsoid, and interdigitation zones.

This report by Staurenghi et al establishes a precedent for streamlining terminology to allow more efficient and collaborative use of the technology. OCT has become indispensible in the diagnosis and characterization of intraocular tumors.[4] Al-Dahmash et al[5] studied the value of enhanced depth imaging SD-OCT for choroidal metastasis and noted that this technology has characteristic features and can detect tumors not visible by ophthalmoscopy. Further progress with OCT is inevitable, and now we have a universal glossary of terms for consistency in scientific observations.

Z. E. Daitch, BA
C. L. Shields, MD

References

1. Huang D, Swanson EA, Lin CP, et al. Optical coherence tomography. *Science.* 1991;254:1178-1181.
2. Toth CA, Narayan DG, Boppart SA, et al. A comparison of retinal morphology viewed by optical coherence tomography and by light microscopy. *Arch Ophthalmol.* 1997;115:1425-1428.
3. Drexler W, Morgner U, Ghanta RK, Kärtner FX, Schuman JS, Fujimoto JG. Ultrahigh resolution ophthalmic optical coherence tomography. *Nat Med.* 2001;7:502-507.
4. Shields CL, Pellegrini M, Ferenczy SR, Shields JA. Enhanced depth imaging optical coherence tomography (EDI-OCT) of intraocular tumors. From placid to seasick to rock and rolling topography. The 2013 Francesco Orzalesi Lecture. *Retina.* 2014;34:1495-1512.
5. Al-Dahmash SA, Shields CL, Kaliki S, Johnson T, Shields JA. Enhanced depth imaging optical coherence tomography of choroidal metastasis in 14 eyes. *Retina.* 2014;34:1588-1593.

Plaque Radiotherapy for Juxtapapillary Choroidal Melanoma: Treatment Complications and Visual Outcomes in 650 Consecutive Cases

Sagoo MS, Shields CL, Emrich J, et al (Moorfields Eye Hosp, London, England; Thomas Jefferson Univ, Philadelphia, PA; Drexel Univ College of Medicine, Philadelphia, PA)

JAMA Ophthalmol 132:697-702, 2014

Importance.—The treatment of juxtapapillary choroidal melanoma is challenging because of the proximity of the tumor to visually important structures.

Objective.—To report the complications of treatment of juxtapapillary choroidal melanoma with plaque radiotherapy.

Design, Setting, and Participants.—In this retrospective case series of patients from the Ocular Oncology Service, Wills Eye Hospital, 650 consecutive eyes with juxtapapillary choroidal melanoma ($\leq$1 mm to optic disc) treated with plaque radiotherapy from October 1, 1974, through November 30, 2005, were studied.

Main Outcomes and Measures.—Kaplan-Meier analysis of rates of radiation complications, secondary enucleation, and visual acuity outcomes.

Results.—The 5-year (10-year) rate of nonproliferative retinopathy was 66% (75%); proliferative retinopathy, 24% (32%); maculopathy, 56% (65%); papillopathy, 61% (77%); cataract, 66% (80%); neovascular glaucoma, 15% (22%); vitreous hemorrhage, 35% (42%); and secondary enucleation, 16% (26%). Visual acuity of 20/200 or worse occurred in 54% (87%), and loss of more than 5 lines of Snellen visual acuity was found in 45% (78%).

Conclusions and Relevance.—Among this case series, plaque radiotherapy for juxtapapillary choroidal melanoma commonly led to retinopathy and papillopathy, but globe retention was 84% at 5 years. Vision loss should be anticipated in 45% by 5 years. Plaque radiotherapy remains a suitable choice for the treatment of juxtapapillary melanoma with a high globe retention rate.

▶ Juxtapapillary choroidal melanoma is challenging to treat because of its proximity to the optic disc. Although enucleation was once the treatment of choice for juxtapapillary melanoma, current techniques can provide globe and possibly some vision salvage. One such treatment is custom-designed notched plaque radiotherapy. In 1994, De Potter et al from Wills Eye Hospital reported plaque radiotherapy as an alternative to enucleation with the former exhibiting a lower risk for metastasis, particularly in older patients.[1] The challenge with this technique is the difficulty in accuracy of radiotherapy design and the precarious surgical placement of the device at the optic nerve, deep within the orbit.[2] In 2008, Sagoo et al from Wills Eye Hospital noted that a custom-designed plaque radiotherapy device with a specific notch to partially enwrap the optic disc within the orbit was effective for even more advanced juxtapapillary melanoma that had grown into an epipapillary tumor.[3] They found that notched plaque offered better control than a standard round plaque.

Although several reports have compared the survival rates of various treatments for choroidal melanoma, there is relatively little in the literature on visual outcomes. Plaque radiotherapy for juxtapapillary choroidal melanomas may offer tumor control but with expected poorer visual outcome compared with melanoma more remote from the disc. Irradiation of tumors at the disc leads to papillopathy with eventual optic atrophy and vision loss.[4]

In this report, the authors evaluated complications following plaque radiotherapy in 650 consecutive cases of juxtapapillary choroidal melanoma. They found that the 5-year rate of nonproliferative retinopathy was 66% and of papillopathy was 61%. Five-year visual loss of more than 5 Snellen visual acuity lines was detected in 45% of cases and poor visual acuity of less than 20/200 in 54%. Although the visual outcomes appear undesirable, the globe was saved in 84% of cases, and all patients otherwise would have had enucleation. Thus custom-designed plaque radiotherapy is effective for juxtapapillary melanoma with tumor control and high rate of globe retention, but long-term visual acuity is reduced.

A. Badami, BS
C. L. Shields, MD

References

1. De Potter P, Shields CL, Shields JA, Cater JR, Tardio DJ. Impact of enucleation versus plaque radiotherapy in the management of juxtapapillary choroidal melanoma on patient survival. *Br J Ophthalmol.* 1994;78:109-114.
2. Finger PT, Chin KJ, Tena LB. A five-year study of slotted plaque radiation therapy for choroidal melanoma: near, touching or surrounding the optic nerve. *Ophthalmology.* 2012;119:415-422.
3. Sagoo MS, Shields CL, Mashayekhi A, et al. Plaque radiotherapy for juxtapapillary choroidal melanoma overhanging the optic disc in 141 consecutive patients. *Arch Ophthalmol.* 2008;126:1515-1522.
4. Shields CL, Shields JA, Cater J, et al. Plaque radiotherapy for uveal melanoma. Long-term visual outcome in 1106 patients. *Arch Ophthalmol.* 2000;118:1219-1228.

Chromosome 3 Status Combined with *BAP1* and *EIF1AX* Mutation Profiles is a Strong Prognostic Indicator for Uveal Melanoma

Ewens KG, Kanetsky PA, Richards-Yutz J, et al (Univ of Pennsylvania, Philadelphia; Moffitt Cancer Ctr, Tampa, FL; et al)
Invest Ophthalmol Vis Sci 55:5160-5167, 2014

Purpose.—Uveal melanoma (UM), the most common intraocular tumor in adults, is associated with a high burden of mortality due to distant metastasis. Somatic mutations in *GNAQ*, *GNA11*, *SF3B1*, *EIF1AX* and *BAP1* have been identified in UM. The aim of this study was to determine the prognostic value of these mutation(s) in UM metastasis.

Methods.—Taqman assays were used to screen for specific mutations in *GNA11*, *GNAQ* and *SF3B1* in 116 UM samples. Standard Sanger sequencing or next-generation sequencing methods were used to screen exons 1 and 2 of *EIF1AX* and all exons of *BAP1*. The association of gene mutations with tumor characteristics, chromosome-3 copy number and metastatic status were analyzed by logistic regression.

Results.—Somatic mutations in exons 4 and 5 of *GNAQ* and *GNA11* were present in a mutually exclusive manner in 82% of tumors. There were 11 (10%) tumors with mutations in *SF3B1*, 18 (16%) with *EIF1AX* and 56 (50%) with BAP1 mutations. In univariate analysis, mutation in *BAP1* was associated with increased risk of metastasis (6.3-fold), while *EIF1AX* mutation decreased the risk by 7.9-fold. Multivariate logistic regression indicated tumors with chromosome-3 monosomy/*BAP1*-mutation/*EIF1AX*-normal were associated with 45.6-fold risk for metastasis compared to tumors with chromosome-3 disomy/*BAP1*-normal/*EIF1AX*-mutation.

Conclusions.—The results of this analysis suggest that chromosome-3 status and tumor size remain the most significant predictors of metastasis; however combining information on these variables with the presence of mutations in *BAP1* and *EIF1AX* further refines the odd ratio for risk of metastasis.

▶ Uveal melanoma (UM) is a rare and extraordinarily malignant tumor, with high rate of metastasis and death, even from a tumor measuring only 3 or 4 mm in thickness. This tumor represents one of the most serious and deadliest tumors found in the human body. The most common site of metastasis from uveal melanoma is to the liver. Factors predictive of metastasis include large tumor size, ciliary body location, extraocular extension, and intrinsic genetic mutations, including abnormalities in chromosomes 3, 6, and 8 as strongly predictive of metastasis. Investigators are searching to further identify specific genetic causes of UM and prognostic indicators for metastasis. Recently, somatic mutations in 5 genes were named to be associated with UM including G-protein α-subunits *GNAQ* and *GNA11*, tumor suppressor gene *BAP1*, splicing factor *SF3B1*, and the X-linked translation initiation factor *EIF1AX*.

In this report, Ewens et al from the University of Pennsylvania, in conjunction with the Ocular Oncology Service at Wills Eye Hospital of Thomas Jefferson University, examined the presence of mutations in *GNAQ*, *GNA11*, *BAP1*, *SF3B1*, and *EIF1AX*, in addition to the status of chromosome 3 and other prognostic factors in 116 UM patients. Their goal was to explore the prognostic value of these mutations for UM metastasis. They found that *GNAQ* and *GNA11*, 2 G-protein α-subunits, were present in 82% of UM, but this was not prognostic of metastasis. Their findings are comparable to previous findings that indicated 80% of UM carry mutations in *GNAQ* and *GNA11*.[1] It is thought that these mutations are involved in early melanoma development because they are found in all stages of tumor progression. Mutant copies of *SF3B1* were found in 10% of tumors and showed no significant link to metastasis. Mutations in *EIF1AX* were found in 16% of tumors, and this mutation was surprisingly found to serve a protective role, with a 7.9-fold decrease in risk for metastasis. Analysis of mutations in *BAP1*, a chromosome 3 p-linked tumor suppressor protein, showed 56 of 116 tumors (48%) contained *BAP1* mutations, and 43 of these 56 tumors (77%) demonstrated metastatic disease. Of these, 42 (98%) displayed chromosome-3 monosomy. This supports the conclusion that recessive *BAP1* mutations are revealed when 1 normal copy of chromosome 3 is lost. Harbour et al previously recognized that 84% of aggressively metastatic UM contained inactivating somatic mutations in *BAP1*, suggesting that loss of *BAP1* is an essential event in late progression of UM.[2]

Ewens et al concluded that examination of the status of chromosome 3 and tumor size, in conjunction with analysis of mutations in *BAP1* and *EIF1AX*, can help to further determine the risk of metastasis in UM.

M. Sivalingam, BA
C. L. Shields, MD

References

1. Van Raamsdonk CD, Greiwank KG, Crosby MB, et al. Mutations in GNA11 in uveal melanoma. *N Engl J Med.* 2010;363:2191-2199.
2. Harbour JW, Onken MD, Roberson EDO, et al. Frequent mutation of BAP1 in metastasizing uveal melanomas. *Science.* 2010;330:1410-1413.

Intra-arterial Chemotherapy for Retinoblastoma in 70 Eyes: Outcomes Based on the International Classification of Retinoblastoma

Shields CL, Manjandavida FP, Lally SE, et al (Thomas Jefferson Univ, Philadelphia, PA; et al)

Ophthalmology 121:1453-1460, 2014

Objective.—To analyze our 5-year experience of intra-arterial chemotherapy (IAC) for retinoblastoma as primary or secondary therapy.

Design.—Retrospective interventional case series.

Participants.—A total of 70 eyes of 67 patients.

Intervention.—Ophthalmic artery chemotherapy infusion under fluoroscopic guidance was performed using melphalan (3, 5, or 7.5 mg) in every case, with additional topotecan (1 mg) and/or carboplatin (30 or 50 mg) as necessary.

Main Outcome Measures.—Tumor control and treatment complications.

Results.—The mean patient age at IAC was 30 months. The treatment was primary in 36 eyes and secondary in 34 eyes. Those primary therapy eyes were classified according to the International Classification of Retinoblastoma (ICRB) as group A (n = 0), B (n = 1), C (n = 4), D (n = 17), or E (n = 14). The secondary therapy eyes had failed previous intravenous chemotherapy (n = 34) in every case. Each eye received a mean of 3 IAC sessions per eye (median, 3; range, 1–7 sessions). After IAC with a mean follow-up of 19 months, globe salvage was achieved in 72% of primary-treated cases and in 62% of secondary-treated cases. Specifically, primary therapy achieved globe salvage for group B (100%), group C (100%), group D (94%), and group E (36%). Of all 70 eyes, complete regression was achieved for solid tumor in 48 of 51 eyes (94%), subretinal seeds in 40 of 42 eyes (95%), and vitreous seeds in 34 of 39 eyes (87%). After each catheterization (n = 198), the main complications included transient eyelid edema (5%), blepharoptosis (5%), and forehead hyperemia (2%). More lasting complications included vitreous hemorrhage (2%), branch retinal artery obstruction (1%), ophthalmic artery spasm with reperfusion (2%), ophthalmic artery obstruction (2%), partial choroidal ischemia (2%), and optic neuropathy (<1%). Over the past 3 years, the combined incidence of ophthalmic, retinal, and choroidal vascular ischemia was reduced to 1%. There was no patient with stroke, seizure, neurologic impairment, limb ischemia, secondary leukemia, metastasis, or death.

Conclusions.—Five-year experience with IAC indicates that this technique is remarkably effective for the management of retinoblastoma as both a primary and a secondary treatment.

▶ Retinoblastoma is a dangerous ocular malignancy, with high risk for metastasis if untreated. Relatively early detection and treatment has led to survival of 97% or better in the United States. Management options for retinoblastoma include enucleation, intravenous chemotherapy, intra-arterial chemotherapy, and established methods such as laser photocoagulation, thermotherapy, cryotherapy, plaque radiotherapy, and external beam radiotherapy.[1]

Intra-arterial chemotherapy (IAC) has recently risen as an exceptionally powerful treatment option for retinoblastoma. IAC involves selective ophthalmic artery infusion with local high-dose chemotherapy. This requires collaboration of a team of neurosurgeon/interventional neuroradiologist, pediatric oncologist, and ocular oncologist. The technique involves placement of a thin catheter into the femoral artery up to the internal carotid artery and then reaching the orifice of the ophthalmic artery to pulse chemotherapy into the vessel that reaches the eye.[2,3] The benefits of IAC include powerful local control and minimal systemic toxicity. Complications can range from eyelid edema to orbital congestion to vascular compromise of the ophthalmic retinal or choroidal vessels.[4]

In this study by Shields et al, the 5-year experience with IAC for retinoblastoma, based on the International Classification of Retinoblastoma (ICRB), is provided. The ICRB groups eyes with retinoblastoma from least (A) to most (E) advanced based on tumor size, seeding, and hemorrhage.[5] Globe salvage was achieved in 72% of eyes treated with primary IAC. Specifically, primary IAC globe salvage was achieved in 100% for groups B and C eyes, 94% in group D eyes and 36% for group E eyes. Among the group E eyes that failed and came to enucleation, the main retinoblastoma was controlled, but recurrent subretinal or vitreous seeds were the main reason for enucleation. For those eyes treated with IAC as a secondary measure, globe salvage was achieved in 62% of eyes. Overall, in all cases with secondary IAC, tumor control was achieved in 93% of eyes, subretinal seed control in 89%, and vitreous seed control in 89%.

Great strides have been made in the management of retinoblastoma, particularly in advanced eyes with extensive tumor. IAC allows delivery of chemotherapy to save eyes that once would have been enucleated. The future is even brighter because the addition of intravitreal melphalan could lead to even higher globe salvage with possible preservation of vision.

P. G. Iyer, MPH
C. L. Shields, MD

References

1. Shields CL, Shields JA. Retinoblastoma management: advances in enucleation, intravenous chemoreduction, and intra-arterial chemotherapy. *Curr Opin Ophthalmol.* 2010;21:203-212.
2. Shields CL, Ramasubramanian A, Rosenwasser R, Shields JA. Superselective catheterization of the ophthalmic artery for intraarterial chemotherapy for retinoblastoma. *Retina.* 2009;29:1207-1209.
3. Abramson DH, Dunkel IJ, Brodie SE, et al. A phase I/II study of direct intraarterial (ophthalmic artery) chemotherapy with melphalan for intraocular retinoblastoma: initial results. *Ophthalmology.* 2008;115:1398-1404.
4. Shields CL, Bianciotto CG, Jabbour P, et al. Intra-arterial chemotherapy for retinoblastoma: report No. 2, treatment complications. *Arch Ophthalmol.* 2011; 129:1407-1415.
5. Shields CL, Shields JA. Basic understanding of current classification and management of retinoblastoma. *Curr Opin Ophthalmol.* 2006;17:228-234.

Ocular melanoma and the BAP1 hereditary cancer syndrome: implications for the dermatologist

Martorano LM, Winkelmann RR, Cebulla CM, et al (Univ Hosps, Cleveland, OH; Ohio Univ, Athens; The Ohio State Univ, Clolumbus; et al)

Int J Dermatol 53:657-663, 2014

Ocular melanoma is a rare subtype of melanoma, which includes uveal melanoma (UM) and conjunctival melanoma. UM is associated with an increased risk of cutaneous melanoma (CM) in addition to mesothelioma, skin lesions such as epithelioid atypical Spitz tumors, and other internal malignancies due to a germline mutation of the BRCA1-associated protein 1 (*BAP1*) gene. Such familial risks are important for dermatologists to recognize when screening patients with a history of UM for CM and other malignancies. Molecular genetics further help to elucidate the connections between UM and CM by revealing similarities and differences in important mutations among the melanoma subtypes. Both UM and CM have been shown to harbor germline mutation of *BAP1*. However, somatic mutations in either *GNAQ* or *GNA11* are unique to UM tumors and could be used as potential markers to differentiate UM from metastatic CM and act as direct therapeutic targets. However, CM-associated *BRAF* and *CDKN2A* mutations are rare in UM. This review addresses the clinical features, pathogenesis, and current treatment options of UM, focusing on UM and the *BAP1* cancer syndrome to raise awareness of ocular melanoma and its greater role in the predisposition to a hereditary cancer syndrome.

▶ Cutaneous malignant melanoma is responsible for more than 70% of deaths from skin cancer, accounting for approximately 8000 Americans annually. Furthermore, skin melanoma accounts for more than 90% of all melanoma cases, with ocular melanoma representing only 5%. Ocular melanomas generally arise from melanocytes in the uvea (choroid, ciliary body, or iris), and rarely in the conjunctiva.[1] Uveal melanoma (UM) has a poor prognosis with mortality of 50%. The poor prognosis correlates with increasing melanoma thickness.[2] Researchers and physicians have long sought to identify genetic and molecular pathways responsible for the development of UM, metastatic risk, and association with cutaneous melanoma (CM).[3,4]

In this review, Martorano et al look at the relationship between UM and CM and the genetic factors that influence this relationship. They assert that genetics are the driving force of UM development. Somatic mutations in the G-proteins (GNAQ or GNAII), specific to UM, have been detected in 83% of their 186 UM samples and serve as an early event in malignant transformation. GNAQ mutations can lead to constitutive activation of the MAP kinase pathway and set the stage for further somatic mutations of tumor suppressor genes. *BRCA1*-associated protein I (BAPI) is a tumor suppressor gene that Martorano et al identified in 84% of metastasizing UMs. They found that both UM and CM can have germline mutations of BAPI. Inherited defects in BAPI increases a patient's risk of developing UM, CM, and other malignancies. Germline mutations in BAPI have been identified in a small group of patients with UM and are correlated with more aggressive cancer phenotypes.

How is this information clinically relevant? Martorano et al concluded that because UM and CM have been shown to have germline mutations in BAPI and higher frequencies of CMs are found in patients with UM, dermatologists should screen for a family history of cancer in patients with UM. The incidence of UM has remained stable, but the incidence of CM continues to increase. Similarly, ophthalmologists should be aware of the cutaneous findings because patients with UM are at a higher risk for developing CM, especially those with a *BAP-1* mutation.

Early detection of mutations in BAPI is essential in the management of patients with UM, CM, or both to allow detection of other malignancies at an early point. Martorano et al recommend that dermatologists understand the relationship between germline BAPI mutations and screen patients with a history of UM for CM and other malignancies. There is hope to increase awareness of uveal melanoma and its role in the predisposition of hereditary cancer syndrome.

E. B. Elimimian, MPH
C. L. Shields, MD

References

1. Grin JM, Grant-Kels JM, Grin CM, Berke A, Kels BD. Ocular melanomas and melanocytic lesions of the eye. *J Am Acad Dermatol.* 1998;38:716-730.
2. Shields CL, Furuta M, Thangappan A, et al. Metastasis of uveal melanoma millimeter-by-millimeter in 8033 consecutive eyes. *Arch Ophthalmol.* 2009;127: 989-998.
3. Shields CL, Shields JA. Ocular melanoma: relatively rare but requiring respect. *Clin Dermatol.* 2009;27:122-133.
4. Garbe C, Eigentler TK. Diagnosis and treatment of cutaneous melanoma: state of the art 2006. *Melanoma Res.* 2007;17:117-127.

Use of Topical Ice for Local Anesthesia for Intravitreal Injections

Lindsell LB, Miller DM, Brown JL (Univ of Cincinnati, OH; Cincinnati Eye Inst, OH)

JAMA Ophthalmol 132:1010-1011, 2014

Background.—The incidence of a true allergy to topical anesthetics is difficult to quantify because many episodes are adverse reactions rather than true hypersensitivity. Few instances are encountered in clinical practice, since topical anesthetic allergy likely affects less than 1% of the population. For patients with such an allergy, an alternative anesthetic technique is needed. A patient with a history of severe allergy to local anesthetics was given intravitreal injections using an effective alternative.

Case Report.—Woman, in her 60s, had lost vision in her right eye and reported having experienced anaphylaxis or a severe anaphylactic reaction to lidocaine. Visual acuity was 20/200 OD and 20/20

OS. She was found to have moderate drusen, retinal pigment epithelium atrophy, and temporal perifoveal subretinal hemorrhage with pigment epithelium detachment and subfoveal fluid in the right eye. The left eye had moderate drusen and retinal pigment epithelium atrophy. The diagnosis was neovascular age-related macular degeneration in the right eye and drusen without neovascularization in the left. The treatment chosen was intravitreal bevacizumab. Ice topical anesthesia was used to perform this procedure.

Before the povidone-iodine was instilled, an ice pack was created using a sterile glove filled with small ice cubes or chips. This was applied to the closed temporal aspect of the inner eyelid for 1 or 2 minutes, when the patient reported the eyelid was sufficiently numbed. The patient was asked to look up and one glove finger filled with ice was applied directly to the inferotemporal bulbar conjunctiva for about 2 minutes to achieve anesthesia, after which the injection was given.

Analysis.—Local anesthetics can be classified as esters or amides and cross-reactivity between these classes is rare but not impossible. Sensitivity to an agent does not imply that the patient will also be sensitive to other agents in the same class. If the patient does not respond to the anesthetic with an anaphylactic reaction, the practitioner may consider a trial of anesthetic from the opposite class or refer the patient for skin patch testing to confirm a true allergy or the safety of using an alternative anesthetic. In addition, the patient may be reacting to the anesthetic or the preservative, with the latter often being a para-aminobenzoic acid (PABA) metabolite allergy, which manifests as sensitivity to both classes of anesthetic. A preservative-free anesthetic can be used for patients with PABA allergy.

If the patient is truly allergic to local anesthetics or simply afraid because of a previous severe reaction, ice may be an effective alternative. Analgesia using ice is achieved through its ability to slow or reduce nerve conduction through cooling as well as produce localized vasoconstriction. Ice anesthesia occurs quickly and is sustained for 5 to 10 minutes or longer, which is more than long enough to perform an intravitreal injection.

Conclusions.—Ice analgesia is a simple, inexpensive alternative to the use of topical anesthetic agents. Patients with allergic symptoms or fear of developing such symptoms can be managed with ice anesthesia for many short procedures.

▶ Documented use of ice as a local anesthetic dates back to the 18th and 19th centuries.[1] Examples include chilling a limb before amputation or applying a rabbit's bladder with ice and salt inside for dental procedures. The use of these methods was warranted and necessitated because of the lack of other effective alternatives at the time, but it also did not suffer from the side effects and adverse reactions that our modern anesthetics can cause. Currently, ophthalmologists face a unique challenge when it comes to providing appropriate local anesthetic to diverse patient populations and in diverse clinical settings. There continues to be potentially painful procedures in our field such as intravitreal injection for retinal conditions. Hence, there is an interest in anesthetic alternatives.

Traditional local anesthetics, such as topical proparacaine 0.5%, or proparacaine 0.5% with 4% lidocaine-soaked cotton tipped swabs, and 3.5% lidocaine gel, have been shown effective in preventing pain during intravitreal injections in most patients.[2] If there is a mild allergic reaction to an anesthetic then an agent from the opposite class (eg, ester or amide) may be tried. Ester anesthetics are metabolized to a para-aminobenzoic acid (PABA) metabolite, whereas preservatives prepared with amide anesthetics are metabolized to PABA itself. Therefore, patients with PABA allergies would benefit from either lidocaine or topical ice anesthesia. Lindsell et al present a case in which the patient had an adverse reaction to lidocaine and was further treated with only topical ice as anesthesia preceding intravitreal injections.

In such precautionary cases, topical ice can be an effective alternative. To achieve adequate local anesthesia with topical ice, a sterile glove filled with small ice cubes or ice chips is to be applied to the closed temporal aspect of the lower eyelid and held in place for 1 to 2 minutes. After the patient claims numbness, the patient should look upward while one of the glove fingers filled with ice is directly applied to the inferotemporal bulbar conjunctiva and held in position for 2 minutes. In this instance, the patient described minimal to no discomfort with this method. Analgesia achieved from topical ice appears to be multifactorial. Factors contributing to its anesthetic quality include slowed nerve conduction, vasoconstriction that reduces pain substance release, and endorphin release potentiation. This technique is simple and inexpensive, which lends implications for its use in situations in which patient allergies exist and clinical settings in which financial or other limitations might exist.

B. M. Lawson, BS
C. L. Shields, MD

References

1. Zimmer M. History of anaesthesia: early forms of local anaesthesia. *Eur J Anaesthesiol.* 2014;31:1-12.
2. Davis MJ, Pollack JS, Shott S. Comparison of topical anesthetics for intravitreal injections: a randomized clinical trial. *Retina.* 2012;32:701-705.

Expanding the Clinical Phenotype of Hereditary *BAP1* Cancer Predisposition Syndrome, Reporting Three New Cases

Pilarski R, Cebulla CM, Massengill JB, et al (The Ohio State Univ, Columbus; et al)

Genes Chromosomes Cancer 53:177-182, 2014

The clinical phenotype of *BAP1* hereditary cancer predisposition syndrome (MIM 614327) includes uveal melanoma (UM), cutaneous melanoma (CM), renal cell carcinoma (RCC), and mesothelioma. However, the frequency of the syndrome in patients with UM and the association with other cancers are still not clear. In this study, we screened 46 previously untested, unrelated UM patients with high risk for hereditary cancer for germline mutation in *BAP1*. We also studied four additional patients with a personal or family history suggestive of *BAP1* hereditary cancer syndrome. We identified three patients with germline pathogenic mutations (c.2050 C>T, pGln684*; c.1182C>G, p.Tyr394*, and c.1882_1885delTCAC, p. Ser628Profs*8) in *BAP1*. Two of these three patients presented with UM and the third with a metastatic adenocarcinoma likely from a hepatic cholangiocarcinoma. Reported family histories included UM, mesothelioma, RCC, CM, and several other internal malignancies. The results of this study confirm the association between germline *BAP1* mutation and predisposition to UM, mesothelioma, CM and RCC. However, other cancers, such as cholangiocarcinoma and breast carcinoma may be part of the phenotype of this hereditary cancer predisposition syndrome. In addition, the results support the existence of other candidate genes in addition to *BAP1* contributing to hereditary predisposition to UM.

▶ Uveal melanoma is the most common primary cancer of the eye,[1] and it is rarely associated with familial predisposition.[2,3] More recently, it has been found that individuals with germline mutations of the BRCA1-associated protein 1 (*BAP1*) gene on chromosome 3p21 have an increased risk of developing uveal melanoma (UM), as well as malignant mesothelioma (MM), cutaneous melanoma (CM), renal cell carcinoma (RCC), and melanocytic *BAP1*-mutated atypical intradermal tumors (MBAITs).[4] The classic findings of *BAP1* hereditary cancer predisposition syndrome are still relatively new, and ongoing investigation continues to define the complete phenotypic spectrum of cancers associated with *BAP1* germline mutations.

In this report, Pilarski et al evaluated 46 patients presenting with UM and 4 patients with a personal or family history suggesting *BAP1* hereditary cancer predisposition syndrome. Of the 50 patients, 3 were reported to have germline pathogenic mutations in *BAP1* (6%). The patients with a germline mutation in the *BAP1* gene reported a history of cancers that included UM, MM, CM, and RCC, supporting previous studies regarding the presentation of *BAP1* hereditary cancer predisposition syndrome. These patients also reported other types of cancer, such as hepatic cholangiocarcinoma and breast carcinoma. A family history of breast, pancreatic, and ovarian cancers were additionally found in the first- and second-degree relatives of the 3 patients with the germline *BAP1* mutation.

Pilarski et al concluded that other cancers, such as cholangiocarcinoma and breast carcinoma, might also be added to the phenotype in germline *BAP1* mutations. Further research into this mutation, along with the host and environmental factors that lead to malignancy in different organ systems, should be explored.

These authors suggest that patients with known germline BAP1 mutation should be evaluated as follows:

1. Annual ophthalmological examinations beginning at age 11 years.
2. Annual dermatological examinations starting at age 22 years.

3. Adherence to the American Cancer Society screening guidelines for other types of cancers.
4. Follow-up with primary care physicians for signs and symptoms of other cancers.

At present, it is important for ophthalmologists to understand the relationship between *BAP1* hereditary cancer predisposition syndrome and the increased risk of developing UM and other cancers.

R. House, BA
C. Shields, MD

References

1. Shields CL, Manalac J, Das C, Ferguson K, Shields JA. Choroidal melanoma. Clinical features, classification, and top 10 pseudomelanomas. *Curr Opin Ophthalmol.* 2014;25:177-185.
2. Harbour JW, Onken MD, Roberson EDO, et al. Frequent mutation of BAP1 in metastasizing uveal melanomas. *Science.* 2010;330:1410-1413.
3. Höiom V, Edsgärd D, Helgadottir H, et al. Hereditary uveal melanoma: a report of a germline mutation in BAP1. *Genes Chromosomes Cancer.* 2013;52:378-384.
4. Carbone M, Ferris LK, Baumann F, et al. BAP1 cancer syndrome: malignant mesothelioma, uveal and cutaneous melanoma, and MBAITs. *J Transl Med.* 2012;10:179.

Effect of Selumetinib vs Chemotherapy on Progression-Free Survival in Uveal Melanoma: A Randomized Clinical Trial

Carvajal RD, Sosman JA, Quevedo JF, et al (Memorial Sloan-Kettering Cancer Ctr, NY; Vanderbilt Univ Med Ctr, Nashville, TN; Mayo Clinic, Rochester, MN; et al)
JAMA 311:2397-2405, 2014

Importance.—Uveal melanoma is characterized by mutations in *GNAQ* and *GNA11*, resulting in mitogen-activated protein kinase pathway activation.

Objective.—To assess the efficacy of selumetinib, a selective, non-adenosine triphosphate competitive inhibitor of MEK1 and MEK2, in uveal melanoma.

Design, Setting, and Participants.—Randomized, open-label, phase 2 clinical trial comparing selumetinib vs chemotherapy conducted from August 2010 through December 2013 among 120 patients with metastatic uveal melanoma at 15 academic oncology centers in the United States and Canada.

Interventions.—One hundred one patients were randomized in a 1:1 ratio to receive selumetinib, 75 mg orally twice daily on a continual basis (n = 50), or chemotherapy (temozolomide, 150 mg/m^2 orally daily for 5 of every 28 days, or dacarbazine, 1000 mg/m^2 intravenously every 21 days [investigator choice]; n = 51) until disease progression, death, intolerable adverse effects, or withdrawal of consent. After primary outcome analysis, 19 patients were registered and 18 treated with selumetinib without randomization to complete the planned 120-patient enrollment. Patients in the chemotherapy group could receive selumetinib at the time of radiographic progression.

Main Outcomes and Measures.—Progression-free survival, the primary end point, was assessed as of April 22, 2013. Additional end points, including overall survival, response rate, and safety/toxicity, were assessed as of December 31, 2013.

Results.—Median progression-free survival among patients randomized to chemotherapy was 7 weeks (95% CI, 4.3-8.4 weeks; median treatment duration, 8 weeks; interquartile range [IQR], 4.3-16 weeks) and among those randomized to selumetinib was 15.9 weeks (95% CI, 8.4-21.1 weeks; median treatment duration, 16.1 weeks; IQR, 8.1-25.3 weeks) (hazard ratio, 0.46; 95% CI, 0.30-0.71; $P < .001$). Median overall survival time was 9.1 months (95% CI, 6.1-11.1 months) with chemotherapy and 11.8 months (95% CI, 9.8-15.7 months) with selumetinib (hazard ratio, 0.66; 95% CI, 0.41-1.06; $P = .09$). No objective responses were observed with chemotherapy. Forty-nine percent of patients treated with selumetinib achieved tumor regression, with 14% achieving an objective radiographic response to therapy. Treatment-related adverse events were observed in 97% of patients treated with selumetinib, with 37% requiring at least 1 dose reduction.

Conclusions and Relevance.—In this hypothesis-generating study of patients with advanced uveal melanoma, selumetinib compared with chemotherapy resulted in a modestly improved progression-free survival and response rate; however, no improvement in overall survival was observed. Improvement in clinical outcomes was accompanied by a high rate of adverse events.

Trial Registration.—clinicaltrials.gov Identifier: NCT01143402.

▶ Uveal melanoma is the most common intraocular tumor in adults and carries a serious prognosis. Of all cases of uveal melanoma, approximately 50% develop metastatic disease and prognosis following metastasis is poor. To date, there are no systemic therapies approved to treat metastatic uveal melanoma. These tumors are often associated with oncogenic mutations in the *GNAQ* or *GNA11* genes, both of which normally encode for essential proteins in the mitogen-activated protein kinase (MAPK) pathway. Disruption of this pathway disturbs normal cell division, leading to abnormal cell proliferation. Selumetinib is an orally active agent that has been demonstrated to inhibit the MAPK pathway, which should theoretically improve outcomes in uveal melanoma patients. Thus far, selumetinib has been investigated in both preclinical and clinical settings to determine efficacy for non-small cell lung cancer, thyroid cancer, and uveal melanoma.

In this report, Carvajal and associates performed a randomized, controlled, phase 2 clinical trial that compared selumetinib to chemotherapy in patients with metastatic uveal melanoma. The treatment group was limited to chemotherapy-naive patients because previous studies had shown that the efficacy of selumetinib decreased when administered to patients who had received chemotherapy. Selumetinib was administered with randomization to 50 patients and administered without randomization to 19 patients, and temozolomide or dacarbazine was administered with randomization to 51 patients. Progression-free survival was shown to be 15.9 weeks with selumetinib and 7 weeks with chemotherapy. The 4-month progression-free survival rate was 43.1% with selumetinib and 8.5% with chemotherapy. However, overall survival was not significantly improved, and treatment with selumetinib was associated with a high rate of adverse events.

Carvajal et al provide further validation of Patel et al,[1] who also suggested that advanced uveal melanoma can respond to systemic therapy, a finding that had not been demonstrated with any other drug to date. The promising results of this current report suggest that in addition to uveal melanoma, other advanced malignancies caused by mutations in the MAPK pathway may also show a similar response to therapies that inhibit this pathway. The authors plan to confirm their conclusions in ongoing phase 3 clinical trials of this drug.

J. E. Landy, BA
C. L. Shields, MD

Reference

1. Patel M, Smyth E, Chapman PB, et al. Therapeutic implications of the emerging molecular biology of uveal melanoma. *Clin Cancer Res*. 2011;17:2087-2100.

12 Pathology

Eyelid Sebaceous Carcinoma: Clinicopathologic and Multiparametric Immunohistochemical Analysis That Includes Adipophilin

Jakobiec FA, Mendoza PR (Massachusetts Eye and Ear Infirmary, Boston; Harvard Med School, Boston, MA)

Am J Ophthalmol 157:186-208.e2, 2014

Purpose.—To evaluate the fine cytopathologic features and immunohistochemistry of eyelid sebaceous carcinoma.

Design.—Retrospective clinicopathologic study.

Methods.—Clinical records and microscopic glass slides of 12 patients diagnosed with sebaceous carcinoma were reviewed. Paraffin-embedded tissue recuts were immunoreacted for epithelial membrane antigen (EMA), Ber-EP4, p53, Ki-67, and adipophilin for cytoplasmic lipid. Invasive growth and intraepithelial spread were analyzed separately. Cytoplasmic and nuclear characteristics were correlated with the results of the immunohistochemical profiling.

Results.—Five patients experienced recurrences, but no metastases or tumor-related deaths were discovered. The nuclei in 11 invasive tumor cells were typically round with finely divided, granular, or smudgy chromatin without prominent margination at the nuclear membrane; they exhibited small punctate nucleoli. Positivity for EMA (both diffuse and focal), p53 (72% of nuclei), and Ki-67 (45% proliferation index) was demonstrated. Adipophilin positivity in vesicular and granular forms was detected in paraffin sections in all invasive tumors, most prominently in moderately differentiated and well-differentiated lesions. Among 9 cases exhibiting intraepithelial extensions, 6 showed mostly granular positivity and 3 vesicular positivity. p53 identified residual atypical intraepithelial cells when conjunctival epithelial sloughing occurred.

Conclusions.—Immunohistochemistry can make significant contributions to the diagnosis of sebaceous carcinoma. p53 and vesicular granular adipophilin positivity were highly reliable in supplementing the routine microscopic diagnosis of infiltrative tumors and both can be used in paraffin sections, thereby obviating cumbersome oil red O staining of frozen sections. The cells found in intraepithelial spread were strongly EMA and p53 positive, with more granular than vesicular adipophilin positivity (Table 3).

▶ There is a wealth of information in this retrospective clinicopathologic study by Jakobiec and Mendoza, the aim of which was to evaluate the cytopathologic

TABLE 3.—Sebaceous Carcinoma of the Eyelids: Helpful Histopathologic and Immunohistochemical Features in Differential Diagnosis

Parameter	Sebaceous Carcinoma	Epidermoid (Squamous) Carcinoma	Basal Cell Carcinoma
Nuclear characteristics	Round, delicate, finely divided, nonmarginated chromatin; punctate nucleolus	Vesicular; marginated chromatin; prominent nucleolus	Small, dark, compact; inconspicuous nucleolus
Cytoplasmic characteristics	Absent peripheral palisading and clefting. variably vacuolated, diaphanous, occasionally eosinophilic	Eosinophilic, uncommon clear cell variant	Scant
Epithelial membrane antigen (EMA)	+	+	−
Ber-EP4	−	−	+
Ki-67 (nuclear pattern)	45%	<25%[a]	<10%[b]
p53 (nuclear pattern)	72%	<50%	<20%[b]
Adipophilin (cytoplasmic pattern)	+	−[c]	−
Androgen receptor (nuclear pattern)[d]	+(100%)	−(100%)	+(40%-60%)

+, Present in > 10% of cells; −, present in < 10% of cells or more often none.

[a]Reference: Ohara M, Sotozono C, Tsuchihashi Y, Kinoshita S. Ki-67 labeling index as a marker of malignancy in ocular surface neoplasms. *Jpn J Ophthalmol* 2004;48(6):524-529.

[b]Sclerosing, infiltrative, and metatypical tumors had values twice as high. Reference: Barrett TL, Smith KJ, Hodge JJ, Butler R, Hall FW, Skelton HG. Immunohistochemical nuclear staining for p53, PCNA, and Ki-67 in different histologic variants of basal cell carcinoma. *J Am Acad Dermatol* 1997;37(3 Pt 1):430-437.

[c]Small collections of adipophilin granules can be present in foci of necrosis.

[d]References: (1) Bayer-Garner IB, Givens V, Smoller B. Immunohistochemical staining for androgen receptors: a sensitive marker of sebaceous differentiation.

Am J Dermatopathol 1999;21(5):426-431. (2) Asadi-Amoli F, Khoshnevis F, Haeri H, Jahanzad I, Pazira R, Shahsiah R. Comparative examination of androgen receptor reactivity for differential diagnosis of sebaceous carcinoma from squamous cell and basal cell carcinoma. *Am J Clin Pathol* 2010;134(1):22-26.

features and immunohistochemistry of eyelid sebaceous carcinomas. Twelve cases of sebaceous carcinomas were included in the study. Representative sections were reviewed from each case, which totaled 119 specimens. Of these specimens, 44 contained histopathologic evidence of sebaceous carcinoma, and 25 of them underwent further immunohistochemical (IHC) analysis with the following IHC probes: epithelial membrane antigen (EBA), Ber-EP4, p53, Ki-67, and adipophilin. Although no controls or examples of other epithelial tumors were included in the study, the authors were able to abundantly highlight histologic and IHC differences between normal and other epithelial tumors with findings in sebaceous carcinoma given their extensive knowledge and experience. A comprehensive description of the histopathologic findings was reported, which was summarized in the invaluable table included here.

Of note, the authors specify the utility of p53 IHC staining in assessing intraepithelial spread from sebaceous carcinoma. After processing and sectioning, the epithelium may be sloughed off in areas with intraepithelial spread, making it difficult to microscopically analyze the specimen. p53 IHC staining could be beneficial in these instances, where positivity, according to the authors, should be regarded "as presumptive evidence of spread of sebaceous carcinoma."

In addition to the helpful histologic descriptions, the article provides a valuable protocol when approaching a case suspicious for sebaceous carcinoma. This protocol includes adipophilin IHC, the utility of which is also highlighted in the study by Milman et al. In summary, when IHC stains are used, EMA and p53 should be performed initially. If either or both are positive, then diagnosis should be confirmed with adipophilin staining. As underscored by others, however, the authors "point out that IHC staining should be performed after careful standard microscopic evaluation raises the prospect of sebaceous carcinoma."

V. Lee, MD

Diagnostic Utility of Adipophilin Immunostain in Periocular Carcinomas

Milman T, Schear MJ, Eagle RC Jr (The New York Eye and Ear Infirmary; New York Inst of Technology College of Osteopathic Medicine; Wills Eye Hosp, Philadelphia, PA)

Ophthalmology 121:964-971, 2014

Purpose.—To determine the efficacy of adipophilin immunohistochemistry in the diagnosis of sebaceous carcinoma of the ocular adnexal region and to provide the guidelines for interpretation of this immunostain.

Design.—Retrospective, histopathologic case series.

Participants.—A total of 25 patients with sebaceous carcinoma, 21 patients with basal cell carcinoma, 22 patients with conjunctival squamous cell carcinoma, 9 patients with cutaneous squamous cell carcinoma, and 5 patients with conjunctival mucoepidermoid carcinoma.

Methods.—Immunohistochemical staining for adipophilin was performed on paraffin-embedded tissues and correlated with hematoxylin–eosin, periodic acid–Schiff (PAS), and mucicarmine-stained preparations. Immunostaining was quantified by light microscopy and with a computerized image analysis system of scanned images. Statistical analysis was performed to compare immunostaining patterns within the tumor categories by stage and grade, between the different neoplasms, and for correlation between light microscopy observations and computerized image analysis.

Main Outcome Measures.—Localization of adipophilin immunostain, intensity of immunostaining, percent of immunoreactive cells, percentages of vacuolar staining and granular staining, and vacuole size.

Results.—Adipophilin expression was observed in 100% of sebaceous carcinomas, 100% of cutaneous squamous cell carcinomas, 95% of basal cell carcinomas, 73% of conjunctival squamous cell carcinomas, and 60% of mucoepidermoid carcinomas. Sebaceous carcinomas demonstrated significantly stronger adipophilin expression, a greater number of intracytoplasmic vacuoles, and larger vacuoles. The specificity and sensitivity of adipophilin immunostaining in the diagnosis of sebaceous carcinoma were both 100% when more than 5% of the staining occurred in vacuoles (<95% granular staining). The diagnostic sensitivity and specificity were 100% and 96%, respectively, when the staining was graded as moderately or strongly intense and were 92% and 85% when the vacuoles were greater than 1.5 μm in diameter.

Conclusions.—Although upregulation of neoplastic steatogenesis is observed in both sebaceous and nonsebaceous carcinomas, the pattern and intensity of adipophilin immunostaining are helpful in distinguishing sebaceous carcinoma from other neoplasms with overlapping histology (Figs 1 and 2).

▶ The purpose of this thoughtful and well-conducted study is to determine the relevance and utility of adipophilin immunohistochemistry (IHC) in diagnosing periocular sebaceous carcinoma. Sebaceous carcinoma is an uncommon malignant epithelial tumor with a propensity for the periocular area. Histologically, sebaceous carcinoma presents as a range from well-differentiated lobulated sebaceous cells with foamy cytoplasm to infiltrating, undifferentiated cells with marked nuclear pleomorphism, hyperchromatism, and minimal intracytoplasmic lipid. Classic presentations of the tumor require only light microscopy for diagnosis and no additional stains. However, poorly differentiated tumors are challenging, such that prior reports in the literature have found that 23% to 77% of cases are misdiagnosed. Accurate diagnosis of sebaceous carcinoma is critical because its management and treatment differs from the management and treatment of other epithelial tumors. Historically, Oil Red O and/or Sudan Black IV were used in aiding the diagnosis of sebaceous carcinoma, but these stains are difficult to perform and require fresh tissue. Since then, several immunohistochemical stains have been used, such as low molecular weight cytokeratins, epithelial membrane antigen, Ber-EP4, and cancer antigen 19-9. However, the development of an immunohistochemical stain against lipid droplet-associated proteins in formalin fixed paraffin embedded tissues, such as adipophilin (adipocyte-differentiation-related protein), opens up an unexplored welcomed frontier. Its utility in sebaceous carcinoma needs to be determined.

The authors conducted a retrospective, histopathologic case series, examining specimens from a total of 82 patients, of which 25 were sebaceous carcinomas, 21 were basal cell carcinomas, 22 were conjunctival squamous cell carcinoma, 9 were cutaneous squamous cell carcinomas, and 5 were mucoepidermoid carcinomas. Normal sebaceous glands and skin served as controls. IHC staining with adipophilin was graded and analyzed by 3 pathologists and with Aperio imaging analysis. As expected, adipophilin staining was found to some degree in all tumor groups. The value of this study, however, lies in the meticulous examination of the degree and pattern of adipophilin staining. Examples of sebaceous and nonsebaceous carcinomas are shown in Figs 1 and 2, which

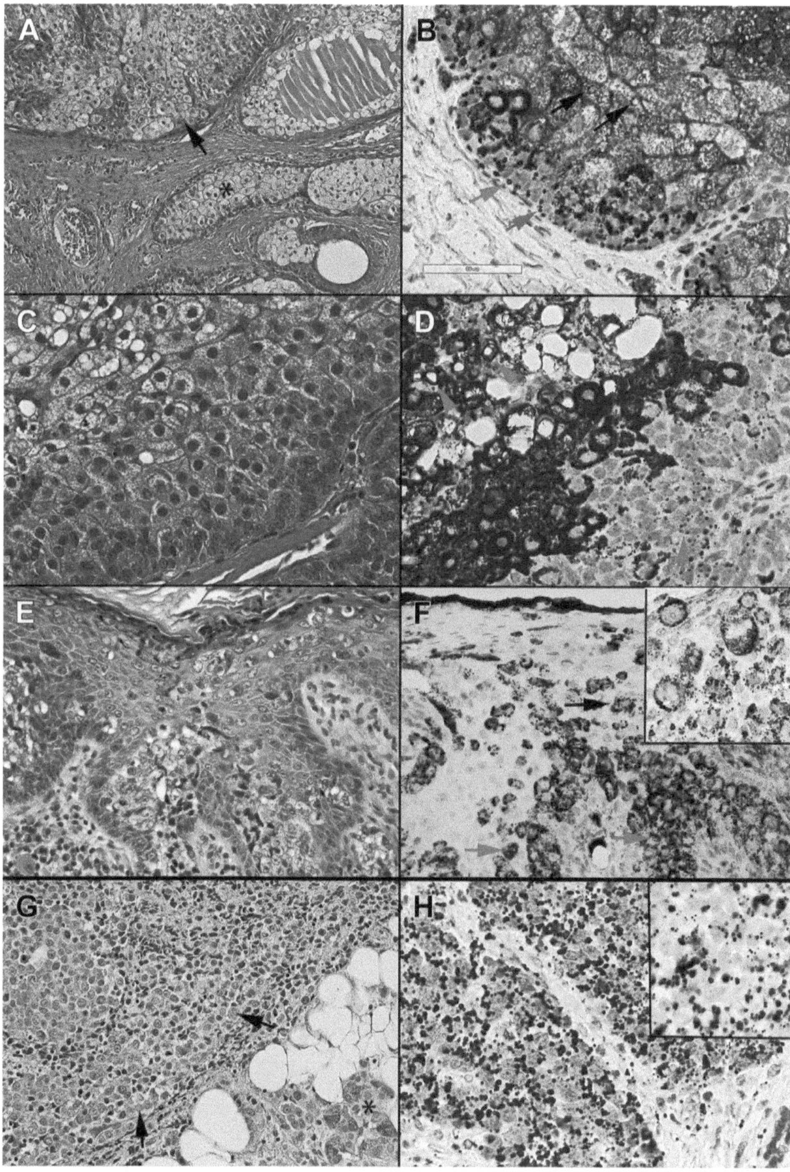

FIGURE 1.—Adipophilin expression in sebaceous carcinoma and normal sebaceous glands. **A,** Nests of well-differentiated sebaceous carcinoma with abundant mature sebocytes (*arrow*) adjacent to the lobules of normal sebaceous glands (*asterisk*) are present. **B,** Within the normal sebaceous gland, adipophilin is expressed as minute vacuoles and granules in germinative cells (*red arrows*), gradually increasing in size with maturation of sebocytes (*black arrows*). **C, D,** Within the well-differentiated sebaceous carcinoma, the adipophilin is similarly expressed as small vacuoles and granules in outer undifferentiated cells (*arrow*) progressing to larger vacuoles in well-differentiated central cells (*arrowheads*). **E, F,** Moderately differentiated sebaceous carcinoma cells infiltrate the epidermis in a pagetoid pattern and demonstrate strong, diffuse immunoreactivity for adipophilin as confluent medium-sized intracytoplasmic vacuoles (*red arrows*) and small vacuoles and granules (*black arrow*). **G, H,** Poorly differentiated sebaceous carcinoma (*arrows*) metastatic to the lymph node and gland (*asterisk*) demonstrates moderate to strong immunoreactivity for adipophilin in nearly all neoplastic cells, manifesting as small vacuoles and granules. Stain, hematoxylin–eosin (**A, C, E, G**); antibody, adipophilin (**B, D, F, H**); original magnification ×50 (A), ×250 (**B, C, D**), ×100 (**E, F, G, H**). For Interpretation of the references to color in this figure legend, the reader is referred to web version of this article. (Reprinted from Ophthalmology. Milman T, Schear MJ, Eagle RC Jr. Diagnostic utility of adipophilin immunostain in periocular carcinomas. *Ophthalmology.* 2014;121:964-971, Copyright 2014, with permission from American Academy of Ophthalmology.)

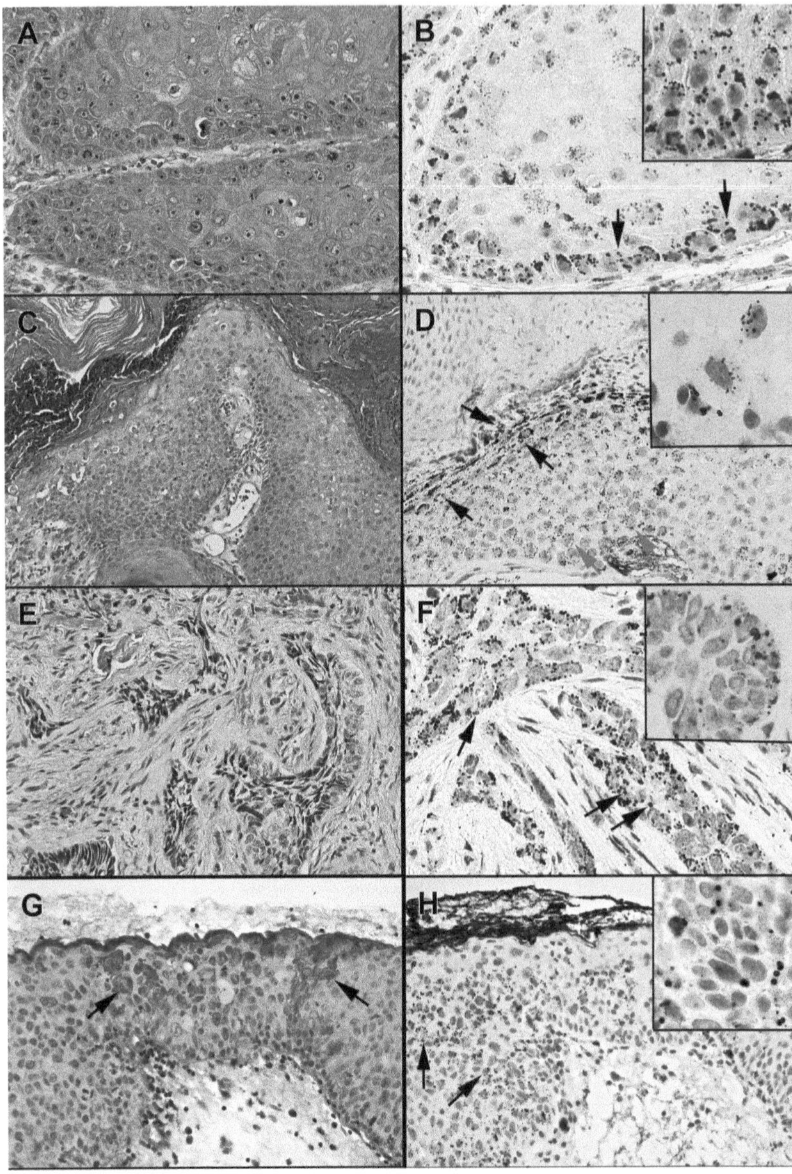

FIGURE 2.—Adipophilin expression in nonsebaceous carcinomas. **A, B**, Well-differentiated keratinizing conjunctival squamous cell carcinoma demonstrates weak to moderate immunoreactivity for adipophilin, predominantly in the neoplastic basal epithelial cells as confluent perinuclear granules and rare small vacuoles (*black arrows*). The neoplastic cells with more prominent squamous differentiation demonstrate minute perinuclear granules (*red arrow*). **C, D**, Well differentiated cutaneous squamous cell carcinoma demonstrates small perinuclear adipophilin vacuoles in the superficial squamous cells and in overlying parakeratin. Most of the neoplastic cells in deeper parts of the tumor demonstrate weak, granular intracytoplasmic immunoreactivity for adipophilin (*red arrows*). **E, F**, Bands of moderately differentiated morpheaform basal cell carcinoma demonstrate focal, weak-to-moderate immunoreactivity for adipophilin in a form of rare small vacuoles (*arrows*) and granules. **G**, PAS—stained preparation after diastase digestion highlights presence of intracytoplasmic mucin in the neoplastic epithelial cells (*arrows*), consistent with mucoepidermoid carcinoma. **H**, Adipophilin immunostain demonstrates weak, focal granular staining that does not appear to correspond to intracytoplasmic mucin. The inset highlights rare vacuoles in the neoplastic cells. Stains, hematoxylin—eosin (**A, C, E**) and PAS postdiastase (**G**); antibody, adipophilin (**B, D, F, H**); original magnification ×150 (**A**), ×250 (**B, F**), ×100 (**C, D, E, G, H**). For Interpretation of the references to color in this figure legend, the reader is referred to web version of this article. (Reprinted from Ophthalmology. Milman T, Schear MJ, Eagle RC Jr. Diagnostic utility of adipophilin immunostain in periocular carcinomas. *Ophthalmology.* 2014;121:964-971,Copyright 2014, with permission from American Academy of Ophthalmology.)

effectively demonstrate the different patterns observed between these 2 groups of periocular carcinomas.

The authors concluded that "the presence of greater than 5% vacuoles and less than 95% granules to be 100% sensitive and 100% specific in distinguishing sebaceous carcinoma from other periocular and ocular carcinomas." In addition, moderate to strong adipophilin immunostaining intensity also supported the diagnosis of sebaceous carcinoma. However, the authors caution that further studies need to be performed in cases of poorly differentiated tumors. This is evidenced in the figures reproduced here, where one can imagine overlap between adipophilin staining patterns between a poorly differentiated sebaceous carcinoma and one of the other periocular epithelial carcinomas. As with any IHC staining, the positive predictive value is only meaningful when there is sufficient suspicion for a diagnosis of sebaceous carcinoma on light microscopy. In these cases, judicious and rational use of IHC staining enhances the diagnostic utility of these additional studies.

V. Lee, MD

Characterisation of retinoblastomas without *RB1* mutations: genomic, gene expression, and clinical studies

Rushlow DE, Mol BM, Kennett JY, et al (Univ Health Network, Toronto, Ontario, Canada; VU Univ Med Ctr Amsterdam, Netherlands; Univ of British Columbia, Vancouver, Canada)

Lancet Oncol 14:327-334, 2013

Background.—Retinoblastoma is the childhood retinal cancer that defined tumour-suppressor genes. Previous work shows that mutation of both alleles of the *RB1* retinoblastoma suppressor gene initiates disease. We aimed to characterise non-familial retinoblastoma tumours with no detectable *RB1* mutations.

Methods.—Of 1068 unilateral non-familial retinoblastoma tumours, we compared those with no evidence of *RB1* mutations ($RB1^{+/+}$) with tumours carrying a mutation in both alleles ($RB1^{-/-}$). We analysed genomic copy number, *RB1* gene expression and protein function, retinal gene expression, histological features, and clinical data.

Findings.—No *RB1* mutations ($RB1^{+/+}$) were reported in 29 (2·7%) of 1068 unilateral retinoblastoma tumours. 15 of the 29 $RB1^{+/+}$ tumours had high-level *MYCN* oncogene amplification (28–121 copies; $RB1^{+/+}$ $MYCN^{A}$), whereas none of 93 $RB1^{-/-}$ primary tumours tested showed *MYCN* amplification ($p < 0{\cdot}0001$). $RB1^{+/+}MYCN^{A}$ tumours expressed functional RB1 protein, had fewer overall genomic copy-number changes in genes characteristic of retinoblastoma than did $RB1^{-/-}$ tumours, and showed distinct aggressive histological features. *MYCN* amplification was the sole copy-number change in one $RB1^{+/+}MYCN^{A}$ retinoblastoma. One additional *MYCNA* tumour was discovered after the initial frequencies were determined, and this is included in further analyses. Median age at diagnosis of the 17 children with $RB1^{+/+}MYCN^{A}$ tumours was

4·5 months (IQR 3·5–10), compared with 24 months (15–37) for 79 children with nonfamilial unilateral *RB1*$^{-/-}$ retinoblastoma.

Interpretation.—Amplification of the *MYCN* oncogene might initiate retinoblastoma in the presence of non-mutated *RB1* genes. These unilateral *RB1*$^{+/+}$*MYCN*^{A} retinoblastomas are characterised by distinct histological features, only a few of the genomic copy-number changes that are characteristic of retinoblastoma, and very early age of diagnosis.

▶ This perspicacious study by Rushlow et al provides a mechanistic clue to the oncogenic driving force in the development of retinoblastomas that do not harbor RB1 mutations. Children with bilateral retinoblastoma constitute about 40% of all cases. According to Knudson's hypothesis, these children carry a constitutional RB1 mutation that predisposes them to retinoblastoma development. The other 60% of children have unilateral, nonfamilial disease. The predominant theory is that mutations in both RB1 alleles cause all cases of retinoblastoma. Therefore, if an RB1 mutation is not elucidated by standard genetic testing, translocations, deep intronic mutations, or alterations in unknown RB1 regulatory regions are suspected. However, 2 independent laboratories recently discovered a possible alternative mechanism in RB1 +/+ tumors, specifically MYCN oncogene amplification. The aim of this study is to further investigate other genetic causes for unilateral retinoblastomas with nonmutated RB1 alleles.

Five clinical laboratories reviewed a total of 1068 cases of unilateral retinoblastomas. Of those cases, 30 were found to harbor no RB1 mutations. Further examination of these RB1 +/+ cases found MYCN amplification in 16 cases. None of the RB1-/- primary tumors tested showed more than 10 MYCN copies, whereas a little more than half of the RB1 +/+ tumors showed high-level MYCN amplification (28-121 copies of MYCN), which was statistically significant.

Clinical correlation found that children with RB1 +/+ MYCNA retinoblastomas presented at a much younger age (average age, 4.5 months) than children with unilateral RB1-/- retinoblastomas (average age, 24 months). In addition, these tumors were often found to be larger and more invasive relative to the young age at presentation. Histologically, RB1 +/+ MYCNA tumors have distinctive histologic features, such as a predominance of undifferentiated round blue cells with large prominent, multiple nucleoli; necrosis; apoptosis; and little calcification. These features are reminiscent of those seen in other MYCNA embryonic tumors, such as neuroblastoma. However, rosettes, nuclear molding, and other features characteristic of RB1-/- retinoblastoma were absent.

The authors estimated from their study that 18% of children with nonfamilial unilateral retinoblastoma diagnosed at age 6 months or younger will have RB1 +/+ MYCNA retinoblastoma. This study supports the idea that the RB1 +/+ retinoblastoma group is likely heterogeneous, harboring other oncogenic mutations besides RB1. Although the authors showed well that MYCN amplification may be a causative mechanism in half of the RB1 +/+ cases studied, further studies need to be performed to elucidate the genetic alterations of the remaining cases.

V. Lee, MD

A new rosette in retinoblastoma

Das D, Bhattacharjee K, Barthakur SS, et al (Uveitis and Neuro-Ophthalmology Services, Guwahati, Assam, India; Sri Sankaradeva Nethralaya, Guwahati, Assam, India)

Indian J Ophthalmol 62:638-641, 2014

Retinoblastoma, the most common primary malignant intraocular tumor of childhood is a great success story in pediatric and ocular oncology. Pathology of retinoblastoma is important to guide the treatment modalities. Differentiated retinoblastoma is commonly seen in younger age group. Since a hundred years, we have been observing two typical true rosettes in retinoblastoma in the form of Flexner-Wintersteiner (FW) and Homer Wright (HW) rosettes and in many occasions pseudorosettes have been documented. In the present case report, a third new type of rosette was identified in a differentiated retinoblastoma which had an unusual anterior segment involvement.

▶ The authors describe a new rosette seen in a case of retinoblastoma in a 2-month-old female infant. Rosettes, in general, refer to a histologic architectural pattern seen in a variety of neural tumors. Cells are typically arranged in a halo or spoke-wheel arrangement that surrounds either a cluster of cytoplasmic processes or empty space. Two classic rosettes have been described in retinoblastomas, Homer Wright and Flexner-Wintersteiner. However, these rosettes are not pathognomonic for retinoblastoma because they are observed in other tumors such as neuroblastomas and pineal tumors.

The new rosette is described as being larger than Homer Wright and Flexner-Wintersteiner rosettes, consisting of a ring of cells surrounding a lumen infiltrated centrally by a collection of basophilic cells (Fig 5 in the original article).

The authors speculate this new rosette may be associated with well-differentiated retinoblastomas with minimal necrosis and anterior segment involvement. More cases with evidence of this rosette need to be studied to establish the significance of this new rosette.

V. Lee, MD

Histology of Müller's muscle observed in quiescent Graves' orbitopathy

Lowinger A, Gill HS, Phan I, et al (California Pacific Med Ctr, San Francisco; Univ of Toronto, Ontario; Kaiser Permanente San Francisco, CA; et al)

Can J Ophthalmol 48:468-470, 2013

Objective.—Histologic examination of Müller's muscle (MM) in patients with clinically significant upper eyelid retraction secondary to Graves' orbitopathy (GO).

Design.—Prospective, single-blinded, comparative experimental study at a single institution.

Participants.—Patients from a single San Francisco Bay Area practice (RZS).

Methods.—Consecutive patients with upper eyelid retraction secondary to GO who underwent surgical correction by transcutaneous mullerectomy were recruited between January and December 2011. An equal number of control MM specimens were gathered in consecutive patients undergoing conjunctivo-MM resection for ptosis correction. A total of 10 specimens in each group was available for analysis. The proportion of fat and fibrosis, as well as inflammatory markers, was studied and graded in both the study and the control group by a masked pathologist. These data were compared between groups using the Student *t*-test.

Results.—No significant difference between the 2 groups of MM specimens was detected.

Conclusions.—Patients with quiescent GO with clinically significant eyelid retraction exhibit normal MM histology.

▶ This study is a prospective histologic comparison of Müller's muscle (MM) from patients with quiescent Graves orbitopathy (GO) and upper eyelid retraction and MM from patients with ptosis. Upper eyelid retraction is the most common manifestation of GO and may cause significant ocular surface problems that can lead to vision loss.[1] Previous studies have shown contradicting histologic findings when examining MM from patients with GO, which include fibrosis, fat infiltration, and presence of mast cells.[2-4] The value of this undertaking lies in elucidating the histopathologic mechanisms leading to MM dysfunction in GO, which is generally perceived as an inflammatory-fibrosis condition. Improved understanding of the underlying pathologic mechanisms may be attained if definitive histopathologic findings can be identified from rigorous studies of histologic specimens. Such findings could lead to more specific and appropriate treatments.

In this study, the authors enrolled 10 consecutive patients with stable Graves disease and clinically significant upper eyelid retraction, who were undergoing transcutaneous müllerectomy, for the experimental group, and 10 consecutive patients with unspecified ptosis undergoing conjunctivo-MM resection were included in the study as the control group. Specimens were stained with hematoxylin and eosin, Masson trichrome, and Giemsa. Specimens were also analyzed with immunohistochemical staining for the presence of T cells (CD3), B cells (CD20), general hematopoietic cells (CD45), monocytes and macrophages (CD68), and mast cells (CD117). The results demonstrated no difference between the experimental and control groups.

There are numerous shortcomings in this study, and the authors detail these well in their conclusion. Nevertheless, the importance of this study lies in these deficiencies, where future studies can be constructed more effectively to minimize these limitations and maximize relevant histopathologic correlations and findings. The control group, for example, should be age matched because fibrosis and fat infiltration may be affected by age. The etiology of ptosis in the control group should be specified and controlled for as much as possible because certain etiologies may have confounding histologic findings. Patients should be further subgrouped according to their GO activity and undergo subanalysis with histologic findings. The study was also not sufficiently powered to reach statistical significance. Future studies should build on this and other studies to achieve more definitive conclusions. Lastly, the authors inadvertently touched on the fascinating association of ptosis with human immunodeficiency virus infection and long-term antiretroviral treatment, which is currently thought to be related to mitochondrial dysfunction in the levator palpebrae muscle, presenting histologically with ragged red fibers.[5,6] This small reference by the authors reaffirms the importance of pursuing rigorous histologic studies to reveal underlying pathologic mechanisms that expand our understanding of disease.

V. Lee, MD

References

1. Ribeiro SF, Garcia DM, Leal V, et al. Graded müllerectomy for correction of graves upper eyelid retraction: effect on eyelid movements. *Ophthal Plast Reconstr Surg.* 2014;30:384-387.
2. Cahill KV, Buerger GF Jr, Johnson BL. Ptosis associated with fatty infiltration of Müller's muscle and levator muscle. *Ophthal Plast Reconstr Surg.* 1986;2:213-217.
3. Cockerham KP, Hidayat AA, Brown HG, Cockerham GC, Graner SR. Clinicopathologic evaluation of the mueller muscle in thyroid-associated orbitopathy. *Ophthal Plast Reconstr Surg.* 2002;18:11-17.
4. Grove AS. Upper eyelid retraction and Graves' disease. *Ophthalmology.* 1981;88: 499-506.
5. Moscato EE, Bloomer MM, Garcia-Kennedy R, Seiff SR. Human immunodeficiency virus-associated blepharoptosis. *Ophthal Plast Reconstr Surg.* 2011;27:360-363.
6. Silkiss RZ, Lee H, Gills Ray VL. Highly active antiretroviral therapy–associated ptosis in patients with human immunodeficiency virus. *Arch Ophthalmol.* 2009; 127:345-346.

Geographic Atrophy: A Histopathologic Assessment

Bird AC, Phillips RL, Hageman GS (Univ College London, England; Univ of Iowa; Univ of Utah, Salt Lake City)

JAMA Ophthalmol 132:338-345, 2014

Importance.—Geographic atrophy (GA) is the major cause of blind registration in Western communities, although, with few exceptions, it is less common than choroidal neovascular disease. The variation of phenotype implies that age-related macular degeneration (AMD) does not follow the same course from one case to another and that phenotyping may be important before initiating a therapeutic trial.

Objective.—To document photoreceptor and retinal pigment epithelium (RPE) cell loss and other changes at the RPE-choroid interface in donated human eyes in which visual loss was deemed to be due to GA.

Design, Setting, and Participants.—Histological study of a consecutive series of eyes donated by individuals previously diagnosed clinically as having GA. Donors were chosen on the basis of available clinical records (from MidAmerica Transplant Services, St Louis, Missouri; the Iowa Lions Eye Bank, Iowa City; and the Utah Lions Eye Bank, Salt Lake City) and selected were those considered to have GA due to AMD. Tissues in the regions of atrophy were examined with light, electron, and autofluorescence microscopy.

Results.—In most of the 37 donors examined, there was marked loss of photoreceptor cells for variable distances distal from the edge of the GA. Rod loss was greater than cone loss. An inverse relationship existed between the quantity of autofluorescent inclusions in the RPE and the thickness of sub-RPE basal laminar deposit. Integrity of the choroid varied from one eye to another and was not related strictly to photoreceptor survival. In some eyes, photoreceptor loss existed in the absence of obvious morphological changes in the Bruch membrane or RPE.

Conclusions and Relevance.—The findings support the view that photoreceptor loss occurs early in AMD in a proportion of cases and imply that photoreceptor-cell loss may contribute to the functional loss recorded in early stages of AMD at least in part. The variation of changes from one eye to another implies that patients selected for a specific prophylactic therapy for early AMD should be chosen on the basis of the characteristics of their disease.

► Classically, geographic atrophy (GA) is a late form of age-related macular degeneration (AMD) and is clinically characterized as a round- or oval-shaped area in the posterior pole, most notable for its sharply demarcated areas of retinal pigment epithelium (RPE) loss. These areas of RPE loss are associated with overlying outer retina loss, through which choroidal vessels become more prominent and visible. Hogan first theorized, later confirmed by Sarks and colleagues, that photoreceptor loss occurred before the loss of RPE cells in areas that later became geographic atrophy.[1-3] Sarks also posited the idea that the loss of the choriocapillaris was a result of the loss of RPE cells, not the cause of it, thereby explaining the typical time course of GA.[2,3]

Although the exact pathological mechanisms of GA are still being sought, the newer imaging modalities of fundus auto-fluorescence (FAF) and high-resolution optical coherence tomography (OCT) have turned the research focus to the junctional area between GA and the surrounding tissue. From these studies, 2 patterns of GA have been revealed in vivo: 1) an abrupt transition from GA to an area of normal outer nuclear layer thickness with integrity of the lines on OCT composing the outer nuclear layer, external limiting membrane, outer segments, ellipsoid zone, and RPE cells and 2) clinically undetectable photoreceptor layer loss with intact RPE cells.[4,5]

It is within this context that Bird and colleagues have their most interesting and relevant findings. The vast majority of patients (32 of 37 in this study, 86%) with vision loss secondary to GA have an undetectable layer of photoreceptor loss with intact RPE that extends up to 1400 microns from the edge of the GA on histologic examination. This leaves only 14% of GA patients with an abrupt transition from GA to "normal" retinal tissue.

The visual implications of these results are rather straightforward; in a majority of cases, photoreceptor cell loss extends far beyond the area of GA, which predates the RPE cell loss and likely explains many of the early visual functional changes seen in patients with early AMD. What is more complicated, however, is the implication this study has for ongoing clinical research. The authors convincingly argue that fundus autofluorescence is not a reliable indicator for the extent of photoreceptor cell loss and should not be used as a primary outcome for clinical trials aimed at preventing GA progression. Future work will be needed to determine whether in vivo imaging will be able to mimic the histopathologic findings and adequately image/quantify these areas of photoreceptor cell loss adjacent to GA for monitoring progression and functional changes in patients with AMD.

B. VanderBeek, MD

V. Lee, MD

References

1. Hogan MJ. Role of the retinal pigment epithelium in macular disease. *Trans Am Acad Ophthalmol Otolaryngol.* 1972;76:64-80.
2. Sarks SH. Ageing and degeneration in the macular region: a clinico-pathological study. *Br J Ophthalmol.* 1976;60:324-341.
3. Sarks JP, Sarks SH, Killingsworth MC. Evolution of geographic atrophy of the retinal pigment epithelium. *Eye (Lond).* 1988;2:552-577.
4. Wolf-Schnurrbusch UE, Enzmann V, Brinkmann CK, Wolf S. Morphologic changes in patients with geographic atrophy assessed with a novel spectral OCT-SLO combination. *Invest Ophthalmol Vis Sci.* 2008;49:3095-3099.
5. Fleckenstein M, Charbel Issa P, Helb HM. High-resolution spectral domain-OCT imaging in geographic atrophy associated with age-related macular degeneration. *Invest Ophthalmol Vis Sci.* 2008;49:4137-4144.

Retinal Cavernous Hemangioma: Fifty-Two Years of Clinical Follow-up With Clinicopathologic Correlation

Shields JA, Eagle RC Jr, Ewing MQ, et al (Thomas Jefferson Univ, Philadelphia, PA; Pennsylvania Hosp, Philadelphia)
Retina 34:1253-1257, 2014

Purpose.—To report long-term follow-up and histopathology of a retinal cavernous hemangioma and to review the literature on this subject.

Methods.—A newborn girl was noted immediately after birth to a have hyphema and vitreous hemorrhage in her left eye. The bleeding recurred throughout childhood and the etiology was not determined. Upon referral at age 22, a large retinal cavernous hemangioma was first recognized and recurrent hemorrhages continued, eventually leading to pain and secondary glaucoma. The patient declined treatment. At age 52, the hemangioma was stable in size, but ocular pain and blindness necessitated enucleation.

Results.—During the 52-year course, the fundus mass did not enlarge, but numerous episodes of hyphema and vitreous hemorrhage led to chronic glaucoma and eventual blindness. The main histopathologic finding in the disorganized globe was a retinal mass composed of large endothelial-lined vascular channels with thin walls, typical of a retinal cavernous hemangioma. The tumor extended anteriorly into the ciliary body, explaining the recurrent hyphemas. Additional chronic features included extensive fibrosis of the entire anterior segment, iris, and retina with proliferative vitreoretinopathy and widespread intraocular hemosiderosis from chronic hemorrhage. The patient has been free of pain since enucleation.

Conclusion.—Retinal cavernous hemangioma is a congenital stationary lesion that can cause recurrent intraocular hemorrhage, fibrosis, glaucoma, pain, and blindness, requiring enucleation. Retinal cavernous should be included in the differential diagnosis of childhood hyphema and vitreous hemorrhage.

► The authors present a unique case report of a patient followed for 52 years for a retinal cavernous hemangioma (RCH), who eventually underwent an enucleation and subsequent histopathologic confirmation of the retinal lesion. This case highlights principal clinical and histologic features of RCH, while also evoking current research focuses under investigation. RCH are typically isolated, unilateral, vascular lesions that may also be syndromic and/or associated with an autosomal dominant inheritance pattern. These lesions tend to be stable over time, exhibiting minimal growth. Rarely, RH can lead to vitreous hemorrhages as in the reported patient. Reports on the histopathology of these tumors are rare,[1] which is understandable given the rarity of the tumor itself. Histopathologic review of this globe revealed a posterior lesion composed of large, cavernous channels filled with blood, measuring about 200 to 500 μm in diameter. Retinal pigment epithelial (RPE) hyperplasia was seen at the base of the lesion with large quantities of soft drusenoid material. Drusen and RPE alterations are associated with many choroidal tumors and disorders. However, the disclosure of iron in this case, along with the presence of drusenoid deposition and RPE changes, underscores the possible significance of iron overload and disorders of the retina and RPE cells, which is an area of active research.[2,3]

V. Lee, MD

References

1. Davies WS, Thumim M. Cavernous hemangioma of the optic disc and retina. *Trans Am Acad Ophthalmol Otolaryngol.* 1956;60:217-218.
2. Lukinova N, Iacovelli J, Dentchev T, et al. Iron chelation protects the retinal pigment epithelial cell line ARPE-19 against cell death triggered by diverse stimuli. *Invest Ophthalmol Vis Sci.* 2009;50:1440-1447.
3. Wong RW, Richa DC, Hahn P, Green WR, Dunaief JL. Iron toxicity as a potential factor in AMD. *Retina.* 2007;27:997-1003.

Choroidal Lymphoma: Clinical Features and Association with Systemic Lymphoma

Mashayekhi A, Shukla SY, Shields JA, et al (Thomas Jefferson Univ, Philadelphia, PA)
Ophthalmology 121:342-351, 2014

Purpose.—To describe the clinical and histopathologic features of choroidal lymphoma (CL) and its association with systemic lymphoma.

Design.—Observational case series.

Participants.—Fifty-nine patients (73 eyes) with CL.

Methods.—Retrospective chart review.

Main Outcome Measures.—Clinical features, histopathology, and systemic lymphoma.

Results.—Of 59 patients with CL, systemic lymphoma was absent in 41 (primary CL; 69%) and present in 18 (secondary CL; 31%). Of 18 patients with systemic lymphoma at presentation, 14 (78%) had known systemic lymphoma and 4 (22%) were diagnosed with systemic lymphoma shortly after presentation. The most common types of systemic lymphoma in patients with secondary CL were diffuse large cell lymphoma (n = 5, 28%), chronic lymphocytic leukemia/lymphoma (n = 4, 22%), multiple myeloma (n = 2, 11%), Waldenstrom's macroglobulinemia (n = 2, 11%), extranodal marginal zone lymphoma (n = 2, 11%), plasmablastic lymphoma (n = 1, 6%), and unspecified non–Hodgkin lymphoma (n = 2, 11%). Compared with patients with primary CL, patients with secondary CL had a shorter mean duration of ocular symptoms (5 vs. 17 months), had less often received steroids before referral (11% vs. 46%), and were more likely to have bilateral ocular involvement (33% vs. 20%). Eyes with secondary CL had a higher rate of poor vision (≤20/200) (46% vs. 12%), iris (20% vs. 4%) or ciliary body (30% vs. 8%) lymphoma, episcleral vascular congestion (40% vs. 16%), anterior chamber reaction (30% vs. 14%), hyphema (15% vs. 0%), vitreous cellular infiltration (30% vs. 4%), and severe media haziness (20% vs. 0%). Secondary CL was morphologically more high grade (50% diffuse large cell lymphoma) compared with primary CL (37% low-grade non–Hodgkin lymphoma, 27% extranodal marginal zone lymphoma). None of the 33 patients with primary CL and subsequent follow-up developed systemic lymphoma during a mean follow-up of 50 months (median, 35 months; range, 2–231 months).

Conclusions.—Secondary CL is morphologically high grade and associated with more severe ocular findings. Patients with CL and no known systemic lymphoma at presentation should undergo systemic evaluation to rule out the possibility of undiagnosed concurrent systemic lymphoma. However, none of the patients with primary CL in our study had late development of systemic lymphoma (Table 4).

► Choroidal lymphoma (CL) is such a rare disorder that it presents as a diagnostic or management dilemma for many ophthalmologists, including retina specialists. This is especially true if there is no known systemic disease at the time of ophthalmic presentation. Mashayehki et al reviewed 59 cases seen at the Wills Eye Hospital for choroidal lymphoma and provide an illuminating discussion of their findings. Clinicians can take several salient points from this article.

Ultrasonography is the most useful, noninvasive, imaging test, and a B scan can show acoustically hollow thickening of the choroid. B scans can sometimes show epibulbar extension as well, but these features should not be confused with choroidal melanoma.

TABLE 4.—Choroidal Lymphoma: Ocular Biopsy and Pathology Results

Feature	All Eyes (N = 44)	Primary Group (n = 30)	Secondary Group (n = 14)
Ocular biopsy, technique*			
Anterior epibulbar biopsy	22 (50)	17 (57)	5 (36)
Transvitreal FNAB of choroids	16 (36)	13 (43)	3 (21)
Enucleation	3 (7)	0 (0)	3 (21)
FNAB of iris/ciliary body	2 (5)	2 (7)	0 (0)
Transscleral choroidal biopsy	2 (5)	0 (0)	2 (14)
Postmortem eye examination	2 (5)	0 (0)	2 (14)
FNAB of vitreous	1 (2)	0 (0)	1 (7)
Lid biopsy	1 (2)	0 (0)	1 (7)
Ocular biopsy, pathologic results			
Low-grade NHL, not further classified	12 (27)	11 (37)	1 (7)
Atypical lymphoid infiltrate	10 (23)	7 (23)	3 (21)
EMZL (MALT)	8 (18)	8 (27)	0 (0)
Diffuse large cell lymphoma	7 (16)	0 (0)	7 (50)
Lymphoma, not further classified	3 (7)	2 (7)	1 (7)
Plasmacytoma	2 (5)	1 (3)	1 (7)
Plasmablastic lymphoma	1 (2)	0 (0)	1 (7)
Inadequate sample	1 (2)	1 (3)	0 (0)

EMZL (MALT) = extranodal marginal zone lymphoma of mucosa-associated lymphoid tissue type; FNAB = fine-needle aspiration biopsy; NHL = non–Hodgkin lymphoma

Data are n (%).

*Five eyes had >1 ocular biopsy.

On presentation, it is notable that 69% of their cases were primary CL, meaning that they did not have previous or coexisting systemic lymphoma and were not diagnosed with lymphoma by systemic evaluation within 6 months of presentation. Cases in which a prior or current history of systemic lymphoma exists or cases in which systemic lymphoma is diagnosed within 6 months of ocular findings were labeled secondary CL. Interestingly, bilateral disease was seen in 20% of primary CL, and 33% of secondary CL cases. Vitreous cells or infiltration was detected in 30% of secondary CL cases and only 2% of primary CL cases. Thus, the majority of the time, no vitritis will be seen.

Although diagnosis of CL can be made with confidence clinically, definitive diagnosis requires histopathologic evaluation. In this series, ocular specimens were most commonly obtained from a biopsy of an anterior bulbar extension of a deeper choroidal lesion, followed by transvitreal needle biopsy of the choroidal infiltrate. Others have used anterior chamber paracentesis and/or vitrectomy in the presence of robust anterior chamber reaction and/or vitritis. Depending on the amount of tissue obtained, histologic examination of suspected lymphoma cases include routine histopathologic review, immunohistochemical staining, and flow cytometry. The biopsy approach and findings are represented in Table 4. Analysis of the histologic findings revealed that eyes with secondary CL were morphologically higher grade than eyes with primary CL. Therefore, necessary precautions should be taken in cases where high-grade CL is diagnosed histologically with no known diagnosis of systemic lymphoma because some of the patients in this series developed systemic lymphoma within 6 months of their ocular findings. It is also imperative for the ophthalmologist to discuss with the ocular pathologist the approach and handling of tissue specimens in these cases before procurement of the tissue.

Currently, it is understood that there are varying degrees of metastatic potential for these lesions. Grossniklaus[1] has pointed out that uveal lymphoid proliferation can have a spectrum ranging from lesions with only reactive hyperplasia to more aggressive lymphoid neoplasms. Consistent with this concept, Mashayekhi et al found that, in contrast to secondary CL, none of their primary CL cases were known to develop systemic disease with a follow-up ranging from 2 to 231 months. In their review of 22 patients with uveal lymphoma seen at the Cleveland Clinic, Aronow et al[2] found that initial systemic imaging demonstrated disease localized to the eye in 77.3% of cases, and none of their patients developed new systemic disease with a median follow-up of 30.3 months. Patients with primary CL, no high-risk histopathology, and no systemic disease found with initial evaluation seem to have a lower risk for systemic involvement. These patients should still have an annual systemic evaluation. In contrast, the patients with more aggressive disease will often present as secondary CL and should be followed more closely.

B. J. Kim, MD
V. Lee, MD

References

1. Grossniklaus HE, Martin DF, Avery R, et al. Uveal lymphoid infiltration. Report of four cases and clinicopathologic review. *Ophthalmology.* 1998;105:1265-1273.
2. Aronow ME, Portell CA, Sweetenham JW, Singh AD. Uveal lymphoma: clinical features, diagnostic studies, treatment selection, and outcomes. *Ophthalmology.* 2014;121:334-341.

Usefulness of a Red Chromagen in the Diagnosis of Melanocytic Lesions of the Conjunctiva

Jiang K, Brownstein S, Lam K, et al (Univ of Ottawa, Ontario, Canada; et al)
JAMA Ophthalmol 132:622-629, 2014

Importance.—Immunohistochemical analyses may assist in the diagnosis of precancerous and cancerous conjunctival lesions.

Objective.—To use Vector Red (VR) to identify an immunologic marker that is sensitive for all melanocytes and another that is sensitive and specific for activated and/or atypical conjunctival melanocytic lesions (MLs).

Design, Setting, and Participants.—Eight specimens each of control lesions (normal conjunctiva and normal uvea as well as choroidal melanoma) and 8 from the diagnostic categories (conjunctival nevus, primary acquired melanosis with mild or no atypia, primary acquired melanosis with moderate to severe atypia, and conjunctival melanoma) that provided sufficient quantity and quality of tissue were available for processing. The specimens were obtained from the Ophthalmic Pathology Laboratory, The

Ottawa Hospital, from 2005 to 2013. The specimens were immunolabeled with human melanoma black 45 (HMB45), melanoma antigen recognized by T cells 1 (Melan-A), S100, and Ki67 using VR and a double panmelanoma cocktail (dPANMEL) using 3,3′-diaminobenzidine (DAB) and VR. The HMB45-immunolabeled specimens were additionally developed with DAB, with and without overnight bleaching with hydrogen peroxide, 4%. Data were collected by 2 pathologists who were masked to sample grouping.

Main Outcomes and Measures.—Differentiation between benign and malignant MLs based on immunomarker profile.

Results.—Immunoreactivity was best visualized in specimens with VR. Melan-A labeled all melanocytes (100% sensitivity; panmelanocyte marker) without discriminating between benign and malignant lesions (0% specificity). Atypical melanocytes were most specifically labeled with HMB45 (96% specificity, 97% sensitivity; atypia marker). In primary acquired melanosis specimens, we found that the percentage of HMB45 ($P < .001$), S100 ($P < .001$), and Ki67 ($P \leq .02$) positivity increased significantly with worsening atypia.

Conclusions and Relevance.—We recommend VR, which rarely requires specimen bleaching, as the standard substrate for immunohistochemical analysis of conjunctival MLs. We found Melan-A and HMB45 to best characterize MLs. In conjunctival MLs, the use of VR with Melan-A and HMB45 provides substantial sensitivity for all melanocytes and for atypical melanocytes, respectively, and reduces specimen-processing time for laboratories performing immunohistochemistry on MLs.

▶ In this retrospective and prospective histologic case series, the authors attempt to identify the most relevant immunohistochemical markers for differentiating malignant melanocytic conjunctival lesions from benign lesions. Concurrently, the authors also propose the use of Vector Red (VR), a red chromagen, for immunohistochemical processing, instead of a brown chromagen, such as 3,3′-diaminobenzidine (DAB), to reduce the abundance of brown pigmentation from the immunostain substrate and innate melanin pigment. This study has tremendous clinical relevance because the task of accurately diagnosing malignant melanocytic conjunctival lesions is critical, given their management and prognostic implications. Immunohistochemical analysis is often used in these cases, and therefore, clarity regarding which immunostains to use is warranted.

The authors included a minimum of 8 specimens from the following diagnostic categories: nevus; primary acquired melanosis (PAM), which was further subcategorized as with no atypia to mild atypia or moderate to severe atypia; and conjunctival melanoma. Normal conjunctiva, uvea, and choroidal melanomas were used as controls. The following immunochemistry stains were performed: double panmelanoma cocktail (dPANMEL), S100, human melanoma black 45 (HMB45), melanoma antigen recognized by T cells 1 (Melan-A), and Ki67. In addition, specimens that were immunostained with HMB45 were processed with VR and DAB substrates, as well as 4% H_2O_2 bleaching or potassium permanganate/oxalic acid bleaching with DAB chromagen. The other markers were developed with VR only. Two pathologists reviewed each case in a masked fashion. The results showed that Melan-A identified all melanocytic cells with 100% sensitivity and specificity, whereas HMB45 highlighted atypical melanocytes with 97% sensitivity and 96% specificity. Statistical significance was achieved with HMB45 staining in differentiating PAM without to mild atypia from PAM with moderate to severe atypia and conjunctival melanoma. Immunoreactivity was best visualized with VR chromagen and did not require bleaching to remove the innate melanin pigment for interpretation. As a side observation, when bleaching was performed, the authors found potassium permanganate/oxalic acid bleaching was effective but led to altered cellular antigenicity, whereas 4% H_2O_2 bleaching was variable at removing pigmentation from the specimen.

The authors concluded that Melan-A and HMB45 outperformed other markers in identifying all melanocytic cells and atypical melanocytic cells, respectively. Although the authors' conclusions are soundly based on statistically significant results, the study presumes accurate initial histologic diagnosis of the cases, which is then confirmed with subsequent immunohistochemical analysis. This presumption can be made because the pathologists analyzing the cases in this study are extremely experienced in analyzing conjunctival lesions. However, this may not reflect the practice of many pathology laboratories where initial interpretations can be varied due to unfamiliarity with conjunctival lesions. An inaccurate initial histologic diagnosis will only be compounded by imperfect immunostains. For example, few of the cases that were considered benign lesions in the study demonstrated positivity with atypical markers. Therefore, importance should be stressed that immunohistochemical analysis cannot replace initial histologic analysis by a pathologist who is experienced at interpreting conjunctival lesions. The authors' ultimate recommendation when approaching melanocytic conjunctival lesions is that diagnosis should be initially made with routine histologic studies (hematoxylin and eosin [H&E] and H&E with bleaching), and if diagnosis cannot be made, then the following immunostains should be employed: Melan-A, HMB45, and Ki67 with VR.

V. Lee, MD

Effective Melanin Depigmentation of Human and Murine Ocular Tissues: An Improved Method for Paraffin and Frozen Sections

Manicam C, Pitz S, Brochhausen C, et al (Johannes Gutenberg Univ Mainz, Germany)

PLoS One 9:e102512, 2014

Purpose.—The removal of excessive melanin pigments that obscure ocular tissue morphology is important to address scientific questions and for differential diagnosis of ocular tumours based on histology. Thus, the goal of the present study was to establish an effective and fast melanin bleaching method for paraffin and frozen mouse and human ocular tissues.

Methods.—Paraffin-embedded and frozen ocular specimens from mice and human donors were subjected to bleaching employing two methods.

The first employed potassium permanganate ($KMnO_4$) with oxalic acid, and the second 10% hydrogen peroxide (H_2O_2). To determine optimal bleaching conditions, depigmentation was carried out at various incubation times. The effect of diluents used for 10% H_2O_2 was assessed using phosphate-buffered saline (PBS), and deionized water. Three different slide types and two fixatives, which were ice-cold acetone with 80% methanol, and 4% paraformaldehyde (PFA) were used to determine the optimal conditions for better tissue adherence during bleaching. All tissues were stained in hematoxylin and eosin for histological evaluation.

Results.—Optimal bleaching was achieved using warm 10% H_2O_2 diluted in PBS at 65°C for 120 minutes. Chromium-gelatin-coated slides prevented tissue detachment. Adherence of cryosections was also improved with post-fixation using 4% PFA and overnight air-drying at RT after cryosectioning. Tissue morphology was preserved under these conditions. Conversely, tissues bleached in $KMnO_4$/oxalic acid demonstrated poor depigmentation with extensive tissue damage.

Conclusions.—Warm dilute H_2O_2 at 65°C for 120 minutes rapidly and effectively bleached both cryo- and paraffin sections of murine and human ocular tissues (Table 1).

▶ The aim of this study is to establish a melanin bleaching protocol for paraffin- and cryo-embedded human and murine ocular tissues. The authors tested various parameters using the most commonly used bleaching protocols, potassium permanganate with oxalic acid ($KMnO_4$/oxalic acid) and 10% hydrogen peroxide (H_2O_2), and compared the bleaching efficiency of each method. Bleaching of pigmented ocular structures and/or lesions is an invaluable tool to the pathologist when evaluating the morphology of cells that are obscured by the presence of melanin granules. Meticulous examination of cellular characteristics is needed in attaining a diagnosis and in grading, in cases of tumors. Therefore, a study that standardizes and optimizes such a vital tool is warranted. The simultaneous evaluation of human and murine samples provides an added benefit to scientific investigators who also use bleaching methods to study ocular tissues.

For mice samples, sections of tissue were obtained from enucleated globes that were either immediately embedded in optimal cutting temperature cryomedia and kept at −20°C or fixed with 4% paraformaldehyde in 0.1 M phosphate buffer saline (PBS, pH 7.4) for 24 hours then embedded in paraffin. For human samples, tissues were fixed in 4% paraformaldehyde and embedded in paraffin. Various conditions, such as temperature, incubation time, and slides, were tested. Bleaching efficiency, tissue preservation, and tissue adherence to the slide were evaluated. The authors found warm 10% H_2O_2 diluted in PBS at 65°C for 120 minutes provided the best results for both human and murine paraffin- and cryo-embedded samples and that tissue best adhered to chromium gelatin-coated slides.

The authors accurately point out that the results from their study are most applicable to routine hematoxylin and eosin (H&E) staining and may not be applicable to other staining methods, such as immunohistochemical staining, or certain experimental conditions. Despite the authors' specificity, they

TABLE 1.—Trouble-Shooting Guidelines for Melanin Bleaching Using Hydrogen Peroxide (H_2O_2) and Hematoxylin and Eosin (HE) Staining

Problem Areas	Trouble-Shooting	Solutions
Tissues detaching from the slides during and after treatment with H_2O_2	a) H_2O_2 treatment is very harsh on tissues. Thus, slides need to be coated or subbed for better adherence.	a) Slide subbing with chromium gelatin.
	b) Under-fixation	b) Paraffin tissues should be fixed for an optimum period of time in 4% PFA prior to routine tissue processing. Cryosections should be post-fixed in 4% PFA before treatment with the bleaching agent.
Faint staining with eosin	a) Eosin is water-soluble. A washing step with water or diluted alcohol after eosin immersion can remove the eosin from tissues.	a) Use anhydrous or 95% ethanol prior to counterstaining with eosin for enhancement and better differentiation of the stain.
	b) The pH of the eosin may be too alkaline i.e. above 5.0 due to a carryover of the bluing solution.	b) Wash the slides thoroughly after the bluing step (if one was used) to ensure there is no residual carryover.
Bleaching incomplete	Diluent for H_2O_2 was deionized water.	Use PBS as diluents.
Over-staining with hematoxylin (the sections look too dark)	a) The tissue sections were stained too long in regressive hematoxylin i.e. Harris', Ehrlich's, and Delafield's.	a) Use an additional step of 2% acid alcohol to remove the excess stain after staining with hematoxylin.
	b) The differentiation step was too short.	b) Adjust the differentiation time by dipping in acid alcohol until the slides start to turn pink.
Tissue sections are too pink	Pinkish color of the stained tissue sections is due to inadequate 'bluing'.	Use a bluing agent e.g. tap water, Scott's solution, ammonia solution in quick dipping motions of slides till they start to turn blue.

Courtesy of C. Manicam, *PLOS One*. 2014.

provide a simple but helpful table for troubleshooting general problems that can arise with bleaching (Table 1). The conclusion from this study differs from the conclusion reached by Jiang et al,[1] which is likely due to the different methodology used in the latter study. The disparate conclusions between the 2 groups nicely exemplify the need to compare, standardize, and optimize histologic techniques, even common ones, to ensure accurate analysis of specimens.

V. Lee, MD

Reference

1. Jiang K, Brownstein S, Lam K, Burns B, Farmer J. Usefulness of a Red Chromagen in the Diagnosis of Melanocytic Lesions of the Conjunctiva. *JAMA Ophthalmology*. 2014;132(5):622.

Consensus Statement on the Immunohistochemical Detection of Ocular Lymphatic Vessels

Schroedl F, Kaser-Eichberger A, Schlereth SL, et al (Paracelsus Med Univ, Salzburg, Austria; Univ of Cologne, Germany; et al)
Invest Ophthalmol Vis Sci 55:6440-6442, 2014

There is currently considerable controversy about existence and classification of "lymphatic vessels" in the eye. Some of the confusion is certainly caused by inappropriate use (or nonuse) of the correct immunohistochemical markers. Many experts in the field expressed the need for a consensus statement, and, in this perspective, authors offer arguments and solutions to reliably continue with immunohistochemical ocular lymphatic research.

▶ Resulting from a discussion at the 2014 annual Association for Research in Vision and Ophthalmology meeting, the authors propose guidelines for histologic, immunohistochemical, and ultrastructural detection of ocular and periocular lymphatics. Although the detection of lymphatics is not frequently performed in clinical pathology, these guidelines may still serve a purpose for ocular pathologists in understanding the pathophysiology of ocular disorders. The eye is traditionally taught as lacking a lymphatic system, which likely contributes to its immunity. However, this immunity appears to be violated in certain conditions and may be associated with lymphangiogenesis, as in cases of corneal inflammatory disorders.[1,2] Given the potential magnitude and scope the presence, activation, and/or development of lymphatics may have on ocular disorders and diseases, recommendations on detecting ocular lymphatics is a valuable tool. The authors provide the following criteria: "(1) the presence/absence of erythrocytes/lymph-like fluid is insufficient to discriminate between lymphatic and blood vessels, (2) the use of more than one lymphatic endothelial marker or a marker panel is recommended for immunohistochemistry in the eye except for regions where the existence of lymphatics is already well established (ie, physiologically in conjunctiva and pathologically in inflamed cornea), (3) the use of markers in ultrastructural analysis is recommended (again except for ocular regions where existence of lymphatics is well established as in conjunctiva and inflamed cornea), and (4) the use of appropriate control tissue and appropriate documentation for detection of blood and lymphatic vessels is recommended." Guidelines such as these will hopefully progress our understanding of ocular disorders and continue the strong tradition of ocular pathologists in illuminating the pathophysiology of ocular diseases.

V. Lee, MD

References

1. Cursiefen C, Chen L, Borges LP, et al. VEGF-A stimulates lymphangiogenesis and hemangiogenesis in inflammatory neovascularization via macrophage recruitment. *J Clin Invest.* 2004;113:1040-1050.
2. Cursiefen C, Schlötzer-Schrehardt U, Küchle M, et al. Lymphatic vessels in vascularized human corneas: immunohistochemical investigation using lyve-1 and podoplanin. *Invest Ophthalmol Vis Sci.* 2002;43:2127-2135.

Immunophenotyping of Paucicellular Samples

Stacchini A, Demurtas A, Aliberti S (Città della Salute e della Scienza, Turin, Italy)

Curr Protoc Cytom 68:9.46.1-9.46.14, 2014

Immunophenotyping of paucicellular samples may represent a diagnostic challenge in the flow cytometry (FC) laboratory routine, as the scarcity of cells limits the number of tests that can be performed. Specimens such as fine needle aspirates (FNA), human body fluids (BF), cerebrospinal fluid (CSF), or ocular fluid (OF) sent for FC investigations in the case of suspicion of lymphoma, or for lymphoma monitoring, may contain very low numbers of cells. In these cases, it is mandatory to obtain the largest amount possible of useful information from a single tube. The basic protocol described in this unit provides a method that combines the use of multiple monoclonal antibodies (MAbs) with a Boolean gating strategy to identify and quantify the main lymphocyte populations, as well as to detect lymphomatous B cells or any aberrant T cell expression, if present, in paucicellular samples.

▶ This is a protocol for flow cytometry of paucicellular samples, which is valuable not only to ocular pathologists but also to general ophthalmologists who submit any specimens that may require cytologic analysis. Flow cytometry (FC) is an ancillary test commonly used in conjunction with conventional cytology, especially in cases of hematologic malignancies such as lymphomas. In ophthalmology, FC has been applied to samples from fine needle aspirates (FNA) and ocular fluids. However, samples from the eye are paucicellular by nature, defined as containing less than 0.3 × 106 total cells. Therefore, care must be taken by the ophthalmologist and ocular pathologist to prevent cellular decay and cell loss from unnecessary steps and time delays. Apoptotic, necrotic, and/or damaged cells produce artifacts on FC and are, therefore, selected out of the analysis. This decreases the number of events that can be analyzed, thereby decreasing diagnostic potential. Therefore, cell viability needs to be high (minimum > 50%) and preserved during the obtaining, transporting, and processing of the specimen.

Although this protocol focuses specifically on using a multiparametric FC with a multicolored-antibody-parameter FC assay, the following general guidelines extrapolated from the protocol can be applied to any paucicellular specimens: For FNA, contents from the syringe, including the needle, should be placed as soon as possible in fresh tissue media (such as the holding media described in the protocol) and transported to the lab or stored at 4°C immediately; for ocular fluids, specimens should be collected in an appropriate vessel, such as a syringe, and transported immediately to the lab. It is critical to have the specimen processed as quickly as possible to avoid cell loss. If this is not possible, fresh tissue media should be added to the specimen at 1:1 ratio and kept at room temperature. Communication between the ophthalmologist and ocular pathologist before obtaining the specimen is therefore critical for minimizing lost time and maintaining the integrity of the specimen. As pointed out by the authors, there is no general consensus to the minimal number of events that must be analyzed for diagnosis or exclusion of malignancy and/or other diagnoses. Usually, the combination of the appropriate clinical setting with discrete cluster of expected FC findings is sufficient for diagnosis.[1] By understanding the parameters of the laboratory tests used in pathology, ophthalmologists and ocular pathologists can work together more effectively to provide outstanding care to our patients.

V. Lee, MD

Reference

1. Barnett D, Louzao R, Gambell P, De J, Oldaker T, Hanson CA, ICSH/ICCS Working Group. Validation of cell-based fluorescence assays: practice guidelines from the ICSH and ICCS - part IV - postanalytic considerations: validation of cell-based fluorescence assays: postanalytic considerations. *Cytometry B Clin Cytom.* 2013;84:309-314.

Article Index

Chapter 1: Cataract Surgery

Chapter 2: Refractive Surgery

Chapter 3: Cornea

Chapter 4: Glaucoma

Chapter 5: Retina

Chapter 6: Uveitis

Chapter 7: Oculoplastic Surgery

Chapter 8: Pediatric Ophthalmology

Chapter 9: Neuro-ophthalmology

Chapter 10: Imaging

Chapter 11: Ocular Oncology

Chapter 12: Pathology

Author Index

A

B

C

D

E

F

G

W

Y

Z

MIX
Papier | Fördert gute Waldnutzung
FSC® C083411

Kolibri 360 GmbH
Ferdinand-Jühlke-Straße 7
99095 Erfurt, Deutschland
produktsicherheit@kolibri360.de